Religion and Medicine

Also by Jeff Levin

Religion and The Social Sciences: Basic and Applied Research Perspectives
(Edited)

Upon These Three Things: Jewish Perspectives on Loving God

Judaism and Health: A Handbook of Practical, Professional, and Scholarly Resources
(Edited with Michele F. Prince)

Healing to all Their Flesh: Jewish and Christian Perspectives on Spirituality, Theology, and Health
(Edited with Keith G. Meador)

Divine Love: Perspectives from the World's Religious Traditions
(Edited with Stephen G. Post)

Faith, Medicine, and Science: A Festschrift in Honor of Dr. David B. Larson
(Edited with Harold G. Koenig)

Religion in The Lives of African Americans: Social, Psychological, and Health Perspectives
(with Robert Joseph Taylor and Linda M. Chatters)

God, Faith, and Health: Exploring the Spirituality-Healing Connection

Essentials of Complementary and Alternative Medicine
(Edited with Wayne B. Jonas)

Religion in Aging and Health: Theoretical Foundations and Methodological Frontiers
(Edited)

Religion and Medicine

A History of the Encounter Between Humanity's Two Greatest Institutions

JEFF LEVIN

With a Foreword by
STEPHEN G. POST

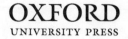

OXFORD
UNIVERSITY PRESS

OXFORD
UNIVERSITY PRESS

Oxford University Press is a department of the University of Oxford. It furthers
the University's objective of excellence in research, scholarship, and education
by publishing worldwide. Oxford is a registered trade mark of Oxford University
Press in the UK and certain other countries.

Published in the United States of America by Oxford University Press
198 Madison Avenue, New York, NY 10016, United States of America.

Library of Congress Cataloging-in-Publication Data
Names: Levin, Jeffrey S., author.
Title: Religion and medicine : a history of the encounter between
humanity's two greatest institutions / Jeff Levin, Ph.D., M.P.H. ;
with a foreword by Stephen G. Post.
Description: New York, NY, United States of America : Oxford University Press, 2020. |
Includes bibliographical references and index.
Identifiers: LCCN 2019044758 (print) | LCCN 2019044759 (ebook) |
ISBN 9780190867355 (hb) | ISBN 9780190867379 (epub) | ISBN 9780190867386 (online)
Subjects: LCSH: Medicine—Religious aspects.
Classification: LCC BL65.M4 L485 2020 (print) | LCC BL65.M4 (ebook) | DDC 201/.661—dc23
LC record available at https://lccn.loc.gov/2019044758
LC ebook record available at https://lccn.loc.gov/2019044759

3 5 7 9 8 6 4 2

Printed by Sheridan Books, Inc., United States of America

*For Dr. Berton H. Kaplan, of blessed memory, a great mentor and friend,
who encouraged my earliest explorations of the interconnections between religion
and medicine*

Contents

Foreword

The perennial interface of religion and medicine has cried out for a truly great book that is both fully comprehensive and consistently deep in its analysis. Levin's *Religion and Medicine* succeeds brilliantly in providing the big picture of this interface. It is far and away the finest scholarly work yet published that combines scientific as well as deeply learned humanistic insights in a text of immense clarity, maturity, and sophistication. One would expect this from Jeff, for his book is the culmination of a lifetime of diligent scholarship for which he is rightly renowned. It is hard to imagine that any one scholar could have made such a pioneering contribution across this interface, but indeed Levin has done so.

Religion and Medicine will appeal to a wide variety of readers: the historian, the medical anthropologist, the epidemiologist, the devotee of randomized controlled studies, the medical educator, the medical ethicist and humanist clinician, the healthcare advocate and policymaker, the comparative religionist, the thoughtful scholar of mind-body medicine, and those wanting to know how and from where the intense altruistic passion that strives for the good of patients arose. Levin's book also points us in the direction of a new American medicine, one that takes into scientifically informed consideration the subjective meanings of the patient as a person experiencing illness and the healing importance of empathic skills, and that finally takes into full account the oft-quoted 1925 statement of Harvard physician Francis Peabody: "For the secret of the care of the patient is in caring for the patient."

I began reading Jeff's manuscript early one February morning in a Stony Brook Medical Center coffee shop and did not return home until very late at night, astonished by the clarity and depth of analysis on each page. My pen had run out of ink for all the underlining and notes that flowed over those hours as my sense of time and place all but disappeared. I immediately called Harold G. Koenig of Duke University, who is one of two other individuals who might be included with Jeff at the very pinnacle of excellence among researchers on religion and health, and who like me has known Jeff from at least the early 1990s. Harold listened patiently as I enthusiastically explained why this book is the best that we may ever have, or could ever imagine having.

Jeff Levin has many talents, but there has to be something more than talent behind this book. For the past nearly forty years Jeff has been enduringly called to this work by a special spiritual vocation that makes him one of the most reliably creative scholars, speakers, and educators of our time. *Religion and Medicine* is nothing less than a work of love for truth, humanity, and healing at its fullest. After reading it, I am convinced that no one—and certainly not myself—could possibly write a foreword that can do this book justice.

A day after reading his manuscript, I emailed Jeff a brief note of congratulations. He wrote back, "Stephen, this was a labor of love . . . a summary of every dimension of this encounter since the beginning of time. I spent a lot of hours, while writing, wondering if I was nuts in taking this on, but am happy with how it turned out. I have always felt there needed to be a single scholarly text that brings everything together and looks at the big picture, and I am grateful that I can leave this one work behind me when I shuffle off some day. Jeff" (email, February 23, 2019). Professor Levin, when you "shuffle off some day," please rest assured that you have created a great work that will take its place among the classics, and know that your readers are deeply grateful. If the great physician William Osler were alive today, given his strong appreciation for the interface of medicine and religion generally and his interest in patients' experience of illness in particular, Jeff's book would most certainly occupy an honored place on his legendary bedside reading table.

We might note that the ancient Hippocratic physicians were unlikely to treat the poor, the contagious, or the dying, and only later in the West under the influence of the three Abrahamic religious traditions do we see emerging the passion for the care of the patient that we hope to find in every good physician today. Levin, who comes from a lineage of notable rabbis and physicians, rightly points to the fact that so many institutions of healing "were birthed by religion, externalizations of its prophetic role to speak out against brokenness and to labor to repair the world." He ends the book with a call to us all to "heal the world"— *tikkun olam* in Judaism—and on each page are found inspiration and insights to do so.

Early on in *Religion and Medicine* Levin covers the history of world religions and the systems of healing that have arisen universally from them, both in the East and in the West. He demonstrates that "the intersections of the faith-based and medical sectors are multifaceted and of long standing." He explores ritual religious healing in the ancient world, drawing on the finest scholarship with discernment and measured interpretation. Hinduism, Buddhism, Judaism, and Islam are amply discussed, as are shamanism and indigenous healing traditions. When Levin turns to healing in Christianity, with its roots in Jesus's role as a healer, he delineates the Christian origins of the first hospitals in the West, for the care of the sick was considered a spiritual calling and responsibility.

Among many other topics, he includes a penetrating analysis of the American New Thought metaphysical perspectives on healing and disease as manifest in the nineteenth century, as well as the health systems that arose from specific religious traditions across the United States, such as the Seventh-day Adventists and Sisters of Mercy. His nuanced discussion of medical missions extends from the pioneering work of Albert Schweitzer to Dame Cicely Saunders, who in 1967 founded the first hospice, St. Christopher's, based entirely on her deeply spiritual Anglican sense of religious calling. Despite the many nursing and social work texts in which Dame Cicely is mentioned, few if any note that she was profoundly shaped in all her trailblazing efforts by prayer and theology, from which emerged her idea of the "total pain" that includes spiritual distress. It is as though we are interested in what she did, but not in *why* she did it. Levin reminds us of such religious promptings, and we do indeed need to notice and acknowledge the passionate work of religious people in creating new healing institutions that expand and enrich medical practice. This includes the emergence of the twentieth-century healthcare chaplaincy movement, involving Harvard physician Richard Cabot and Presbyterian minister Anton Boisen, whom Levin discusses appreciatively.

Chapter 5, "Scientists and Scholars," is the most compelling assessment yet of the movement of scientific study as applied to faith, resilience, coping, and prayer in the face of illness. Levin has been the leading epidemiologic scientist in this area since its serious inception in the mid-1980s; he expands in passing on some of his own research and interpretation while deeply discussing many other key figures.

Also in this chapter, Jeff touches on his own education and work in public health and epidemiology since 1982, when he was a graduate student at the University of North Carolina studying with the renowned epidemiologist Berton H. Kaplan. It was there, in Chapel Hill, that he first came to appreciate Kaplan's research showing that religious attendance affected cardiovascular outcomes in large data sets over time. Kaplan challenged Levin to study how religion influences health, and Levin has devoted his career to the topic ever since.

In 1990 Levin received his first grant from the U.S. National Institutes of Health, and then benefited from the efforts of the private-sector National Institute for Healthcare Research (NIHR), founded by psychiatrist David B. Larson. The NIHR began sponsoring major research conferences and funding further research and education so that "by the 21st century it could be truthfully said that religion and health research has consolidated into a genuine *field*." I had the honor of serving on the NIHR board of directors and working closely with Larson as so many future leaders of this field were brought into face-to-face dialogue and many programs were funded in academic medical centers across America.

Levin notes that the most significant benchmark in the emergence of this field was the 2001 Oxford publication of the *Handbook of Religion and Health*, written by our mutual friends Koenig, Larson, and the gifted psychologist Michael E. McCullough. Levin himself wrote the foreword for the first edition of this masterpiece. If a doctoral student were to approach me about how to get started in this exciting field of research, I would tell that student to read Levin's *Religion and Medicine* and then follow up with the second edition of Koenig's *Handbook of Religion and Health* (from 2012). These two works together provide any serious students with all the essential background they need.

Chapter 6, "Teaching and Training," is the work of someone who has followed medical education very closely over the years. I was uplifted by the section titled "Sir John and David," where Levin pays a high compliment to John Marks Templeton and Larson. Sir John's interest in seeing research and education unfold in this field is nicely summarized, including his belief that "unlimited love" has the power to transform body and mind, and that love is a major part of any truly healing interaction. I had the honor of knowing Sir John for fifteen years, and at his request in 2001 founded an institute to study love, compassion, and healing, with advisers like Levin, Greg Fricchione (director of the Benson-Henry Institute for Mind Body Medicine at Massachusetts General Hospital), Byron Johnson (Levin's colleague at Baylor), and several others.

Levin's great appreciation for the work of Larson and the many pioneer educators that the NIHR brought into the field, including Christina M. Puchalski, is well justified. After that wave of activity, religion and medicine went mainstream in medical schools, in many residency training programs, and in the awareness of clinicians across North America and Europe. Following Larson's sudden passing in 2002, we convened the NIHR board and decided to dissolve that institution in order to transfer the funds to endow the David B. Larson Fellowship in Health and Spirituality at the John W. Kluge Center of the Library of Congress, which remains active to this day. Levin also touches on the annual David B. Larson Memorial Lecture in Religion and Health, ongoing since 2003 and cohosted by Levin and Koenig, which has been delivered yearly by a luminary in the field. As someone involved in the movement from its inception, Levin provides a splendid history and summary of medical education in this area.

Chapter 7, "Prescriptions and Proscriptions," is an enormous contribution to medical ethics. Rarely has anyone given such careful attention to the various religious roots of medical ethics, both ancient and modern. Indeed, the entire modern field of medical ethics emerged from religiously grounded thinkers such as Paul Ramsey, Richard A. McCormick, Rabbi Immanuel Jakobovits, Al Jonsen, Kenneth Vaux, H. Tristram Engelhardt, and Edmund D. Pellegrino. Levin's knowledge of the field of medical ethics and its development at the interface with religions is exceptional.

In Chapter 8, Levin addresses with thoroughness and clarity the rich interface of religion and health policy formation, and the partnership between medicine and religious organizations in this area of healthcare and public health advocacy. Finally, in Chapter 9, he points powerfully to the future choices and challenges that loom as we make the most of the religion and medicine interface. He addresses federal funding of studies in this area and political, professional, ethical, and research challenges, and asks us to foster a future where this interface is understood and recognized for its importance in medicine and healing.

To conclude, each of us has a unique part to play in the healing of the world. Jeff Levin has been a passionate healer all of his life, and this awesome scholarly work, *Religion and Medicine*, points us toward a healing future where we can each benefit from his accumulated knowledge and unwavering commitment to this broad and all-important interface. Professor Levin brings his analytical talent to the interface, but such a splendid legacy emanates not just from his mind but from his heart, and perhaps also from the mystery of the soul.

I know I speak for hundreds and even thousands of researchers and scholars, friends and colleagues, both living and dead, who are forever grateful to Jeff Levin for his life's work. His is a truly astonishing harvest for the betterment of both medicine and religion in their awesome synergy. For those of us still among the living and fortunate enough to have *Religion and Medicine* on our desks, we welcome this tremendous gift for the building of a healthier world.

Stephen G. Post, Ph.D.
Professor of Family, Population, and Preventive Medicine
Head, Division of Medicine in Society
Director, Center for Medical Humanities, Compassionate Care, and Bioethics
The Renaissance School of Medicine at Stony Brook University

Acknowledgments

Religion and Medicine is the culmination of lifelong interests that lie at the interface of religion, broadly defined, and medicine and healing. Within my genealogy are physicians and rabbis—men of science and of faith—as well as psychotherapists and healers. My great-grandfather Rabbi Judah Leib Levin was both a cofounder of Agudath HaRabbonim, the first organization of Orthodox rabbis in the United States, and inventor of the combined adding and subtracting machine. My mother was one of the first cohort of Reiki healers trained and certified in this country. I also had a great uncle who was both a homeopathic physician and a kabbalist, and another great uncle who was president of the Union of American Hebrew Congregations, the governing body of Reform Judaism, as was his father. Another great-grandfather was both a pioneering neurologist and a trustee of Hebrew Union College. I could go on.

This heritage is recapitulated in my academic career. By profession I am an epidemiologist—and married to an epidemiologist—with training in graduate schools of public health and biomedical sciences, yet my undergraduate degree is in religion. Since the early 1980s, my research and writing have focused on the impact of religious participation and spiritual engagement on the physical and mental health of people and populations. How I fell into this unusual career path is a story that I tell later in this book. One might say I was born to it.

While my formal engagement of the broad interface of religion and medicine has been as an academic scientist, analyzing epidemiologic data from large population-based studies, I have come to acknowledge that this may be among the least interesting points of intersection between the domains of faith and healing. No disparagement is meant of those of us who conduct research on this topic. But there is a historical context to this work that extends back centuries and millennia, and there is thus a narrative to unpack that is typically glossed over in articles and books on this subject.

From reading these works one may get the mistaken idea that in the recent past a few doctors and scientists, myself included, for reasons not entirely clear or perhaps for evangelistic motives, woke up one day and decided to hasten the intrusion of faith and subjectivity into the domain of science and reason. To some commentators, this has been a welcome development, a long-needed rapprochement and a remedy to the materialism and reductionism of Western medicine. To others, this development is something quite sinister and destructive. I cannot speak for any of my colleagues, but none of this has anything at all to do with how or why I came to conduct research on religious factors in health, nor why I am fascinated by the larger subject of religion and medicine. Nor does it describe why I have written this book.

As is apparent in the pages that follow, religion has been a part of the story of medicine since the origins of the medical profession and the healing arts. And medicine and healing have been a part of the story of religion since the origins of religion among our earliest human ancestors. Each of these domains or sectors— religion and medicine—represents a significant chapter in the story of the other. Rabbi Immanuel Jakobovits, pioneering figure in medical ethics, put it most succinctly: "Religion and medicine have been in alliance with each other in every land, among all peoples, and almost throughout the entire course of recorded human history."

Institutions of healing and care were birthed by religion, externalizations of its prophetic role to speak out against brokenness and to labor to repair the world, from the first priest-healers to the first hospitals to contemporary developments such as public health missions, the pastoral care profession, and the field of bioethics. The instrumental functions of faith, spirituality, and religious involvement can be seen not just in the research studies spoken of earlier but in ongoing congregational health promotion programs, innovations in medical education, and faith-based advocacy for healthcare policy and reform.

Religion and Medicine tells this story of the encounter between religion and medicine, from its ancient beginnings up through the present day. The book is organized topically, each chapter focusing on a respective point of intersection between the institutions of religion and medicine. No claim is being made that every such intersection is represented here. The history of religious healing, for one, is mentioned only in passing. It is such an enormous topic, including its esoteric dimensions, that it merits its own book-length treatment. I have taught a class on this fascinating subject to medical humanities students at Baylor, and their feedback has been encouraging. But such a book is a project for another time.

Over the past few years, I have lectured on the material in *Religion and Medicine* at several academic medical centers, including Harvard, Duke, Baylor, and Texas. Audiences included physicians, nurses, public health scientists, pastoral care professionals, religious and theological scholars, bioethicists, medical humanities professors, and graduate students in several fields. These presentations were well received and encouraged me to consider expanding this work into a book manuscript.

I am deeply grateful to Cynthia Read, my editor at Oxford University Press, for her kindness and enthusiasm and patience. I was long aware of her gigantic reputation and stature within academic religious publishing, and I owe my good fortune in connecting with her to my Baylor colleague Philip Jenkins. For many years, whenever I would pass along one of my latest medical journal articles, he would invariably tell me that it should become a book and that I should send a prospectus to Cynthia. In 2016 I shared a copy of a paper titled "Partnerships Between the Faith-Based and Medical Sectors: Implications for Preventive Medicine and Public Health," published in *Preventive Medicine Reports* and the topic of my recent lectures, and received the usual response from Philip: send this to Cynthia right away. I am glad that I finally listened.

Besides Philip, my other colleagues at Baylor's Institute for Studies of Religion have been supportive of me throughout this project and my earlier work on this subject. From lending an ear to my ideas to chatting informally as I progressed through the manuscript to more substantive comments, my sincerest thanks are offered to Byron Johnson, Rodney Stark, David Jeffrey, Gordon Melton, and Tommy Kidd. It is a great privilege to be part of such a remarkable and multidisciplinary group of scholars and to read the continual flow of books and articles that come from these brilliant men. I hope that *Religion and Medicine* has earned a place alongside their great works of historical, literary, philosophical, and social science scholarship.

Finally, I reserve my deepest gratitude for the two greatest sources of blessing and goodness in my life. To my dear wife, Lea, whom I love more than I can express in words, I am thankful for her constant support and prayers and for her vast insight and wisdom. And to the *Ribbono Shel Olam*, the Master and Creator of the Universe, I give thanks for the continuing *chesed* (lovingkindness) that sustains me in my life and in my work.

Jeff Levin
Woodway, Texas

1

Conflict and Cooperation

Religion and medicine. What do these two greatest of social institutions have to do with each other?

Religion occupies the domain of spirit, a highly contested space that many contemporaries do not believe exists in objective reality.[1] Medicine is, presumably, the product of science and reason, of empirical study, its truths validated only by observable effects on human physical bodies.[2] To some modern-day reformers, the renewed encounter between religion and medicine—or spirit and body, or faith and reason—is cause for rejoicing, a restoration of an ancient alliance that should never have been torn asunder.[3] To some skeptics and humanists, this encounter is an affront, better left dead and buried in the distant past before the advent of modern Western biomedicine, which presumably exiled superstitious notions of spirituality forever from the science of healing.[4]

A popular internet meme is titled "A Brief History of Medicine." Several versions are floating around, and it goes something like this:

> I have an earache.
> 2000 BCE: Here, eat this root.
> 1000 CE: Here, say this prayer.
> 1850 CE: Here, drink this potion.
> 1930 CE: Here, swallow this pill.
> 1950 CE: Here, take this antibiotic.
> 2000 CE: Here, eat this root and say this prayer.

In a nutshell, this list presents the history of medicine, with a few liberties taken. The trajectory is familiar: from natural remedies and faith healing to modern scientific therapies and, recently, back to natural ("alternative") and spiritual interventions. Not unexpectedly, many leaders of Western biomedicine do not consider this progression particularly savory, viewing with skepticism, suspicion, and alarm renewed interest in the psyche and spirit and in holism.[5] In the 1990s I made a slide out of this meme and for years opened my lecture-circuit talks with it. Depending upon the audience, it elicited a smile, a nod, a laugh, a groan, or a concerned look, and among those who responded negatively there was always a pause as they nervously waited to discover my side on the issue.

Religion and Medicine. Jeff Levin, Oxford University Press (2020) © Oxford University Press.
DOI: 10.1093/oso/9780190867355.001.0001

The history of the encounter between religion and medicine can be traced back thousands of years, from the etiologic beliefs and medical traditions of the ancients—East and West—to the healing ministry of Jesus and the work and writings of myriad later figures: medieval physician-philosophers such as ʻAlī ibn Mūsā ar-Riḍā and Moses Maimonides, Enlightenment-era thinkers like John Wesley and the faith-based fathers of the natural hygiene movement, major nineteenth- and twentieth-century leaders of Western academic medicine and psychiatry, and contemporary pioneers in research on religion and health.

On the whole, the starting point for this discussion dates to centuries before the Common Era. Manly P. Hall,[6] scholar of mysticism, wrote extensively on the pre-Christian origins of therapeutic cults and the esoteric medical and healing practices of ancient mystery schools. He identified the origins of "metaphysical healing" in the ancient "priest-physician-psychologist" (or, in the vernacular, witch doctor), who functioned in part from the trance state and through dream interpretation, able to discern the spiritual mystery of disease.[7] Historian Gary B. Ferngren has documented modalities of healing that existed in Greece, Rome, and the ancient near East.[8] "Healing in the ancient world took a variety of forms," he notes, "some secular and some religious or magical."[9] The etiology of disease, moreover, was given various attributions, including divine (often retributive), demonic, magical, and natural sources of causation.

These systems of medical beliefs and practices, and associated professional roles, evolved centuries before Jesus and the apostles.[10] They were heirs to diagnostic and therapeutic philosophies and traditions prevalent throughout the ancient world. The construction of a uniquely Christian healing tradition was owed in part to existing schools of thought received from the Greco-Roman world, as well as to characteristic Jewish beliefs about longevity, disease risk, mental health and well-being, disease prevention, and healing based on the Torah and teachings of the rabbis.[11] Harold Y. Vanderpool, historian of medicine and religion, described four distinct ways that Jesus healed.[12] He did so through exorcism, that is, casting out demons; through physically healing the afflicted; through the agency of one's faith in God's ability to cure; and through offering forgiveness of sin and, concomitantly, mitigation of the psychologically damaging effects of guilt.

In the East, parallel traditions of religiously informed healing and medicinal systems, influenced by sources as disparate as *Sāṅkhya, Rāja-yoga*, and streams of Buddhism, have flourished for thousands of years in India (*Āyurveda*), Tibet (*Sowa-Rigpa*), and China (*Zhōng Yī*, or traditional Chinese medicine).[13] These healing philosophies have ancient roots yet prosper today in an era when Western biomedicine has spread its influence and hegemony around the globe. Such indigenous traditions of medicine have made inroads in the West, part of the global and cross-cultural currents that have stimulated the growing popularity of integrative medical therapies. This is seen in ascending utilization rates[14] and evolving content of postgraduate medical education curricula.[15] Western physicians-in-training may never incorporate Indian or traditional Chinese elements into their clinical practice, but many now complete their undergraduate and postgraduate medical education at least having read about these systems. This would have been unheard of a generation ago.

For each of the Western monotheistic faith traditions, centuries of theologically informed writing exists on themes related to medical practice, the biomedical sciences, and personal health and wellness. Notable examples are many.

Moses Maimonides's treatises on health, published at the end of the twelfth century, contributed to his fame as a physician,[16] which in his day was as much a source of his renown as his stature as a Talmudic scholar and philosopher. The treatises contained discourses and information on various topics: coitus, hemorrhoids, asthma, poisons, lethal and pharmaceutical drugs, accidents, and "the regimen of health," the latter in an early self-care text emphasizing what today would be termed psychosocial influences on well-being, as well as diet and natural remedies. For example, in Chapter 1 of *The Regimen of Health*, Maimonides offers this advice: "Drinking water following a meal is bad, corrupting the digestion, except when one is accustomed to it. One should not drink anything with the meal, or after it, as long as it is in the stomach, except pure, cold water; it should not be mixed with anything."[17] This prescription could come from a modern-day textbook of naturopathic medicine.

John Wesley's *Primitive Physic*,[18] published in 1791, has been described as "among the earliest medical self-care guides and a foundational text for the subsequent natural hygiene movement."[19] In contrast to Maimonides's text from six hundred years earlier, Wesley, not a physician, brought to bear a wealth of knowledge on natural remedies not necessarily grounded in the medical science of the day. Some material reads like a late-twentieth-century manual of holistic health and living: "The studious ought to have stated times for exercise, at least two or three hours a-day: the one half of this before dinner, the other before going to bed."[20] Some is consistent with regional traditions of folk medical practice at the time: for example, to treat jaundice in children, "Take half an ounce of fine rhubarb powdered. Mix with it thoroughly, by fine beating, two handfuls of good clean currants. Of this give a teaspoonful every evening."[21] Some invokes superstition or is downright bizarre: "In the last stage [of consumption], suck an healthy woman daily. Tried by my Father."[22]

Muslim scholarship on health and medicine dates to the origins of Islam, drawing on passages in both the Qur'ān and *hadīth* literature.[23] In *Health and Medicine in the Islamic Tradition*, Pakistani scholar Fazlur Rahman traces the history of medical science and practice in Islam from its origins in the Muslim canon up to the present day, including discussion of contemporary bioethical issues. These include the usual topics for medical ethics, such as contraception, abortion, sexuality, and end-of-life issues, but also Islamic teachings addressing human dignity. He also describes what he terms "spiritual medicine,"[24] a subject that subsequent scholars pursued.[25] An important theme for Rahman is the "integrality of faith and reason" and an "emphasis on a holistic universe [that] implies that physical health is integrally related to spiritual or moral health."[26] Another prominent theme, in contrast to the self-help-ism of Wesley, is the communal nature of health for Islam, that the "self is an integral unit, part of an integrated moral-physical universe."[27] Accordingly,

> Submitting to the will of God, Islam, is healthful for the individual. It brings the peace of mind necessary for good health. And since the will of God is for humans to create and maintain a just social order, in that very submission humans become instruments of other people's health, for no society could be called just without access to adequate medical care.[28]

Extant Jewish[29] and Muslim[30] folk medical traditions with medieval or earlier origins can be identified, as well as various Christian folk healing traditions, including contemporary syncretisms such as *curanderismo*.[31] The latter is the indigenous folk healing system of Mexico, Mexican-American communities, and expat Mexican communities of Latin America. Syncretic elements in the beliefs and practices of *curanderos* originate in a hybridization between Roman Catholicism brought by the *conquistadores* and indigenous spiritualities and folk medical traditions existing in the New World. In many instances, for a particular nosological category (*mal ojo, maleficio*) or specialty role (*espiritualista, yerbera*), "formal Roman Catholic elements inform or define the ritual,"[32] which is otherwise rooted in native spiritual or folk medical beliefs and practices.

Discussion of religion in Western biomedicine dates to at least 1835, when Amariah Brigham, a founder of the American Psychiatric Association, published *Observations on the Influence of Religion upon the Health and Physical Welfare of Mankind*.[33] His measured conclusion was that "religious worship and the cultivation of devotional feelings, are beneficial to man, when not carried to an unreasonable extent."[34] This was followed over several decades by a steady stream of writing by clergy and theologians and by psychologists and physicians,[35] whose collective work defined the emergence in the first half of the twentieth century of what became known as the "religion and health movement."[36]

Representative works associated with the movement include Episcopal priest Elwood Worcester and colleagues' *Religion and Medicine*,[37] University of Chicago divinity professor Charles T. Holman's *The Religion of a Healthy Mind*,[38] pastoral care pioneer Carroll A. Wise's *Religion in Illness and Health*,[39] pastoral theologian Seward Hiltner's *Religion and Health*,[40] Lutheran theologian Paul Tillich's essay, "The Relation of Religion and Health,"[41] and pastoral psychologist Wayne E. Oates's *Religious Factors in Mental Illness*.[42] Also significant was establishment of the Blanton-Peale Institute, founded in 1937; the Academy of Religion and Mental Health, founded in 1954 as an academic wing of the institute; and the peer-reviewed *Journal of Religion and Health*, founded in 1961 by the institute. The academy sponsored annual symposia with published proceedings for the next decade.[43]

Modern research and scholarship by academically credentialed experts at the intersection of religion and medicine, broadly defined, has been ongoing for over a century. The earliest work dates to the beginning of Western biomedicine, from esteemed figures in medicine and published in the most prestigious medical journals. No matter the perceptions of this subject matter by later in the twentieth century—as marginal, unscientific, unsound, and unsavory—speculation early on about the impact of religious beliefs and practices, of faith, and of the domain of spirit on health and healing of body and mind was an acceptable topic for scholarly reflection and attracted some of the best minds in medicine.

Notable contributions included John Shaw Billings's analysis of fertility, mortality, and sociodemographic data on American Jews, published in 1891;[44] Sir William Osler's famous essay "The Faith That Heals," published in the *British Medical Journal* (*BMJ*) in 1910;[45] and Alice E. Paulsen's remarkable three-part series on religious healing, published in the *Journal of the American Medical Association* (*JAMA*) in 1926.[46] Other notable essays include contributions to a special issue of *BMJ* that appeared alongside Osler's article,[47] a book review that appeared in an earlier volume of the same journal,[48] and an editorial on "divine healing" that appeared in *Science* in 1892.[49] Even the American Medical Association has been formally wrestling with this subject for sixty years.[50]

In recent decades, institutional alliances have emerged and flourished between the religious and medical sectors. These include establishment of the field of bioethics, the healthcare chaplaincy profession, congregational disease prevention and health promotion programs, academic centers and institutes devoted to medical research and education on spirituality, and much more. Unpacking this history—both ancient and more recent—involves weighing competing narratives about relations between the institutions of religion and medicine, at times characterized by conflict and other times by cooperation. Religion has been viewed, alternately, as a malevolent force in medicine and healing, as a complementary second calling among prominent physicians, and as a source of wisdom underlying systems of medical practice and healing. Let us examine these in order.

Religion as a Malign Force in Medicine

The encounter between religion and medicine, for much of the past millennium and currently still, is marked by contention and controversy. Indeed, simply uttering or reading the phrase *religion and medicine* or its equivalents—*faith and medicine, faith and healing, spirituality and medicine*, and so on—evokes strong responses from earnest people within science and medicine, not necessarily positive, and for good reason. Brandeis sociologist Wendy Cadge has characterized the historical encounter as "a messy story,"[51] notable for the lurid imagery it evokes. A couple of historical examples are most familiar.

The European plague pandemic of the 1340s, known as the Black Death, was the most famous and devastating population-thinning event in human history. As much as half to two-thirds of Europe's population was decimated, probably due to contact with black rats (*Rattus rattus*) infected by vector fleas carrying the *Yersinia pestis* bacterium. Anecdotal evidence suggests that Jews experienced lower mortality than other populations, perhaps due to observance of ritual laws related to hygiene and to social isolation that limited contagion. Accordingly they were widely scapegoated for having caused the outbreak,[52] such as through poisoning of wells, and campaigns of genocide occurred throughout Western Europe, especially in France, Spain, Belgium, Switzerland, Austria, and Germany.[53] This accusation was reinforced by forced confessions, extracted under torture.[54] "The ridiculousness of the charge," according to Oxford historian Cecil Roth, "should have been apparent even to fourteenth-century credulity, for the plague raged virulently even in those places, such as England, where the Christian population was absolutely unadulterated, and elsewhere the Jews suffered with the rest."[55]

Another dark episode in European history was the witch trials beginning in the fifteenth century and the subsequent hanging or burning of women under suspicion of various "magical" practices, including natural healing.[56] Margot Adler, in her history of contemporary neopaganism, summarized this thesis: "the persecutions were used to destroy the power of midwives and healers and bolster the emerging medical profession."[57] According to Adler, recent scholarship has questioned the salience of these motives. Moreover, according to Rodney Stark, the number of victims has been highly inflated, and attribution of this crime primarily to the Roman and Spanish Inquisitions is historically inaccurate.[58] Still, the events did happen, if on a smaller scale, and the witch hunts are still referenced by critics of institutional Western medicine as a metaphor warning of the dangerous hegemony of allopathic physicians who claim a monopoly on healing.[59] That is, just as the church in early modern Europe burned witches for heresy, according to this narrative, so, too, does the "Church of Modern Medicine" persecute nonbelievers and medical heretics.[60]

A few contemporary examples of this messy history can be added to the list.

In the early years of television in the 1950s, among the most popular and ubiquitous offerings were professional wrestling and faith-healing televangelism. These two art forms had more in common than either likely wishes to admit. Christian evangelists with healing ministries dated to the earliest years of radio, the most prominent being Aimee Semple McPherson.[61] Oral Roberts established a television presence in the 1950s,[62] and Kathryn Kuhlman, a successor to McPherson, found a weekly audience for *I Believe in Miracles* beginning in the 1960s.[63] Others joined them on the air in subsequent decades, with national and regional followings. These included Leroy Jenkins, Reverend Ike, Ernest Angley, Peter Popoff, and Benny Hinn, whose healing crusades and miracle services, *This Is Your Day* TV show, and appearances on both Christian and secular news and interview shows made him a media celebrity.

Each of these names has been associated with scandal. Popoff was exposed by skeptic James Randi as guilty of fraud in his healing services,[64] Jenkins went to prison for multiple felony convictions,[65] and Roberts was the subject of a famous exposé by a disgruntled former lieutenant found nearly beaten to death following publication of his book.[66] This is not a blanket indictment, of course, of every person who believes that he or she has a healing gift, but the lure of celebrity and riches has drawn individuals into this occupation whose earnestness may be questioned. Outside of their loyal core audience, TV faith healers on the whole have done much to color public perceptions of religion's place in medicine and impart an air of disrepute.

Since the 1970s, when elective abortion was decriminalized in the United States, acts of violence have been committed against family planning clinics and individual abortion providers. These include bombing, arson, murder, assault, and property crime. Hundreds of other threats were made, but not acted on.[67] Motives for violence include people and groups intent on making a political statement against government funding of reproductive health services,[68] as well as individuals and organizations claiming a religious imprimatur for their actions.[69]

Pro-life groups, on the whole, including faith-based organizations (FBOs), have unequivocally denounced such violent acts.[70] But radical antiabortion activists, notably Randall A. Terry of Operation Rescue, have seemed halfhearted or ambivalent in their condemnation.[71] Population data from the 1980s showed, however, that the incidence of clinic bombings was actually lower in areas where Catholics, Baptists, or Mormons—denominations with strong pro-life views— were proportionally more numerous,[72] but this is an ecologic-level finding and inconclusive. Other research evidence suggests that clinic violence, regardless of motives, tends to reduce utilization rates only modestly and for a limited time, and thus is "ultimately unsuccessful in obstructing the market for abortions [*sic*] services."[73] This underscores that the impact of religion on violence against reproductive health providers and on subsequent abortion rates may be more complex than how it is often depicted, notwithstanding the religious identity of many individual perpetrators.

An ongoing concern among healthcare policymakers in the United States is misinformed consumers who substitute sketchy New Age therapies for validated medical treatment. This idea has been reinforced in the medical literature for many years.[74] As alienation from mainline religion is often coupled with attraction to antiestablishment views about other social institutions (including politics and the environment), so the narrative goes, this may condition a general skepticism of mainstream science and medicine. Use of alternative therapies may of course be for affirmative reasons: the "philosophical congruence" between a holistic, body-mind-spirit worldview and alternative medicine.[75] J. Gordon Melton and his associates noted that the "New Age and Holistic Health movements in theory exist independently, but they are united philosophically by one central concept: that the individual person is responsible for his or her own life and for seeking out the means of transformation needed to achieve a better quality of life."[76]

New Age beliefs in combination with an absence of scientific or clinical training, however, may indeed heighten the likelihood of falling for the claims of charlatans whose pitch resonates with these lay consumers and reinforces their worldview. A recent example is the antivaxxers who oppose routine immunization against childhood diseases, such as measles, on specious grounds related to faith in "natural healing" and to a famous hoax perpetrated in 1998 by Andrew Wakefield, a now delicensed British physician who published faked data purportedly linking the MMR vaccine to autism.[77] Media coverage of this incident caused a significant decline in immunization rates throughout the United Kingdom and the United States. Ten of his twelve coauthors subsequently withdrew their names from the paper and it was retracted from the journal where it was published, but it took rates of vaccine coverage several years to recover.[78]

For some of these examples of religious malevolence extending into the domain of medicine or healing, especially occurring centuries ago, the historical accuracy of tacit accounts may be questionable. Such emotionally charged circumstances are subject to exaggeration, but these events were and are nonetheless real and have been documented as such. Accordingly, associated lurid images are part of the accepted story of the encounter between religion and medicine, and dominate public discourse on the subject. They have contributed to the jarring uneasiness that so many of us feel when we hear or see words such as *religion, spirituality, faith, prayer,* or *God* used in juxtaposition to words like *medicine, health, healing, healthcare,* or *the body.* But these negative images tell only part of the story.

Religion and Medicine as Complementary Callings

An entirely different narrative is possible for the religion-medicine encounter, one more positive and hopeful. As recently noted, this alternative narrative "does not negate these troubling images, but offers a more complete and accurate picture of the fullness of the ways that the worlds of religion and faith, on the one hand, and of medicine and healthcare, on the other, have encountered each other throughout history."[79] For some faith traditions, relations between people and institutions associated with religion and medicine have been characterized more by cooperation, mutuality, and shared values.[80] In certain traditions, the "encounter" has even occurred within the same person.

Take, for example, the religious tradition with which I am most familiar. In Judaism, many of the greatest rabbinic sages were also men of medicine and science.[81] Three in particular were among the most learned and historically significant commentators on the Jewish Scriptures and rabbinic canon.

Moses ben Maimon, also known as Maimonides and the Rambam, was a twelfth-century Spanish rabbi, physician, and philosophical theologian.[82] He was his era's preeminent exegete of Torah and Talmud, wrote extensively on Jewish law and on philosophical theology, and as noted earlier, was the most celebrated Jewish medical figure of his day, authoring numerous texts on health and medical topics.[83] The following century, Moses ben Nachman forged a similar path, from a similar professional background, as Maimonides. Also known as Nachmanides and the Ramban, he was a Catalan rabbi, physician, and philosopher[84] whose influential Torah commentary is still in print and widely used.[85] Ovadiah ben Yaacov Sforno was a sixteenth-century Italian rabbi, physician, and philosopher.[86] He wrote works of religious philosophy and, like the Ramban, is best known for his popular Torah commentary.

This phenomenon can still be observed today in Abraham Twerski, American rabbi and psychiatrist,[87] and Avraham Steinberg, Israeli rabbi, neurologist, and bioethicist.[88] Unlike the previous troika of sages, men of both medicine and religion who emphasized rabbinic scholarship in their published writing, each of these contemporary Jewish scholars is most known for his medical works, although these are heavily informed by *halachah* (Jewish law) and Jewish religious principles and by their rabbinic learning.

Another example, not from medicine but from science and mathematics: my great-grandfather Rabbi Judah Leib Levin.[89] Born in 1863 in Lithuania, he studied at the famous Volozhin Yeshiva and Kovno Kollel and received *s'michah* (rabbinic ordination) from both Rabbi Isaac Elchanan Spektor and Rabbi Naphtali Zvi Yehuda Berlin (known as the Netziv), among others. After marrying and coming to the United States before the turn of the century, his biography contains a very unusual dual accomplishment: in 1901 he cofounded Agudath

Ha-Rabbonim, the oldest rabbinic organization for traditional Orthodox rabbis in the United States,[90] and in the following year he filed the first of three patents culminating in invention of the combined adding and subtracting machine, on display since 1938 in the permanent collection of the Smithsonian Institution.[91] "Religion" and "science" coexisted easily within the *parnassah* (livelihood) of this one accomplished person.

Rabbi Levin was not unique in this regard. The peer-reviewed academic journal *B'Or Ha'Torah* publishes papers on the physical and biological sciences, mathematics, and technology, including medicine and public health, from a Torah-observant perspective by Orthodox Jewish scientists and physicians.[92] The journal is sponsored by the Jerusalem College of Technology, and at the time of this writing has published its twenty-fifth volume. The moral: significant figures in science or technology or medicine may also be accomplished people of faith, and significant religious leaders may be accomplished in medical or scientific or technological fields. There is no inherent reason why this should not be so.

The most familiar twentieth-century Christian exemplar of this complementary calling is Albert Schweitzer: physician, philosopher, theologian, minister, professor, and medical missionary.[93] Moreso even than the rabbinic figures just described, Schweitzer was equally celebrated for his great works in medicine and religion. He was ordained to the Lutheran ministry, received a Ph.D. in theology from the Sorbonne, and in 1906 published his most famous work, on the historical Jesus.[94] That same year, in answer to a personal call to evangelize the gospel through a healing ministry, he began medical school in Strasbourg. Upon graduation, he established a missionary hospital at Lambaréné, in French Equatorial Africa (later Gabon), which became his life's work and for which he was awarded the Nobel Peace Prize in 1952.

A notable example from Islamic history is ʿAlī ibn Mūsā ar-Riḍā, an eighth- and ninth-century Persian Shia imam and descendant of the Prophet Muhammad. Like Maimonides, he wrote works of religion and of medicine.[95] Respective examples include a major collection of Shia *hadīths* and the most influential medical textbook of his era. The former, *al-Sahīfa al-Riḍā*, contains 240 sayings addressing a variety of topics: prayer, morality, good manners, family matters, dietary advice, and more.[96] The latter, *Al-Risalah al-Dhahabiah*, also known as the Golden Treatise, is considered the greatest Islamic medical work of its time.[97] According to a modern biographer, the treatise "contains general programs necessary for putting right man's body and protecting it from diseases, so it is regarded as the main base of preventive medicine in these times and as a great means of improving health."[98] This includes material on cardiology and neurology, and anatomy, physiology, and pathophysiology of organs and body systems, from the perspective of humoral medicine. Despite advances in biomedicine since its writing, ar-Riḍā's medical writing "continues to enjoy the reputation it had when it first appeared, and has continued to rouse interest in scholars of Medical Science."[99] Importantly, he was not alone among significant medieval contributors to Islamic medical thought.[100]

Throughout India for centuries, itinerant holy men and women have traveled the countryside offering spiritual instruction, healing the sick, and performing seeming miracles. These include teachers from established spiritual lineages, such as *swāmīs* (Hindu religious teachers) and ordainees of monastic orders, many of whom established major institutions, as well as obscure *sādhus* (ascetic renunciants) of Hindu or Jain origin and other miscellaneous saints.[101] Paramahansa Yogananda, for example, is best known as a twentieth-century teacher who brought *kriyā yoga* to the West and authored *The Autobiography of a Yogi*.[102] Less widely known is that he also produced a volume on techniques of healing, including preventing and curing physical disease, which relied upon spiritual attainments such as faith, control over the life energy, and "obedience to God's physical laws [as] the method for avoiding bodily ills."[103] Examination of Mahāyāna Buddhist texts has suggested that the origins of Indian medicine, centuries before the Common Era, may lie in "the work of heterodox ascetics rather than from brāhmaṇic intellectuals and that the significant growth of Indian medicine took place in early Buddhist monastic establishments."[104] This provocative thesis underscores the overlapping (and probably inseparable) narratives of religion and medicine in the history of the Indian subcontinent.

Africa is home to numerous cultures, ethnicities, language groups, spiritual traditions, and systems and philosophies of healing. It is wrong to speak of native African healers as a single category, due to the diversity of religious antecedents.[105] In the Bantu communities of sub-Saharan central and southern Africa, the indigenous healing tradition is grounded in the idea that "the interconnected fates of healthiness and of affliction or misfortune are traced to a central source of power (or life) in God and nature. This source of life is mediated by middle-range spirits, ancestors, and consecrated priests who maintain contact with or receive inspiration from that source."[106] In Kongo society, this translates into an etiologic spectrum encompassing numerous possible causal agents of disease: *nzambi* (God), *bisimbi* (nature and nature spirits), *bakisi* (disease spirits), *bankuyu* (ghosts), *bakulu* (ancestor shades), and *bandoki* (witches).[107]

Therapeutic modalities, likewise, are multifaceted, incorporating what people in the West would consider both religious and medical interventions. The *sangoma*, or traditional Bantu healer, exemplifies the inseparability of these etic categories within an indigenous context.[108] Diagnosis may be through altered states of consciousness, spirit possession, out-of-body experiences, divination, dreams, or other ritual psychic means (*femba*). Medical treatment (*muti*) includes use of faith, placebos, and distant healing, as well as plant and animal substances with known pharmacological properties.[109] The fluidity of a professional space incorporating both spiritual and biomedical elements creates ongoing conflict and tension between native healers and conventional medical practitioners, development agencies, and government regulatory bodies.[110]

In *Honoring the Medicine*, Ken "Bear Hawk" Cohen explains that Native American healing "is based on a spiritual philosophy of life"[111] that guides healers and enables discernment of specific healing powers in nature, including in visions, rituals, sacred spaces, herbs and plants, and the life energy that permeates all creation. In other words, the work of a healer is an intrinsically spiritual calling. Cohen makes this clear in his description of the spiritual transmission of teachings and rituals related to healing, which he terms "transcribing the ineffable."[112] He goes on: "Many aspects of Native American healing are still closely guarded oral tradition. Specific techniques of healing, sacred songs, and healing rituals are received directly from elder healers, from spirits encountered during vision quest, and as a result of initiation into secret societies."[113]

In many traditions throughout the world, distinctively religious and medical professional roles cannot easily be differentiated; they are inseparable. Anthropologist George Murdock's cross-cultural ethnographic research using data on 139 societies from the Human Relations Area Files reveals the ubiquity of theories of supernatural causation for illness and disease.[114] These include theories of mystical, animistic, and magical causation involving fate, ominous sensations, contagion, mystical retribution, soul loss, spirit aggression, sorcery, and witchcraft. These concepts of etiology are not the sole province of "primitive" societies but are distributed across the world's cultures.[115] Murdock concludes that his evidence "reinforces the conclusion that supernatural causes of illness far outweigh natural causes in the belief systems of the world's peoples."[116] Are practitioners of the healing arts in these instances practicing medicine? Practicing religion? Both? Does it matter?

Religion as Underlying Systems of Medicine

Yet another take on the encounter between religion and medicine is possible. A correlation can be observed within particular cultures between respective religious traditions and systems of healing. More specifically, beliefs and practices of religions and spiritual paths underlie the "therapeutic knowledge" within associated indigenous medical traditions. The concept of therapeutic knowledge is used by philosophers of medicine and medical anthropologists in reference to the distinctive body of medical knowledge, both diagnostic and therapeutic, underlying respective systems, philosophies, or schools of healing or medical practice.[117] According to philosopher James A. Marcum, diagnostic knowledge is based on discursive knowledge, grounded in logic and seeking to provide rational understandings of the "how" of a medical case presentation or disease.[118] Many examples of a correlation, historically and contemporarily, between such knowledge and associated religious beliefs and worldviews can be identified across faith and wisdom traditions.

Āyurveda, the ancient healing system of India, is rooted in the Vedic religious tradition, elements of which are said to have originated over five thousand years ago.[119] Many of its basic etiologic and therapeutic principles derive from *Sāṅkhya*, one of six schools of Hindu philosophy, whose founder, the semimythical sage Kapila, described three *gunas*, or "universal qualities that pervade all creation."[120] These are *sattva* (positive quality; purity, clarity, perfection), *rajas* (mixed quality; will, action, struggle), and *tamas* (negative quality; inertia, darkness, blindness).[121] In *Āyurveda*, there is a parallel distinction among three *doshas* (characteristic body-type qualities), which predominate alone or in combination within each person. These are known as *vata* (composed of space and air), *pitta* (composed of fire and water), and *kapha* (composed of water and earth). These constitutional types have associated physiological and pathophysiological profiles, as well as lifestyle, dietary, emotional, and stress-response inclinations. Clinical assessment, diagnosis, and treatment in *Āyurveda* are grounded, in part, in differentiating these types.[122] An observable connection between *gunas* and *doshas* is significant for this discussion inasmuch as it points to an underlying influence of the spiritual on the physical.

Also thousands of years old, traditional Chinese medicine (in Mandarin, *Zhōng Yī*) is based on a set of fundamental concepts that inform understandings of disease etiology, diagnosis, and treatment.[123] The two polarities of *yin* (inactive, cold, dark) and *yang* (active, hot, bright) are intrinsic characteristics enabling differentiation of "all physiological functions of the body, as well as the signs and symptoms of pathological change."[124] The five-element theory (*Wu Xing*) distinguishes among five basic substances from which the universe is constructed: wood, fire, earth, metal, and water. This concept likewise "explains the relationships between the human body and the external environment as well as the physiological and pathological relationships among the internal organs within the human body."[125]

Significantly, both the *yin-yang* and five-elements concepts derive from Taoism, which provides a conceptual and explicitly spiritual foundation for traditional Chinese medicine, similarly to how *Sāṅkhya* underlies *Āyurveda*. The Chinese connection is closer still: the importance of the Taoist *qi* (vital life force) and *jīng luo* (network of meridians) along which it flows through the body for purposes of diagnosis and treatment bears a strong resemblance to the centrality of the yogic *prāna* (life force or energy) that moves along *nāḍīs* (channels) for the practice of Indian medicine.

As in India and China, in Tibet the indigenous religious tradition of *Vajrayāna* or Tibetan Buddhism gave rise to a sophisticated medical system, known as *Sowa-Rigpa*.[126] Also influenced by contact with earlier Hindu and Buddhist therapeutic traditions and Persian and Greek humoral medicine, incorporating elements from each, Tibetan medicine is essentially sui generis.[127] In Tibetan medicine, principles of etiology, diagnosis, treatment, and disease prevention originate in material from an Indian text imported into Tibet in the eighth century, known as the *rGyud-bZhi*, or Four Tantras. A central theme is imbalance, which coheres with the Buddhist view of falling out of balance—physically, mentally, or spiritually—as a primary cause of suffering. Imbalances occur in the context of a triad of essential and interdependent elements: *chi* (space), *schara* (energy), and *badahan* (matter). Restoration of balance, whether physical or mental, entails a multifaceted regimen including not only diet, medicinals, and bodywork, but also cultivation of spirituality,[128] such as through virtuous behavior and meditative practices.[129]

In the medieval Islamic world, the indigenous tradition of medicine and healing known as *Unani* (Arabic for "Ionian"), or *Unani-tibb* (Greek medicine), evolved syncretically from multiple influences, primarily Greek humoral medicine.[130] It emerged and took form as a function of the Arab world's location at the crossroads of various trade routes, synthesizing content from the Greco-Roman civilization, Persia, India, and even China, as well as from existing folk healing traditions in the region. *Unani* diagnosis, etiology, and treatment are based, fundamentally, on the system of four humors—*dam* (blood), *ṣafrā'* (yellow bile), *saudā'* (black bile), and *balgham* (phlegm).

Unani was effectively codified by eleventh-century Persian physician Avicenna, in his classic work *The Canon of Medicine*.[131] Largely influenced by Galen, Avicenna posited associations between respective humors and temperaments (blood = sanguine; yellow bile = choleric; black bile = melancholic; phlegm = phlegmatic), and also described qualities (hot, cold, wet, dry) with nosological significance. Health and disease are functions, in part, of balance or imbalance among humors. In *Unani*, religious elements in Islamic culture modified the preexisting system, such that "medieval Islamic medicine was not simply a conduit for Greek ideas, which is the stereotypical picture, but it was a venue for innovation and change."[132] Today, *Unani* remains popular in South India and is undergoing a renaissance throughout the Muslim world,[133] recently receiving an imprimatur from the World Health Organization.[134]

An important dimension of the teachings of the New Thought religious movement of the nineteenth and twentieth centuries were beliefs and practices related to healthy living, prevention of disease, and healing.[135] New Thought evolved from Mary Baker Eddy's Christian Science[136] under the direction of several individuals, including former Eddy follower Emma Curtis Hopkins.[137] A line can be drawn from precursors to New Thought—such as Phineas Quimby's mesmerism, Ralph Waldo Emerson's transcendentalism, and Emanuel Swedenborg's revisioning of Christianity[138]—all the way through to present-day body-mind-spirit therapies such as mindfulness meditation.[139] Sylvester Graham's hygienic movement, and its successor, Herbert M. Shelton's natural hygiene ("orthopathy") movement, evolved from or parallel to New Thought and its precursors, as did so many other health-focused religious organizations, including Ernest Holmes's Science of Mind and Charles Fillmore's Unity.[140] A similar dynamic was observed in a study of respective modern-day successor movements to New Thought and natural hygiene—the emerging New Age spirituality of the 1970s and 1980s and what was once referred to as *holistic health*.[141] The ascendancy of New Age healing was a product, in part, of spiritual antecedents, including the rise of new religious movements, antidualistic themes in popular critiques of science, and antiestablishment sentiments regarding religion, medicine, and other social institutions.[142]

In some instances, correspondences between religion and medicine—or between spirit and body—are not merely implied, but explicit and intended. A notable example involves the work of the famous "sleeping prophet," Edgar Cayce, founder of the Association for Research and Enlightenment.[143] Cayce was a Christian and a Sunday school teacher who, early in life, began exhibiting psychic gifts, which initially disturbed him. Throughout several decades, he gave more than fourteen thousand trance readings—over nine thousand containing detailed information on etiology, diagnostics, or treatment for specific medical conditions and individual cases.[144] This channeled information has been compiled and studied, and a therapeutic system has evolved around the readings.[145] According to a leading practitioner, from the Cayce perspective the experience of healing is "a process of attuning ourselves, our energies, to our true nature, that of becoming companions, co-creators with the Father-God."[146] Cayce is widely considered a father of modern holistic medicine,[147] and the eclectic philosophy communicated through his readings has contributed to ongoing interest in researching spirituality within the field of integrative medicine.

Even further afield, esoteric groups and new religious movements posit worldviews that may encompass unique perspectives on diagnosis, therapy, and healing.[148] My own research has documented explicit and characteristic teachings pertaining to anatomy, physiology, nosology, etiology, pathophysiology, and therapeutic modalities across esoteric philosophies and schools. These include kabbalistic, mystery school, gnostic, brotherhoods, Eastern and Western mystical, shamanic, and New Age traditions.[149] The religious influence on medicine manifests itself in both exoteric and esoteric contexts.

Besides the idea that religious content—beliefs, especially, and other teachings—underlie traditions of diagnosis and treatment, there is another way in which religion underlies medicine. Physicians and other healers manifest an externalization of the prophetic calling to go forth—*lech l'cha*, as God instructed Abraham[150]—to labor for redemption of the world. This calls to mind the Jewish concept of *tikkun olam* (repairing the world),[151] which is often translated from Hebrew, significantly, as "healing the world." It also brings to mind another Jewish concept—the Lurianic kabbalistic idea of "redeeming the sparks," the notion that the purpose of life is to labor to awaken the spark of *kedushah* (holiness), of divine light, lying dormant within every unit of God's creation and, through this act of liberation, to contribute to the collective redemption.[152] The extent to which medical practitioners work to heal broken bodies and minds and restore them to function suggests that medicine can itself be a "sacred vocation."[153]

Circling back to the internet meme cited at the start of this chapter: So where do I come down on the issue broached here? Do I accept the first narrative, that religion has been, at times, a malign force in medicine? Or do I acknowledge that it has made a significant contribution to medicine and to the life and work of individual medical practitioners, both historically and still today? Not to be evasive, but my answer is that each narrative contains truth, so none cancel out the others. But since the first theme—religion and medicine as a disturbing juxtaposition of concepts—has received so much attention, not undeservedly, this book instead focuses on the counterarguments: religion and medicine as complementary callings and religion as underlying medicine. Alliances between religion and medicine have offered, and continue to offer, much to uplift the human condition. The encounter has been at least as much for the good as for the harmful, and offers great benefit moving forward.

Institutionally, the encounter between religion and medicine has been many-sided and many-layered. The story of religion and medicine has been dynamic and evolving, and remains so in the present. The numerous intersections and interconnections between these two great institutional domains offer productive opportunities for cooperation and collaboration in service to the promotion of health and prevention of disease.[154] I elaborate upon these historical and contemporary alliances in this volume.

The Takeaway Point

It may be a bit early in the book for this, but here, in advance, is the takeaway point:

The intersections of the faith-based and medical sectors are multifaceted and of long standing.

Nobody would seriously assert that the formal relations between the institutions of religion and medicine are now or ever have been wholly collegial, at least since the emergence of modern Western medicine in the nineteenth century. As this book shows, however, guarded alliances have existed, even flourished, over that same time period. That such relations have coexisted alongside the more contentious examples described earlier "underscores the nuanced complexity of the encounter between religion and medicine, and suggests that the overall relationship cannot be captured by a single adjective or pithy phrase."[155] Nor do the positive aspects of this encounter overrule or negate the negative images. Both aspects are real. But because the negative has received more play—by historians, scientists, journalists, and popular writers—*Religion and Medicine* makes the case that the tacit view is one-sided and does not accurately map onto the reality of the situation, especially in the present day. There is another, more positive story to tell.

Among the earliest efforts to chart the impact of religion on human health was a review by Kenneth Vaux, published in the journal *Preventive Medicine* in 1976.[156] This article was ground zero for scholarly attention to this subject within the health sciences, and was influential for subsequent research seeking to understand how and why religiousness, broadly defined, seems to influence population rates of health and illness. Vaux's insightful essay provided a baseline for later efforts to explore this subject in the thousands of published studies that followed.[157]

Up to now, the academic discourse on connections between faith or religion and health or medicine has largely been taken up by investigations of empirical data on a putative impact of religious participation on physical and mental health.[158] This has occupied my own efforts since the early 1980s.[159] But other octaves or dimensions to this conversation have mostly been neglected, foremost among these the dynamic interactions between religion and medicine at an institutional level. Mapping these interconnections, these institutional linkages, is the topic of *Religion and Medicine*. My hope is that this effort stimulates wider discussion of the complex interrelations between these two great institutions.

2

Healers and Healthcare

As we have observed, the encounter between religion and medicine is multilayered and goes back to the beginning of human history. The origins of medicine, as an institution and domain of professions and practitioners, are found in the origins of religion. The earliest healers were priests or shamans or magicians. According to French sociologist Émile Durkheim, the first religious prescriptions and proscriptions were "the first form of hygienic and medical interdictions."[1]

From the earliest human awareness of its presence, explained Durkheim, "The soul has always been considered a sacred thing; on this ground, it is opposed to the body which is, in itself profane. . . . It inspires those sentiments which are everywhere reserved for that which is divine."[2] The human soul contains what is "regarded as a spark of the divinity," and so "in a certain sense, there is divinity in us."[3] From this perspective, the physical vehicle, the body, partakes of and is enlivened by the divine presence. There is no ministering to the body without ministering to the soul. Among Durkheim's "primitives," there was thus no need for society to evolve a separate category of medical practitioners.

The complementarity of beliefs, practices, professions, and institutions that emerged around religion and medicine is a theme already touched on. Moving forward in time, one can observe this mutuality and these shared functions made manifest throughout the world, across cultures, across wisdom and faith traditions, and across diverse schools and philosophies of healing up into the Common Era. For much of history, it has not been easy to trace distinct "religion" and "medicine" threads. The beliefs and ideations, ritual behaviors, practitioner roles, and associated institutions of medicine and of religion are identical or at least overlapping. Relative to the temporal sweep of human history, it is only recently that we see the words *religion* and *medicine* as defining separate domains of life.[4]

This view of the complementarity of religion and medicine in the ancient world is reflected in the writing of twentieth-century pioneers in pastoral theology. In a representative example from Rupert E. Davies, Methodist minister and lecturer at Bristol University, the contrast with the worldview of modern scientific medicine is apparent:

> . . . in the simpler forms of human society, no distinction is made between the various parts of life; life is a unity, and religion embraces and permeates the

Religion and Medicine. Jeff Levin, Oxford University Press (2020) © Oxford University Press.
DOI: 10.1093/oso/9780190867355.001.0001

whole. There is nothing which is particularly religious, but there is nothing which is outside religion. Similarly, there is no separation of the mind from the body, no special treatment for the one as distinct from the other; each man is a unity, and the society to which he belongs is a unity.[5]

These words were written in 1962, just before dissatisfaction with the anti-septic materialism of Western medicine was beginning to be aired by proponents of an older, more humanistic approach to healing.[6] Interestingly, this was the same time period when the increasing prominence of secularism and naturalism in the zeitgeist of academic theology and religious studies began to meet resistance. This countermovement was characterized by church historian Martin E. Marty and *Christian Century* contributing editor Dean G. Peerman as "the recovery of transcendence"[7] and by sociologist Peter Berger as "the rediscovery of the supernatural."[8] In short order, these back-to-the-beginnings movements in healing and spirituality evolved in the 1970s into characteristic forms of medical practice (holistic medicine) and psychotherapy (transpersonal psychology). The religious and medical domains were both reconstituting themselves, once again in a more harmonious complementarity, in reaction to the stark dualism of the prevailing worldview.

Scholars have documented religious influences on the origins of the healing arts, the practice of healing, emergence of scientific theories of diagnosis and treatment, and establishment of professions and institutions devoted to healing.[9] The history of medicine, in one sense, is the history of the institutionalization of a once priestly role into a rationalized secular profession housed within specialized facilities,[10] many originating in religious bodies but now operating as businesses. This is as true for psychiatry as for medicine, for the care of the mind as for the body.[11]

The growth of these institutions, including clinics, hospitals, medical research labs, and pharmaceutical manufacturers, has created an enormous commercial sector that today conflicts with the work of independent healers, who function more closely to earlier modalities of delivering healing and medical care. In tracking emergence of these large meta-institutions through the centuries, one observes a continued tension between healers, often manifesting spiritual gifts and shepherding healees toward wholeness through rituals and sacraments, and politically sanctioned commercial concerns, whose original reason for being threatens to become subsumed under a business model prioritizing a corporate bottom line above relief of suffering.

This historic transformation of the organization and practice of medicine from an externalization of the ministry of religions to a rationalized, bureau-cratized, and legally regulated sector of the economy exemplifies German sociologist Max Weber's famous description of the *routinization of charisma*, the transformation and neutering of the germinal spark of insight or revelation present at the establishment of an institution or idea. According to Weber, "The genuine charismatic situation quickly [gives] way to incipient institutions, which emerge from the cooling off of extraordinary states of devotion and fervor."[12] It may sound cynical, but this is a reasonable depiction of medicine's journey from a service rendered by ritual healers to a product marketed and administered by third-party corporate entities backed by government sanction. Weber went on to explain that as routinization continues, "the original doctrines . . . are intellectually adjusted to the needs of that stratum which becomes the primary carrier" of the original message.[13]

To be fair, present dysfunctions and conflicts within Western medicine should not detrimentally color our reading of the past three millennia of medical progress. Establishment of defined professional roles for practicing healing and of localized institutions to care for the sick were among humankind's most constructive innovations. These developments were religiously sponsored from the beginning.[14] Later, spreading globally, across faith traditions—in the pagan world, in Christianity, in Islam, in the East—institutional medical care remains today largely an expression of religious outreach, even if this fact is mostly invisible to the general public.

In the Beginning

In *Healing and Restoring*, religious historian Lawrence E. Sullivan's edited volume documenting the history of medicine within the world's religious traditions,[15] the religious origins of the healing arts are in full view across faiths: in Buddhism, Hinduism, Islam, and the native spiritual traditions of Africa, the Caribbean, Polynesia, and the Americas. A companion volume reinforces the same point for Judaism and the spectrum of Christian denominations.[16] Sullivan hints at the religious ancestry of medicine: "Cultures throughout the world have noticed such similarities in form or function between processes of the human body and structures of the universe. . . . Medical lore warehouses these human evaluations of self, history, and cosmos."[17] Such observations, he suggests, "are not antiquarian curiosities,"[18] but provide insight about beliefs, practices, and experiences of contemporary people in their encounter with medicine.

The earliest humans experienced physical hardships, including hunger, disease, injuries, and concomitantly shorter life expectancy than today. They sought to understand their condition and deduce what to do about it. This was no different than how they sought to understand nature and the environment in which they lived, the world they inhabited, and the cosmos they could see when they looked upward. Accordingly, they constructed a divine cosmos inhabited by gods and other beings and powerful forces believed responsible, in part, for the bodily condition they found themselves in and whom they could call upon or persuade or appease, in some fashion, to receive relief.

The folks who could best negotiate these matters were the first priest-healers. Their facility extended to discerning how and why invisible beings and forces did what they did to affect the lives and bodies of their compatriots, and they were able to discern what to do about this to restore things to their previous state of equilibrium and wholeness. They also served as agents for their tribe or clan, seeking to appease the cosmic and divine forces or helping sick folks reestablish their lives in harmony or right relationship with the wishes of these forces or with nature or the energy of the cosmos. The first of these functions was about "diagnosis"—determining the etiology of disease states; the second was about "treatment"—the specific therapies and interventions prescribed and behaviors proscribed.

The labor of these healers—call them priests, shamans, magicians, sorcerers, trance-channels, mystics—required a working familiarity with the realities of the spirit domain. This could be obtained through noetic or liminal experience, such as via the dream state, trances or other altered states of consciousness, or out-of-body travel, or through divination, which took many forms. Historian of religions Mircea Eliade characterized the shaman of the Paleolithic period as "a specialist in ecstasy."[19]

An insightful description of the spirit journey of the shaman-healer is provided by Scottish religious scholar Ninian Smart in his *Dimensions of the Sacred*:

> It is typical of the shaman to feel that he or she is dismembered, perhaps by ancestors or by wild animals or by other supernatural spirits. His flesh is cut off, and he is reduced to a skeletal state. But he rises up from death and travels to supernal worlds, to heavens to see god, to infernal lands to find the dead. Through such voyages he becomes in some ways a pure spirit and he can travel through the air and perform wonderful deeds. As the wounded healer he can heal; as one who has known death he can overcome death and help those in states of dire sickness. Having celestial knowledge, he can advise his community.[20]

Such experiences, Smart explains, "suggest to individuals who undergo them . . . that divine spirits are entering them. They feel the god within. Such a power source gives the individual a vigor and perception which may help the community. . . ."[21]

In *The Idea of the Holy*, German theologian Rudolf Otto described the divinatory experience as "cognizing and recognizing the holy in its appearances."[22] "Does such a faculty exist," he asked, "and, if so, what is its nature?"[23] He added that such experiences begin with "the fact that a man encounters an occurrence that is not 'natural,' in the sense of being inexplicable by the laws of nature. Since it has actually occurred, it must have had a cause; and, since it has no 'natural' cause, it must (so it is said) have a supernatural one."[24] The ability to have such experiences, draw such conclusions, and communicate them to others provided the authority to negotiate such realms for oneself and as a representative of others.

The diagnostic and therapeutic wisdom received during the liminal experiences of these proto-shamans informed their work as mediums—mediators between clanspeople and the spirit world—and healers. Among cultures in the developing world, throughout the past century and still today, this work continues. A common theme is that disease is a function in part of demonic possession and that methods exist to drive these forces away, so long as the afflicted person is willing to endure treatment. In *The Golden Bough*,[25] his classic work on religion and magic, Scottish anthropologist Sir James Frazer notes that a commonly observed function of priests and sorcerers throughout the world was "to summon or exorcise spirits for the purpose of averting or dispelling sickness."[26] He provides several colorful examples.

Frazer describes a ritual healing act of the Apalai Indians of South America. Villagers presented themselves to be stung painfully by large black ants fastened onto palm leaves, which were then applied to "their faces, thighs, and other parts of their bodies."[27] When the intended effect was not severe enough, the recipients would cry out, "More! More!"[28] until "their skin was thickly studded with tiny swellings like what might have been produced by whipping them with nettles."[29]

He reported similar rituals in Amboyna and Uliase ("sprinkling sick people with pungent spices, such as ginger and cloves, chewed fine, in order by the prickling sensation to drive away the demons of disease which may be clinging to their persons"[30]) and Java ("a popular cure for gout or rheumatism is to rub Spanish pepper into the nails of the fingers and toes of the sufferer; the pungency of the pepper is supposed to be too much for the gout or rheumatism, who accordingly departs in haste"[31]). An especially severe example was observed on the Slave Coast of West Africa:

> . . . the mother of a sick child sometimes believes that an evil spirit has taken possession of the child's body, and in order to drive him out, she makes small cuts in the body of the little sufferer and inserts green peppers or spices in the wounds, believing that she will thereby hurt the evil spirit and force him to be gone. The poor child naturally screams with pain, but the mother hardens her heart in the belief that the demon is suffering equally.[32]

Traversing the interstitial space between observable and invisible worlds has always been treacherous. Specialized healers with knowledge of this mysterious space were and still are relied upon for their expertise, gained through numinous experience. Medical historian Christian Deetjen noted that since earliest times, "Primitive man was constantly surrounded by inimical forces."[33] Accordingly, reliance was placed upon "medicine men [who] used their power gained by observation of the mysterious forces of nature . . . to cure various diseases and troubles. . . ."[34] Deetjen noted further that religion and medicine and the sha-manistic arts (which, writing in 1934, he termed "witchcraft") "form a trinity which is as old as the human race. It is impossible to separate them completely even to this day."[35]

This observation about the persisting inseparability of religion and med-icine among indigenous shaman-healers was still considered valid over half a century later. In 1990 medical anthropologist Michael James Winkelman published a remarkable cross-cultural study of shamans and other "magico-religious" healers from all major regions of the world and from 1750 BCE until the present,[36] taken from the Standard Cross-Cultural Sample, a well-known ethnographic data resource of 186 cultures.[37] He observed across his sample, and across specializations of healers (e.g., medium, priest, sorcerer/witch), commonalities of shamanic practice. For example, "Examination of the ac-tual procedures employed by the shaman, shaman/healer, and medium indi-cate that they all deliberately utilize trance induction procedures that would affect the patient as a part of their healing ceremonies. . . . Magico-religious healing practices are universally associated with ASC [altered states of con-sciousness] induction procedures because they are effective in facilitating extrasensory awareness and healing."[38] Considerable fascination with these systems of medicine and associated techniques exists today among physicians, anthropologists, and laypeople interested in non-Western healing and in spir-itual and metaphysical exploration.[39]

Religious Healing in the Ancient World

Almost as long ago as when the first healers appeared, specialized roles were instituted for them within indigenous religious systems. In some traditions, dedicated places were established as loci for the practice of healing. Religious institutions were instrumental in establishing these locations, as early as the second half of the first millennium before the Common Era. The "profession-alization" of healing practitioners and identification of recognizable healing locales—whether natural sites or constructed edifices—were a worldwide phe-nomenon, extending from the Indian subcontinent to China and the rest of Asia, and from the Greco-Roman world to the indigenous peoples of the Middle East.[40]

The earliest textual evidence of Indian medicine is found in the Hindu *Vedas*. This is expertly documented with encyclopedic thoroughness by Indologist Kenneth G. Zysk. "A distinctive part of Vedic medicine was its pharmacopoeia,"[41] Zysk notes, and the hymns of the *Atharvaveda* and *Ṛgveda* contain many examples of "botanical wisdom"[42] and folk healing traditions. The foundation of Vedic medicine was "belief in a multitude of benevolent and malevolent deities or spirits that populated the cosmos and caused good and bad effects in the human realm."[43] Accordingly, "The medicine of the Vedic Indians is inextricably connected with their religion and must not be considered in isolation from it."[44]

Beginning around the ninth century BCE, an emerging "paradigm shift" regarding healing in Vedic antiquity saw a "forthright denigration of medicine by the priestly order and the brāhmaṇic hierarchy [which] resulted in the healers' exclusion from the orthodox ritual cults because of the defilement they incurred from contact with impure people with whom they found fellowship."[45] Excommunicated healers, according to Zysk, became wandering ascetics, and "[u]nencumbered by the strictures of brāhmaṇical orthodoxy . . . acquired a radically different view of the world and humankind's place in it, fostered by their intense meditative discipline."[46] This conflict gave rise to the distinct worldview of the emerging medical philosophy of *Āyurveda*, based on a view of healing as restoration of an ideal state of harmony and equilibrium. It also influenced development of healing traditions among the first Buddhist monks, which evolved from this same paradigm shift.

Upon the emergence of Buddhism in the sixth century BCE, according to historian of religions Joseph Mitsuo Kitagawa, a characteristic "impulse to care" was cultivated by monks across various Buddhist factions and subdivisions.[47] This was expressed through emotions of lovingkindness (*mettā*) and compassion (*karuṇā*) toward others, and sympathetic joy (*muditā*) over others' happiness.[48] Tending to the sick was an explicit value, pursued for the greater purpose of reducing suffering. This reflected a core distinctive of Buddhist teaching, its application to the domain of wellness and illness deriving from the beginnings of the religion. "According to the canonical tradition," noted Kitagawa, "the Buddha was concerned with the health of monks and took a keen interest in medicine."[49]

This idea is well articulated by anthropologist Raoul Birnbaum: "Since illness is a chief cause of suffering in the world, and a special focus of Buddhist teachings is the methodical elimination of suffering, the causes and treatments of disease have been a topic of special interest among many Buddhist thinkers."[50] This knowledge of disease etiology coupled with "the superior healing ability"[51] of many monks were effective tools for Buddhist missionaries. Indeed, it was physician-monks from India and Central Asia who were especially instrumental in bringing Buddhism to China.[52]

Buddhist ideas about healing and medicine extended their reach with the spread of Buddhism throughout subsequent centuries. In *Buddhism and Medicine*, historian of medicine C. Pierce Salguero explains that Buddhist writings, rituals, and material culture regarding disease, healing, and health maintenance were carried by merchants, missionaries, and healer-monks across South, East, Central, and Southeast Asia.[53] Medicine and healing "played a central role in Buddhist proselytism in new lands, and it was often among the chief benefits that was held out to new converts."[54] By the third century BCE, during the reign of King Aśoka, medical institutions providing medical care services and treatments were well established in the Indian subcontinent,[55] and in subsequent centuries fanned out through Asia. These included hospitals for patients with diagnosed mental illness,[56] featuring separate sections for specialized practices and treatments.[57] There is also later evidence of hospital-like monastic structures or infirmaries within monastery compounds and devoted to treatment of sick monks.[58]

Contemporaneously, and closely related to the *Sāṅkhya* philosophy from which *Āyurveda* evolved, was the axial-age emergence of the *yoga* school of Hindu philosophy.[59] The idealized attainment of yogic practice is the attainment of *samādhi*, or consciousness of the divine, achieved through *dhyāna* (meditation). Eliade describes this as "complete comprehension of Being [in which] there is 'undifferentiated' (*asamprajñāta*) enstasis."[60] This state resembles the "oneness" spoken of by the great mystics—the intrinsic recognition that *Adonai echad* ("the Lord is One," in the Jewish *shema* prayer). Significantly, Eliade adds, "It is when he has reached this stage that the *yogin* acquires the 'miraculous powers' (*siddhis*) to which book 3 of the *Yoga Sutra* is devoted."[61] The significance of such a state of consciousness for the work of ascetic or mystic healers is plain.

In Patañjali's *Yoga-Sūtras*, appearing centuries later, the third book, entitled *Vibhuti Pada*, describes these seemingly miraculous *siddhis*, translated by Harvard scholar James Haughton Woods as "supernormal powers."[62] This book contains fifty-six *sūtras* on attainment of diverse powers through specialized meditative techniques. Several may be used for diagnostic or therapeutic purposes, applied to oneself or others. Modern *yoga* teachers discourage pursuit of these powers—they are seen as distractions on one's spiritual path—but they are nonetheless considered real, and biographies of modern *yoga* masters contain stories of their use.

Among those *siddhis* with potential medical application are:

- "direct perception of subliminal impressions" (*sūtra* 15), including intuition of past-life *karma* explaining the condition of the body;

- "constraint upon the form of the body" (*sūtra* 21), including dematerialization or invisibility of the body or shutting down of observers' ability to perceive the body through the gross senses;
- "constraint upon powers" (*sūtra* 24), including gaining the strength of an elephant;
- "constraint upon the navel" (*sūtra* 29), including ability to "discern the arrangement of the body,"[63] such as the state of humors and the body's corporeal elements (skin, blood, flesh, sinew, bone, marrow, and semen);
- "mind-stuff penetrates into the body of another" (*sūtra* 38), including ability to hasten "a slackening of this karma which is the cause of bondage";[64] and
- "perfection of the body" (*sūtra* 45), including miscellaneous feats: atomization, levitation, magnification, extension, and other seemingly supernatural physical and mental capacities, which Woods termed "magic powers" or "perfections."[65]

In China, the system of *Zhōng Yī* evolved over many centuries. Its origins probably lie as far back as the Zhou dynasty, in the eleventh century BCE, and concepts and practices have been traced back even further.[66] Known today as traditional Chinese medicine (TCM), this healing system became informed by a fusion of Taoist ideas, such as the *yin-yang* duality and *Wu Xing* (five-elements theory),[67] and Confucian ethics.[68] TCM was also influenced by contemporaneously evolving principles of *Āyurveda*. Parallels between indigenous Chinese and Indian systems of diagnosis and therapy are observed in shared features of (subtle) anatomy and physiology, such as correspondence between *qi* and *prāna*, respective names for the body's healing energy or vital life force, and between *jīng luò* (aka meridians) and *nāḍīs*, respective names of the channels along which this energy flows. TCM's foundational text is the *Neijing*, or Yellow Emperor's Classic of Medicine, attributed to Huang Di in the third millennium BCE but probably dating to about the third century BCE.[69] It is as much a treatise on esoteric metaphysics and cosmology as a medical textbook.

In the ancient West, around the same time, an indigenous medical tradition was taking root,[70] likewise evolving from a radix of religious influences.[71] It emerged from cross-pollination among various sources localized to the ancient Near East, including Mesopotamians, Babylonians, Egyptians, and Hebrews.

In ancient Mesopotamia and Babylonia, according to Ferngren, "Medicine and magic were equally legitimate in therapy, and the two were used in tandem,"[72] often with the same patient. Accordingly, two professions of healers existed: the *āšipu*, a kind of magician-exorcist-priest, and the *asû*, akin to a modern physician. Their respective practices were "distinct but complementary,"[73] and some individuals served in both roles. The former used divination, such as astrology,

for purposes of diagnosis and prescribed various treatments, including con-
fession, sacrifice, and prayers. The latter was a kind of pharmacist, prescribing
herbal remedies without explicit magico-religious imprimatur, and may predate
the former. According to Ferngren, evidence from Sumer suggests the presence
of the *asû* as far back as 3000 BCE.

Indigenous religion in the region, known as the cradle of civilization, was
polytheistic, disease believed to be caused by demons or divine retribution for
sinfulness.[74] As early as the eleventh century BCE, a diagnostic and prognostic
handbook existed that prescribed treatments entailing both religious and medical approaches. The former included purification rituals, penitential prayers,
and "recitals" directed to a pantheon of demonic forces believed responsible for
cases of disease.[75]

The medical techniques of ancient Egypt are more widely preserved than those
of Mesopotamia due to survival of over a dozen scrolls of medical writing found
on papyri and dating as far back as 2000 BCE.[76] According to Ferngren, Egyptian
medical treatments were more naturalistic than in Mesopotamia, but in other
regards strikingly similar. The Egyptians believed that specific gods protected
against specific diseases,[77] and there was "a strong element of religious treatment
within Egyptian medicine at all periods."[78] This included use of prayers, incan-
tation, hymns, and recitals,[79] as well as healing ceremonies conducted in shrines
and temples.[80] Also similar to Mesopotamia, medical practice was specialized,
and three types of healers existed: the *wabw*, or priest; the *sa.u*, a sorcerer or exorcist; and *swnw*, a physician akin to the Mesopotamian *asû*.[81] In other regards,
the magico-religious elements of Egyptian medicine hearkened back even further, to archaic medical traditions throughout the ancient world, including Vedic
medicine.[82]

Around the same time, the Hebrews were coming to an understanding of disease, but there is not much evidence that they ever evolved a uniquely characteristic system of healing. They borrowed from folk remedies of nearby cultures,
and, if necessary, utilized their healers, while careful to avoid pagan elements.[83]
Ferngren observes that there was "no native medical tradition and hence no native physicians . . . [and] we have no evidence that any systematized therapeu-
tics existed in early Israel."[84] What distinguished the etiological ideas of Hebrews
from those of their neighbors derived from their distinct religious outlook, which
was monotheistic or monolatrous. Belief that humans were created in the image
of God had implications for how the cause and cure of disease were understood.
Jewish monotheism did not imply "a rejection of the supernatural concept of the
causation and cure of disease."[85] Quite the contrary. Disturbances in the relations between human beings and God, such as through sin, were paramount, and
restoring the relationship was essential for health to be recovered.[86] It follows,
notes Ferngren, that defining concepts for the medical worldview of Hebrews

included the polarities of purity/impurity and holiness/defilement, with rituals of purification required for recovery.[87]

The Torah details the "moral or spiritual causes" of disease,[88] which appeared as a consequence of rebellious or unholy behavior and could come as a chastisement from God or as an affliction sent by Satan, as in the case of Job.[89] Disease and its cure were a complex dance among obedience to the commandments (*mitzvot*), faith (*emunah*) and trust (*bitachon*) in God, and attentiveness to breeches of holiness (*kedushah*), which needed repairing before a human body could be returned to wholeness. Jewish Scriptures, including the rabbinic canon,[90] go into considerable detail about the significance of such breaches for disease causation, laying out both natural and ritual approaches for healing recommended by the rabbis. The encyclopedic *Biblical and Talmudic Medicine*, compiled by Julius Preuss, is a veritable textbook of these sources.[91]

For physicians, who came later in Jewish history, "the basic attitude was that healing was in the hands of God and the role of the physicians was that of helpers or instruments of God"[92] Medicine, as a distinct profession, developed as a sacred calling; physicians were as likely to be bioethical or *halachic* decisors as healers, which perhaps accounts for the great number of medieval physicians who were also rabbinic scholars or philosophers. Perhaps for similar reasons, dedicated hospitals, too, came much later in Jewish history, although beginning in the Common Era, halls were set up inside synagogues for the sick to obtain respite.[93]

The encounter between religion and medicine also played out in the Greco-Roman world.[94] Among the foundations of the Western medical tradition was a complex interplay between the polytheism of Greece and Rome and their increasingly scientific approach to medicine, combining theoretical and empirical approaches to diagnosis and treatment.[95] In some ways, the medicine of ancient Greece and Rome were carryovers from neighboring cultures of the ancient Near East; in other ways, they represented a clean break.[96] In both contexts, religion was a source of beliefs and practices underlying vernacular perspectives on healing as well as a contributing feature of the methods used by healing practitioners.

This conjunction of religious and secular streams is ably described by medical historian Vivian Nutton, who notes "the plurality of Greek medicine, in which exorcists, religious healers, root-cutters, folk-healers, and *iatroi* ('healers') coexisted in competition."[97] This coexistence was "relatively amicable,"[98] among practitioners and the general populace. Moreover, Nutton adds, "Belief in divine intervention did not exclude secular healing: those who sought the help of a god for one disease might well consult a healer for another. In turn, few healers rejected the gods."[99] Physicians, in turn, according to Ferngren and theologian

Ekaterina N. Lomperis, "regarded both secular and temple medicine as legitimate means of healing."[100]

In pre-Hippocratic Greece, before the fifth century BCE, beliefs about health, healing, and medicine were similar to those throughout the ancient Near East. Supernatural causation was accepted, as was the etiologic significance of possession, whose mitigation required rituals such as purification to counteract effects of invisible demons (*keres*) and vengeful spirits (*alastores*). Ritual healing was provided by shamans, known as *iatromanteis*, who could deduce the source of personal illness and population-wide plague and provide expiation.[101] A secular class of itinerant healers, *iatroi*, also plied their craft, using natural means to treat diseases, understood to arise through naturalistic etiologies, an approach flourishing with the rise of Hippocratic medicine. This marked the onset of a more scientific age for medicine, built on theories of disease deduced from clinical observation and philosophical speculation.[102]

This era also saw local cults arise around shrines and holy sites, in which gods and heroes, such as Asclepius, were venerated and prayed to for healing.[103] A class of physicians, Asclepiads, facilitated such healings, but were secular in outlook. A notable feature of medicine at that time was that "Hippocratic medicine and temple healing flourished side by side."[104] Through temple pilgrimages, the afflicted obtained healing through consulting oracles, offering sacrifices, or undergoing "incubation" in a special hall known as an *abaton*, hoping for a vision or dream leading to a remission of symptoms. These were ancestors of present-day health spas existing throughout Europe.[105] Also at the temples, patients could receive conventional medical treatment from *iatroi*, who "saw no conflict" in practicing there or in secular settings.[106] According to medical historian Guenter B. Risse, "Miracles were expected, but whether Asclepius always came through is unknown."[107]

Greek physicians, notes Ferngren, "had no philosophical objections to religious healing,"[108] which they considered to complement their own practice. In that regard, healing temples and practitioners were pioneers of today's complementary or integrative medicine, the successor doctrine to the alternative medicine model positing mind-body and spiritual approaches to healing as a substitute for allopathic medicine. Today, as in ancient Greece, legions of physicians and healers are willing to take a more inclusive and expansive view of sources of illness and tools that can be used to alleviate suffering.

In more ways than not, the Roman situation was an extension of the Greek. The earliest physicians in Rome were Greek expatriates in the third century BCE,[109] attracted to practice in a land that had never been serviced by a class of professional practitioners as in Greece. What they found resembled what they had left behind: widespread belief in supernatural causation; etiology attributed to the gods (but largely not to demons[110]); and "medical pluralism"[111] comprising natural healing, such as with herbs, as well as religious healing, conducted at shrines, and magical healing, including use of astrology and divination. These immigrant physicians (*medici*) brought with them from Greece a continuity in nosology, etiology, and therapy.[112]

As Rome conquered surrounding territories, medicine became more eclectic and religious and magical elements multiplied, but, over time, so did more rational approaches. As in Greece, religious healing and folk remedies remained popular, but by the Common Era, after Greek physicians began practicing in Rome, secular and naturalistic forms of medicine predominated, including study of anatomy, pathology, and pathophysiology; use of drug therapy; and practice of sophisticated surgery, including orthopedics.[113] Archaeologists have identified buildings dedicated to medical treatment of the sick,[114] including slaves, and military field hospitals were built throughout the growing empire.[115]

Throughout the ancient world, philosophies and systems of healing arose from religious origins. The religious elements were instrumental in formulation of philosophies of diagnosis and treatment, the rituals and practices of experts filling formal healing roles, and in establishment of institutions for healing under religious auspices, the precursors to what became hospitals. In many ancient cultures, according to classicist Sarah Iles Johnston, "There was no sharp delineation between 'rational' medicine and divine medicine."[116]

The influence of religion is also seen in the ubiquity of perspectives on healing that would today be called *holistic*, although there were limits to the holism of ancient healing traditions. For one, they failed to account for a communal dimension of well-being; disease was a status attached to an individual person and was best dealt with via treatment of respective individuals.[117] This approach was germinal for future evolvement of the healing arts and scientific medicine, but did not anticipate or influence the development of public health. Contemporary alliances between institutions of faith and public health cannot be traced back to the ancient world with any reliability.

Religious Healing in Christianity

At the beginning of the Christian era, healing as practiced in regions where the young church was growing was an extension of what came before. Heavily influenced by Greco-Roman beliefs and practices, the medical and healing philosophy and approach adopted by the first Christians recapitulated existing nosologies, types of diagnoses, etiologic understandings of natural and environmental determinants of disease, and therapeutic techniques in circulation at the time.[118] According to Ferngren, one may observe among the early Christians "a continuity with classical culture in their appreciation of secular medicine."[119]

Religious believers were willing "to accept the natural causation of disease and to think that commonly encountered diseases were susceptible of treatment by natural means."[120]

At the same time, Jewish perspectives on the cause and cure of disease, as well as other folk beliefs and practices prevalent in the ancient Near East, contributed to how followers of the early church approached ill health. Judea at the time of Christ, explains Nutton, hosted a mélange of healing options, a disparate collection of ideas and practitioners including itinerant healers practicing ritual magic and holy men preaching observance of the *mitzvot* as the path to health.[121] Still, Ferngren's survey of historical evidence suggests that early Christians were more likely to turn to physicians and contemporary medical care than to ritual healers promising supernatural miracles.[122]

While the emerging Christian church may have adopted a perspective about health and medicine in continuity with what came before, the healing ministry of Jesus as depicted in the Gospels was a decided break with norms of the day, if not altogether sui generis. In *Healing and Christianity*, Episcopal priest Morton Kelsey asserts that "Jesus spoke and acted from a consistent and well-developed point of view which was new and quite at variance with the mainstream of Judaism and of official Greek and Roman religion."[123] His healing ministry functioned through charismatic authority, through pronouncements and actions of one widely believed to exhibit supernatural gifts. Aside from traveling and teaching, there is hardly anything that Jesus did more often than cast out demons and heal the afflicted. To Christians he is the Son of God and the Lord and Savior of humankind; by occupation, he was primarily an exorcist and healer.[124] Almost a fifth of the verses in the Gospels, notes Kelsey, are devoted to healing.[125]

This is not to say that influences on Jesus or precursors to his way of healing have not been proposed. In *De Vita Contemplativa* Philo described a monastic order of healers known as the Therapeutae, believed to be an offshoot of the Essenes.[126] According to Philo, Therapeutae resorted to fasting and prayer and "process an art of medicine more excellent than that in general use in cities (for that only heals bodies, but the other heals souls which are under the mastery of terrible and almost incurable diseases . . .)."[127] New Age and esoteric writers connect Jesus to the Essenes and/or Therapeutae,[128] speculating that he was an initiate or even leader. This literature depicts the Therapeutae as "more contemplative than the practical Essenes, and their monastic self-reflection is speculated to be an influence on the Gnostics, whose own sacred writings contain references to healing that are resonant with psychodynamic theories and the kinds of inner work characteristic of transpersonal and humanistic therapies."[129] However, much of what is popularly believed about the Therapeutae, especially derived from writings of modern neo-Essene groups,[130] is speculative at best or apochryphal.[131] For perhaps good cause, an essay in the *Harvard Theological Review* referred to them as the "so-called Therapeutae."[132]

The apostles carried on the healing work of Jesus, in his name and by his authority, beginning after Pentecost as described in the book of Acts.[133] Just as did their master, they healed physical and mental illness, restored the blind and lame, and cast out demons. In so doing, these efforts were not conducted in fidelity to a particular method of healing, such as a specific ritual or spiritualized technique. "This was not magic where healers manipulated spiritual energy for their goals," explains Kelsey, "but rather human beings used as instruments by the healing, loving spirit of God."[134] Some modern scholars have resisted an "existential, theological interpretation of Jesus and his work as a healer,"[135] preferring to lump in Jesus and his followers with other magical and religious healers of the day whose rituals produced cures, presumably, through invoking a psychosomatic response. But this may be more a case of personal skepticism about God and faith on the part of such scholars, and thus a concomitant tendency to reject any textual evidence suggesting a nonmaterialistic model of reality and, by extension, healing.

Such a skeptical explanation for the healing miracles of Jesus and the apostles does not seem to fit with accounts of severe afflictions and associated healings preserved in the New Testament, nor with normative Christian understandings of these stories as inspired and canonical. Leprosy, withered limbs, palsy, blindness, deafness, and even death (as with Lazarus[136])—these do not seem to be garden-variety infirmities amenable to healing through simple suggestion or placebo. This default view of these apparent miracles bespeaks a naturalistic bias in reading such accounts, as well as substantial doubt about the authenticity and veracity of these texts. My own instinct, as both a medical scientist and religious believer (although not a Christian), is to accept these stories as earnest depictions of real events and then try to understand how and why they might have occurred based on the best evidence from knowledgeable biblical scholars and current wisdom on the salutogenic or healing process.

In the centuries that followed, Church Fathers developed theories of disease and healing that incorporated spiritual elements coexisting alongside natural etiologies and methods and that were instrumental in the spread and assimilation of Christianity into diverse cultures.[137] The extensive patristic literature contains many gems on this subject, such as this "theory of disease" propounded in the fourth-century Clementine homilies:

> Whence many, not knowing how they are influenced, consent to the evil thoughts suggested by the demons, as if they were the reasoning of their own souls . . . . and do not know that they themselves are held captive by the deceiving demons. Therefore the demons who lurk in their souls induce them

to think that it is not a demon that is distressing them, but a bodily disease, such as some acrid matter, or bile, or phlegm, or excess of blood, or inflammation of a membrane, or something else. But even if this were so, the case would not be altered of its being a kind of demon.[138]

A less pessimistic, more nuanced view is advanced by Christian apologist Origen of Alexandria in the third century. He favored the medicine of the day, especially natural remedies, and advocated its substitution for pagan practices still in wide use among Christians. These, he asserted, constituted a grave heresy and reflected poorly on Christianity in the eyes of critics, such as Greek philosopher Celsus:

> For since the science of medicine in useful and necessary to the human race, and many are the points of dispute in it respecting the manner of curing bodies, there are found, for this reason, numerous heresies confessedly prevailing in the science of medicine among the Greeks, and also, I suppose, among those barbarous nations who profess to employ medicine.[139]

While Origen endorsed medicine and did not reject its use for healing maladies of natural cause, he also asserted, clarifies Ferngren, that "the more spiritual Christian should rely solely on God for healing and avoid the use of physicians and medicines."[140] Renouncing medicine for prayer was seen as an expression of asceticism for individuals seeking a closer walk with God,[141] akin to the Nazirite vow or to vows of celibacy or poverty—not required, but gainfully accepted in order to forge a deeper relationship with the Source of Being and offer public testimony to the faithfulness of the Christian deity. On this latter point, some dispute now exists among Christian scholars over whether healing legitimately may serve such a purpose or, instead, is prohibited because the scriptural mandate to heal expired with the apostles.[142]

Over subsequent centuries, the institutional church, East and West, established formal liturgies for sacramental healing and reconciliation. "In the deuterocanonical tradition," notes Greek Orthodox priest Stanley Samuel Harakas, "prayer to God and recourse to the physician are not contradictory, but supplementary practices, providing the normative foundation for the Eastern Orthodox Church regarding the relationship of faith and medicine."[143] Accordingly, both "the encouragement of liturgical approaches to healing, [and] the approval of the medical profession . . . appear repeatedly in the subsequent history of the Orthodox Church. . . ."[144] Orthodox Christianity thus can be seen to have pioneered the contemporary movement toward "integral healing" nearly two millennia ago.[145] This subject is the theme of a recent edited volume on healing in the Orthodox Church,[146] which includes an insightful essay on historical precedents for synergy among medicine, sacrament, and *diakonia*,[147] the latter restated in Roman Catholic tradition as the preferential option for the poor.

In Catholicism, celebrating a sacrament entails at least a couple of essential elements: *epiclesis* (invocation of the Holy Spirit) and *anamnesis* (remembrance of God's mighty works).[148] These elements reify the Eucharistic experience and ensure and affirm the "real presence" of Jesus Christ in the Eucharistic species, the body and blood consumed during Mass. This presence is reinforced spiritually and psychologically through language comprising signs and symbols that "*make present* the reality they symbolize,"[149] including images, songs, the sign of the cross, silence, movement, incense, and specific liturgical colors.[150]

Through the sacrament of anointing the sick, the Catholic Church also fulfills its mission as a sacramental healer. This includes providing benefits to the recipient: healing; strengthening of body, mind, and spirit; forgiveness of sins; preparation for eternal life; and conjoining the suffering person to the crucified Christ.[151] It also implies a church exercising its pastoral role as agent of redemption for the world. In the context of healing, this includes exercising a prophetic voice to speak out for more just models of healthcare delivery, new types of preventive care, and health education and a healthy environment.[152] Such advocacy is consistent with the church's historic mission to exhibit "a charitable concern for their [members'] (and humans' generally) earthly well-being."[153]

This socially conscious extension of the church's mission to care for the needs of the sick is not just an outgrowth of modern-day progressive political ideology or praxis. It dates to the first centuries of the Christian era. "Concern for the poor and their health," according to Harakas, "was a significant priority in Byzantine society during this period."[154] Saint Basil the Great, archbishop of Caesarea in the fourth century, established his famous *Basiliad* just outside the city. Known also as the City of Charity, it consisted of a hospital, hospice, leper colony, poorhouse, homeless shelter, orphanage, school, soup kitchen, and more,[155] and "his monks were expected to go and minister to the poor and sick of the city."[156] Basil's pastoral compassion, exemplified by his service to the sick, was emulated by monks in the centuries following,[157] through rules of monasticism laid out in his *Asketikon*.[158]

Hospitals are not the only religious institutions where healing arts have been sponsored and promoted by the institutional church. The enduring popularity of pilgrimage sites and shrines throughout the Christian world is a reminder of the persistence of healing as a vital concern among Christians and the meaningful way in which believers commune with their church and connect with God. These sites exist throughout Europe, many dating back centuries or more.[159] Often associated with widely publicized Marian apparitions, as at Fátima, Lourdes, and Medjugorje, such shrines have become loci in which seemingly miraculous cures are reported.[160] The possibility of being healed from serious afflictions reinforces belief "that all creation is God's domain, that divine action can be evidenced in the natural,"[161] and accounts for why these sites continue to thrive as pilgrimage and tourist centers.

Both institutional medicine and the institutional church have maintained an uneasy relationship with healing shrines, and efforts to validate reported cures are ongoing but inconsistent. The gold standard is the Lourdes Medical Bureau, established in 1883 and still in operation, whose protocol calls for suspected cures to be referred to the International Lourdes Medical Committee for investigation.[162] A comprehensive analysis of case reports from the Lourdes archives found a total of sixty-seven cures acknowledged by the Catholic Church since 1862, but not a single cure certified from 1976 through 2006.[163] "The Lourdes cures," the investigators found, "have now shrunk to a trickle."[164] Among those that pass muster, attribution to naturalistic mechanisms—for example, as "part of a neuropsychiatric phenomenon"[165]—is tempting and may seem obvious, but how then to account for "cures such as the instantaneous healing of bones or lesions [that] could not be attributed to the mind alone"?[166]

The popularity of healing shrines and pilgrimage sites underscores the presence of ongoing conflict and negotiation between institutional churches and mainstream medicine over purported healings occurring outside the aegis of either party. Miracle cures attributed to places of Catholic pilgrimage are complicating factors for church governance, impacting its public image and relations with mainstream institutions such as the medical sector. This is not unlike the everpresent enthusiasm for faith healing at the margins of some mainline Protestant denominations, a continuing source of vexation for church leaders not wishing to alienate their more charismatic or evangelical members, typically the most committed and located in places experiencing the greatest church growth.[167] Presently, Christian churches continue to deal with touchy issues, exemplified by miracle claims, that in a previous era may have been labeled heresy or apostasy.[168] Western medicine must deal with this same matter—healing occurring outside its control—and descriptions of its struggle to sanction such phenomena have used identical language, of heresy and apostasy, to characterize these efforts.[169]

Religious Healing in New Thought

A parallel tradition of religious healing arose in the Christian world of the nineteenth century. The religious traditions out of which its characteristic medical and health-related principles emerged were unorthodox. Likewise the modalities and principles of healing propounded were unorthodox, even by the outré standards of religious healing. Significantly, this movement, which came to be known as New Thought, originated simultaneously with the advent of scientific medicine in the West, also in the nineteenth century. But while other forms and systems of healing described up to now were expressions or extensions of beliefs or worldviews of respective religions, in this instance the religious worldview itself was a primary expression of a radically unorthodox perspective on the human body, the nature of health and the causes of disease, and how and why healing occurs.

Antecedents of this new movement were many.[170] These include the "animal magnetism" of Franz Anton Mesmer,[171] the transcendentalism of Ralph Waldo Emerson,[172] and ideas about the mental origins of disease and healing proposed by Phineas P. Quimby.[173] Back in time from there, threads go in various directions—to the alchemist and astrologer known as Paracelsus,[174] to Swiss mystic Emanuel Swedenborg,[175] to German exorcist Johann Gassner,[176] and to the esoteric Hindu and Buddhist texts that inspired Theosophists later in the nineteenth century.[177] Forward in time, the most important downstream figure was Mary Baker Eddy, who broke with Quimby and founded Christian Science.[178] Her greatest rivals were the Dressers, Julius and Annetta and son Horatio, like Eddy formerly in the Quimby camp. They challenged her primogeniture and teaching authority, offering a form of "mental healing" less antagonistic to Quimby's original version.[179] Eddy's former disciple, Emma Curtis Hopkins, established her own movement[180] and is most responsible for popularizing the phrase New Thought in the early twentieth century.[181] Hopkins, in turn, had many students, some of whom formed their own groups still in existence.

Not surprisingly for a movement with such diverse influences and impacts, there was (and is) no single New Thought ideology. The history of the movement—if indeed it can be considered a single movement, which is debatable—and the history of the characteristic systems of religious healing that were taught is the history of a series of syncretisms and discipleships and disavowals. It is a story of innovators and eccentrics drawing creatively on multiple sources and then contentiously breaking with one's teacher or master to go in a different direction, until they themselves were broken with by their own students. Horatio W. Dresser, for example, referred to New Thought as "the liberal wing of the mental-healing movement,"[182] which hints at ongoing contention over orthodoxy and schism. The story of New Thought is endlessly fascinating and a much underchronicled epoch of nineteenth-century American religion (and medicine),[183] but too complicated to unpack in more than passing detail here.

The substance of the many schisms and founding of new groups revolved around concepts and ideas pertaining to the nature or reality of disease and relative contributions of mind, soul, spirit, energy, and God or Christ—and beliefs about the same—to the state of the body and to becoming restored to health or wholeness.[184] A closer look at three important figures bears this out.

To Quimby, for example, the starting point for this discussion was Mesmer, but he moved beyond mesmerism to formulate his own theories and approaches. In his biographical commentary in the published edition of Quimby's manuscripts, which he edited, Dresser quotes Quimby in referring to mesmerism as "one of the greatest humbugs of the age."[185] Why? Because, notes Dresser, "the human mind is amenable to suggestion, as we now say; [and] there are subjects capable of being put into a state which we now call hypnosis; and . . . the alleged magnetic, electrical or mesmeric effects are not mysterious at all, but *are the results of the action of mind on mind.*"[186] It is thus all about "the influence of thought" and "there is no such process as 'mesmerism' [nor] 'magnetic healing.'"[187] At the same time, Quimby asserted, "There could be no mesmeric or magnetic science of healing, any more than there exists a medical science: the one true science is spiritual."[188] For good reason, religious historian Catherine L. Albanese remarked on "the roughshod construction" of Quimby's writings, resulting in a "confused, but still commanding, theology of healing."[189] Also, for good reason, Quimby has been described as akin to a Native American shaman.[190]

Eddy, by contrast, rejected the reality of disease, even of the physical. "Theology and physics," she states, "teach that both Spirit and matter are real and good, whereas the fact is that Spirit is good and real, and matter is Spirit's opposite."[191] In other words, matter is neither good nor real. Or in Porterfield's restatement, "Eddy went further than Quimby to claim that disease and death did not really exist at all, but were erroneous beliefs that caused pain when people accepted them."[192] For Eddy, then, her "Christian Science Mind-healing" implied a different connotation of *mind* than Quimby or Mesmer or the others. Healing is attained through healing prayer, whereas the "mind is not a factor in the Principle of Christian Science,"[193] at least in the sense of an independent "healing agent,"[194] as in faith healing. Yet prayer alone is also inadequate: it "cannot change the unalterable Truth . . . but prayer, coupled with a fervent habitual desire to know and do the will of God, will bring us into all Truth."[195]

In *Scientific Christian Medical Practice*, Hopkins puts her own spin on these matters. She offers her first "lesson in Truth," which is "the first idea with which mind everywhere, in all ages, has begun when proclaiming that outside of, and greater than any power exhibited by anything in nature, or in man, is a being called God."[196] What this somewhat opaque statement implies for healing is unpacked further in her chapter "The Word of Faith": "Cures are the works of Truth. Cures or works are wrought by faith. That which we have faith or confidence in is our mental character quality, and goes through our thoughts, through our writings, through our speech, to others."[197] Regarding disease etiology, Hopkins also advances an idea that anticipates by decades both psychosomatic medicine and numerous New Age writers: "It is not yet known very widely that certain religious beliefs make sickness."[198] Accordingly, healing is dependent in part upon affirming the correct thoughts, not quite the same idea as taught by Quimby and Eddy. On this point, too, Hopkins is again almost impenetrable: "Remember this: Even healing is not healing, because Mind needs no healing. Our saying that Mind is given its freedom is also a statement of appearance only. For as God is free, so Mind is free."[199]

All these ideas taken together, in their various and competing forms, were referred to by physician, psychologist, and philosopher William James as the "the Mind-cure movement,"[200] which he equated with New Thought.[201] Its characteristic outlook on life, well-being, and healing was part of what he meant by his famous description of "the religion of healthy-mindedness."[202] This he described as religion in whose adherents is an innate "tendency which looks on all things and sees that they are good,"[203] in contrast to religion of "the sick soul,"[204] which he defined as the opposite. Regarding the importance of mind-cure, James noted, "The medical and clerical professions in the United States are beginning, though with much recalcitrancy and protesting, to open their eyes."[205] It is speculative how much James influenced or was influenced by Horatio Dresser, who was his student at Harvard.[206]

Following Hopkins, various religious organizations sprang forth that, despite considerable differences in ideology, especially regarding healing, shared genealogical roots with early precursors to New Thought and were thus directly or indirectly influenced by Eddy. It is not difficult to connect the dots from Eddy and Hopkins to Religious Science aka Science of Mind,[207] Divine Science,[208] Unity,[209] even Jewish Science,[210] as well as the Emmanuel Movement,[211] itself a key precursor of the modern pastoral care profession.[212]

Other organizations influenced by New Thought received additional inspiration from Eastern wisdom traditions, both directly, from *Vedānta* and *yoga*, and indirectly as read through the teachings of Western groups such as Theosophy and Anthroposophy.[213] A notable example of a group exhibiting all of these influences is Alice Bailey's Lucis Trust, an esoteric organization promoting the Spiritual Hierarchy, a group of discarnate entities also known as the Ascended Masters or Great White Brotherhood. In *Esoteric Healing*, Bailey was critical of organizations that sprung up around New Thought and related groups (which she called "cults"), on account of their contentious attacks on mainstream medicine, while conceding that such groups "are in fact the custodians of needed truths."[214]

Two other New Thought founders exemplify a multiplicity and fluidity of influences and offshoots in the realm of healing. Warren Felt Evans, a Methodist minister and Quimby follower, was influenced by Swedenborg, Hindu and Buddhist teachings, and Theosophy.[215] He founded Mental Science, an atheist/

agnostic branch of the New Thought family tree, and wrote several books on mental healing.[216] Christian D. Larson, a Unitarian teacher, was a former Christian Scientist and later involved in Religious Science, whose founder, Ernest Holmes, was influenced by his writings. Like Evans, Larson is remembered in part for books on mental healing.[217]

Additional Christian movements that strongly emphasize healing or wellness are located on the same New Thought family tree. These include—*among many others*—spiritualism; the positive-thinking movement of Norman Vincent Peale and those who followed; faith healers from Aimee Semple McPherson and Kathryn Kuhlman to Benny Hinn; the prosperity gospel of John and Joel Osteen; Oral Roberts's seed faith; Kenneth Hagin's Word of Faith movement; and modern-day Pentecostal and charismatic Christianity.[218] Non-Christian therapeutically oriented descendants of New Thought include the I AM movement, New Age healing, alternative medicine, and contemporary energy healers.[219]

If a connection of New Thought to the charismatic and prosperity gospel movements seems like a stretch,[220] consider that Christian anticult author Constance Cumbey once wrote a book asserting that televangelist Pat Robertson was among the leading forces promoting the New Age movement.[221] This assessment was based on account of his featuring guests and authors involved in holistic health and wellness centers, and his promotion of healing through spiritual gifts such as "words of knowledge." This odd assertion about the Baptist founder of television's *The 700 Club* underscores the complex and contested history of intertwined elements, including even Pentecostal and charismatic Christianity, all leading back through various routes to New Thought, explicitly or implicitly.

Perhaps the leading contemporary apostle of New Thought was Louise Hay, book publisher and Religious Science practitioner, who built a self-help empire around identifying "metaphysical causations" of illness and providing healing affirmations.[222] For example, cancer is caused by "Deep hurt. Longstanding resentment. Deep secret or grief eating away at the self. Carrying hatreds"; it is remedied by affirming, "I lovingly forgive and release all of the past. I choose to fill my world with joy. I love and approve of myself."[223] Hay's work influenced generations of clairvoyant "medical intuitives" who followed her, including bestselling author Carolyn Myss, who first came to public attention through her work with Duke-trained neurosurgeon C. Norman Shealy, founder of the American Holistic Medical Association.[224]

New Thought is the closest thing to a common source of today's integrative medical worldview, regardless of the particular therapeutic system or modality. Its defining principles, especially a salient influence of mental ideations, lie at the core of contemporary understandings of etiology, diagnosis, and treatment for many complementary and alternative practitioners across professions—including physicians, nurses, allied health professionals, bodyworkers, and

energy workers—of many stripes.[225] The ancient religion-medicine complementarity, in the form of New Thought and its descendants, underlies many
species of humanism and holism present in Western medicine. More so than
other examples given in this chapter, New Thought is both an explicitly religious
movement and an explicitly healing-oriented movement. It represents the fullest restoration of what Dresser was referring to when he described the "original
Christianity" of the early church and Gospels era as "a religion of healing."[226]

Hospitals and Healthcare Systems

If one doubts that Christian churches, collectively, constitute a religion of healing,
one need only observe the extensive denominational branding of medical care
institutions. So many hospitals, healthcare systems, medical care organizations,
and provider practices incorporate the name of a respective Christian denomination in their formal corporate name or that of particular buildings or structures.
Consider today how many medical centers are branded as Catholic, Lutheran,
Baptist, Methodist, Presbyterian, Episcopal, Adventist, Mennonite, LDS, and so
on. Within Roman Catholicism, religious orders own and operate community-
based hospitals, regional academic medical centers, and healthcare facilities of
almost every type,[227] often reflected in the names of these institutions as well.
This is not an exclusively Christian phenomenon: Jewish-branded hospitals
exist in the United States, as well as Buddhist hospitals throughout Asia, Hindu
hospitals in India, and Muslim hospitals throughout the Middle East.

Since the founding of the earliest hospitals in the West by the major Abrahamic
traditions nearly a millennium ago, religious movements have been at the forefront of providing medical care to the public. The establishment and continued
operation of religiously led healthcare systems speaks to their dual vocation or
purpose, of "mending bodies, saving souls,"[228] reflective of the prophetic, pastoral, and charitable mission of institutional religions. Specifically,

> The presence of religiously branded hospitals, clinics, and care facilities in
> most communities speaks to a ubiquitous understanding that God's love can
> and must be externalized, through the agency of religious institutions, to meet
> worldly needs of human beings, including and especially health and healthcare
> needs.[229]

With the rise of scientific medicine in the nineteenth century, the dynamics
of religiously operated medical care institutions were altered. Historians have
described how the evolution of medicine from speculative art to empirical science led to an inevitable secularization of medical theory and laicization of

medical care delivery.[230] Increasingly, as well, the religious value system of these institutions has been preempted by federal mandates governing practice standards. Since expansion of these programs in the United States with the advent of Medicaid and Medicare, it has been "often difficult to distinguish religious from secular hospitals—except perhaps for their names and, in Catholic institutions, their distinctive policies related to reproduction."[231] Now, even the latter point of religious identity may be obsolete, in light of ongoing legal debate over the nondiscrimination mandate within the Affordable Care Act that continues to adjudicate competing claims of religious liberty (on the part of Catholic providers) and access to care (on the part of patients).[232]

The largest religiously operated medical care provider in the United States is the Adventist Health System.[233] It is among the largest nonprofit healthcare systems in existence, with nearly eighty thousand employees working at forty-six hospital campuses in nine states. In its corporate statement on identity and values, foremost among the core principles is its "Christian Mission," defined as service "in harmony with Christ's healing ministry."[234] This principle is reinforced in its institutional mission statement: "Extending the Healing Ministry of Christ."[235] Results of a recent study of providers sampled system-wide suggests that the Adventist Health System has been successful in maintaining its corporate vision in the face of secularizing trends that have challenged other religiously based healthcare systems.[236] The study concluded that a "significant proportion of Adventist Health System providers and staff favor engaging in spiritual practices with patients,"[237] and do so, including praying with patients, sharing religious beliefs, and encouraging more active religious participation among patients. There is also considerable provider support for a screening spiritual history at intake, not yet a system-wide standard.[238]

As the Adventist Health System has grown into a multi-institutional corporate entity, it has shifted away from the distinctively eclectic health- and healing-related principles of Ellen G. White, nineteenth-century founder of the Seventh-day Adventist Church.[239] These included strict dietary practices, such as vegetarianism, as well as aversion to drug therapy and promotion of light and water therapy.[240] Since mid-century, "The distinctiveness of Adventist medicine lay less in its therapies than in its customs, motives, and philosophical justification."[241] To the extent that it has succeeded in maintaining these values in the changing healthcare environment, the Adventists have been more effective in facing such challenges than Catholic and other Protestant healthcare systems.

The presence of a desire to serve, individually and corporately—and concomitants that such a value mandates, as far as service to others—can be found in the vision and mission statements of hospitals across the religious spectrum, not just among Christian-owned institutions that use such language explicitly, such as Seventh-day Adventists. In *Radical Loving Care*, Erie Chapman, founder of the Baptist Healing Trust, advocates building what he terms *Healing Hospitals*. He offers the following description:

> A Healing Hospital is about loving service to others. It is about recognizing something that has increasingly been forgotten in a flood of the complex technology and magic-bullet drugs that now dominate America's hospitals. . . . A Healing Hospital is not built with bricks and mortar. It is built with people who have Servant's Hearts, or a passion to serve, and who know that the fundamental relationship between caregiver and patient can be understood as a Sacred Encounter. It can be created in any healthcare setting where leaders and staff join together in a new commitment to what we call Radical Loving Care— creating a continuous chain of caring light around each and every patient.[242]

This beautiful statement remains an ideal, not yet fully realized in any large healthcare system that I am aware of at present. But it is a wonderful ideal. Who would not want to experience the patient role in such an institution if, heaven forbid, one were facing hospitalization? Significantly, it is a faith-based vision. The language Chapman uses to describe his vision is unlikely to appear in the mission statement of a secular or public hospital, which might be required by law to eschew such wording and even associated underlying concepts.

Hospitals and healthcare systems founded and operated by religious concerns are freer to serve as confessing institutions, to borrow a theological term, and function explicitly and openly according to a "higher" or more transcendent calling: a servant's heart, sacred encounter, radical loving care, and so on. For some institutions, this may be primarily lip service, especially after the passage of time—in some instances, many decades since their founding. But other institutions are able to maintain fidelity to their calling, despite increasing political and economic pressures brought to bear on medical care providers, including complexities of regulatory oversight regarding standards and delivery of care, reimbursement, and liability. Some institutions and creative providers do so by opting out of the system altogether.

Hunter "Patch" Adams is a family physician (and professional clown and social activist) whose dissatisfactions with conventional medical care and the fee-for-service system led him to establish a free hospital and healthcare community, the Gesundheit Institute Teaching Center, on over three hundred acres in rural West Virginia. Adams became famous after his portrayal by actor Robin Williams in a movie that offered a semifictionalized account of his life and work, based in part on his book, *Gesundheit!*[243] The main hospital building has been a work in progress for over forty-five years and is based on a variation of the commune model, envisioned as hosting a multidisciplinary team of providers offering a spectrum of alternative and conventional medical care without accepting insurance nor charging fees. Gesundheit is not an explicitly religious-based healthcare organization, in the sense of other institutions described in this chapter. But it exemplifies many of the same dynamics, except that the underlying worldview expressed in its statement of vision exemplifies both metaphysical and humanistic ideals in support of political communitarianism. Adams is open to any alternative therapies that can prove useful clinically,[244] including spiritual modalities, and be utilized alongside conventional medical care.[245]

Other faith-based institutions operate fully within the normative healthcare system—and from mainline religious perspectives—and manage to remain true to religious values. Some Jewish hospitals, for example, include within their mission statement explicit reference to *tikkun olam*[246] and *tzedakah*,[247] the latter of which is usually translated as *charity* but more accurately connotes *justice*. These values may be considered Jewish equivalents to the Adventist mission to extend the healing ministry of Christ, noted above. A unique version of this phenomenon is seen in the example of the Jewish Hospital–Mercy Health, in Cincinnati, the first Jewish hospital in the United States and currently part of Mercy Health, a large Roman Catholic healthcare ministry and medical care system. The hospital's mission statement captures this shared vision:

> The Jewish Hospital is a community hospital faithful to its Jewish heritage and grounded in the Jewish and Catholic traditions of service to the community. Our purpose is to reveal God's love for all, especially the poor and vulnerable, through the delivery of compassionate health care services and the education of health care professionals.[248]

The hospice movement is another example of a faith-based healing ministry that grew to become a multifaith, multi-institutional sector of the healthcare delivery system. Its roots lie in facilities for the terminally ill operated by the Knights Hospitaller in the fourteenth century (and perhaps before that with Roman Catholic crusaders of the eleventh century), who established places of respite for the dying.[249] Modern-day hospices provide palliative care to chronically and terminally ill people, whether in dedicated residences, within hospitals or skilled nursing facilities, or at a patient's home. The modern hospice movement was founded by Dame Cicely Saunders, whose St. Christopher's Hospice, established in London in 1967, was described by her biographer as "the incarnation of a religious ideal—Cicely's religious ideal,"[250] reflecting her Anglican and evangelical background. An organized Jewish hospice movement, associated with the work of Rabbi Maurice Lamm,[251] operates with its own characteristic religious values. These are grounded in each human being's endowment with "a spark of divinity" on account of God's creation; this "divine image" in turn grants each of us "innate value."[252]

In the present, intersections of the religious and healthcare domains are diverse, taking many unusual forms across the spectrum of spiritual and faith traditions and involving a diversity of healing settings. Faith-healing revivals featuring charismatic Christian pastors draw enormous audiences throughout sub-Saharan Africa, and miraculous works have been reported, including resurrection of the dead.[253] One of the founders of the Roman Catholic charismatic renewal movement was Francis MacNutt, a former priest who established the influential Christian Healing Ministries and became one of the world's leading authorities on healing prayer.[254]

Spiritism has become one of the largest religious denominations in Brazil,[255] and the country is populated by numerous spiritist healers, including the controversial trance medium and psychic surgeon João de Deus (John of God).[256] Unexpected cross-pollination can been observed as well: Columbia University cardiothoracic surgeon Mehmet C. Oz first came to public attention after inviting a Reiki energy healer named Julie Motz into the operating room to assist during surgery.[257] The latter is another example, incidentally, of the reach of New Thought concepts into places where, one would presume, they would never otherwise extend.

A significant challenge for the future of continued religion-healthcare rapprochement will be for religious institutions to negotiate and manage the implied conflict between its sponsored medical care institutions and those among its clergy and members who offer equivalent services outside the system. MacNutt, for one, felt compelled to leave the priesthood in order to start his own organization, and anyway, his services of prayer for the healing of disease, exorcism of demonic spirits, and deliverance from homosexuality would likely gain little traction in today's politically retreating Catholic hospital systems. At the same time, many leaders within religiously run healthcare institutions would affirm that a living faith summons them to discipleship and outreach in order to manifest the prophetic charge to call the world out of its sinful complacency and to repair and heal the world's people and institutions. Fidelity to pastoral and missional traditions that gave birth to ministries of healing and redemption can be found both within and outside of formal religious institutions, and both within and outside of established healthcare institutions.

3

Missions and Ministries

Many of us are familiar with the story of Albert Schweitzer.[1] In 1913, after graduating from medical school, he left for French Equatorial Africa and founded his famous missionary hospital at Lambaréné. During World War I he was brought back to Europe where he and his wife spent time in an internment camp in France, suspected of German sympathies.[2] Following the war and recovery from illness, he returned to Africa and remained there for most of the rest of his life, unwilling to leave his work behind even to receive his Nobel Peace Prize in 1953. He is remembered today as a kind of medical Mother Teresa.[3]

Schweitzer's work as a healer was an extension of his pastoral call to serve the needy. In turn, he defined his work as a pastor as labor in service to healing the afflicted. Both roles, pastor and healer, were expressions of his ethical worldview, which he called "reverence for life."[4] For Schweitzer, this was "not a theory or a philosophy but a discovery—a recognition that the capacity to experience and act on a reverence for all life is a fundamental part of human nature, a characteristic that sets human beings apart from the rest of the natural world."[5] In his autobiography, he elaborated:

> Affirmation of life is the spiritual act by which man ceases to live thoughtlessly and begins to devote himself to his life with reverence in order to give it true value. To affirm life is to deepen, to make more inward, and to exalt the will to live.[6]

In his dual life as minister and healer, tending to people whom he served at Lambaréné, Schweitzer had many epiphanies about the meaning and purpose of life, and his insights have become canonical for those called to medical missions. Of special significance was his understanding that the calling to serve is redemptive—not just for those being served but for the server and society as a whole.

> One can save one's life as a human being, along with one's professional existence, if one seizes every opportunity, however unassuming, to act humanly toward those who need another human being. In this way we serve both the spiritual and the good. Nothing can keep us from this second job of direct human service. So many opportunities are missed because we let them pass by.[7]

Religion and Medicine. Jeff Levin, Oxford University Press (2020) © Oxford University Press.
DOI: 10.1093/oso/9780190867355.001.0001

There was little inherently conflictual for Schweitzer in negotiating his multidimensional path as theological scholar, pastor, and physician. These callings were complementary, and in his work he took inspiration and instruction from the example of Jesus, who "when He called His disciples, required from them nothing more than to follow Him."[8] When his vision of serving in Africa became fully crystallized in his mind, Schweitzer was excited at the prospect of what lay ahead, as it provided an opportunity to live out his Christian witness in a way that honored his multiple talents. It also enabled him to live a missional life whose focus transcended the default orthodox and pietistic approach to missions, which, he lamented, consisted of "preaching the gospel in the pagan world" in hopes of converting heathen natives.[9] As a liberal Christian, this did not appeal to him, and he was concerned that he would not be supported by official missionary organizations. But, no matter, he was secure in his calling:

> I wanted to be a doctor so that I might be able to work without having to talk. For years I had been giving of myself in words, and it was with joy that I had followed the calling of theological teacher and preacher. But this new form of activity would consist not in preaching the religion of love, but in practicing it. Medical knowledge would make it possible for me to carry out my intention in the best and most complete way, wherever the path of service might lead me.[10]

Simultaneously functioning in the medical and religious worlds, Schweitzer did more than anyone to define the popular imagery of the medical missionary. Part selfless humanitarian, part entrepreneur, part community organizer, part pastoral figure—all of these roles coalesced in Schweitzer, creating an idealized vision of the servant doctor called to a life in missions. That this image may be overstated does not seem to matter by now; the caricature is indelibly drawn.

On the flip side, Schweitzer had his critics. He was accused of being morally paternalistic, supportive of views that smacked of colonialism and imperialism, and on record as expressing authoritarian political and economic positions such as opposition to African self-determination.[11] According to the contrarian view, he could be imperious, as a religious figure was more scholar than pastor, and in his hospital work was increasingly brand-conscious, overly concerned with fundraising, and not much of a physician.[12] To critics on the far left, he was racist and corrupt, and his hagiographers were guilty of a collective work to soothe the "liberal conscience"[13] One recent assessment of Schweitzer titled "Icon, Scoundrel, Prophet, Paradigm?" suggested that each descriptor may be partly valid.[14]

True, false, or exaggerated, no matter—these images too have reinforced negative connotations of missions work on the part of secular critics of Christian evangelization. Notwithstanding that this presents a distorted vision of missionaries as ideologues and opportunists using medical aid work as a cover for nefarious attacks on indigenous cultures or religion—something that does not map out against twenty-first-century medical missions work, nor against the work of Schweitzer—again, these images have taken root. Ironically, it could be argued that "Schweitzer was not a typical missionary, if he was a missionary at all."[15] For one, he made little effort to learn any local languages or communicate directly with his patients. At most, he was "a sympathetic bystander,"[16] whose religious beliefs and missions work, respectively, manifested a confounding "coexistence of liberal and conservative elements."[17] He was, simply, a liberal Christian medical doctor called to treat the sick in a far-off land, for reasons related to intrinsic psychodynamics on which we can only speculate a century downstream.

The history of Christian efforts to meet needs of the medically underserved and vulnerable, at home or overseas, is more nuanced than either of these polarized characterizations of Schweitzer. Moreover, the work of medical missionaries is but one piece of a larger phenomenon whereby medical professionals and religious professionals serve in each other's respective world, in partnership or on their own, in order to attend to the physical, psychological, and spiritual needs of people dealing with health challenges. This includes medical care missions operating through religious organizations, pastoral care ministries operating in healthcare settings, and people of faith serving as counselors or therapists and delivering spiritually grounded psychotherapy.

This larger story involves religiously committed individuals—physicians, nurses, clergy, psychologists, laypeople—called to serve through missional work in faraway parts of the world or in clinical settings closer to home. This includes service through ministries of caring that function within hospitals and other healthcare and patient settings in communities throughout the United States. Also included is service delivered through other forms of faith-based counseling in community-based clinical practices in which clients may present with various challenges not limited to physical illness or disability.

For practitioners, all of these avenues of assistance speak to a common ethos that values labor offered up in service to those in need in the name of a higher, spiritual ideal that calls one to come to the aid of others. These forms of service also present the possibility of challenges arising out of a conflict of mission— the implied threat of individuals from one domain or sector operating in another: invading alien turf, one might say. For physicians and nurses working for faith-based relief organizations, clergy making patient rounds in hospitals and clinics, and religious psychotherapists treating patients undergoing mental health or spiritual crises, it is not uncommon to be confronted by conflict or confusion over professional roles, institutional priorities, chain-of-command authority, or decision-making styles.

The motives of providers also may be called into question, and even if pure and innocent, unintended consequences may result. Missionary expansion of respective religions across national and cultural borders, for example, has been described as "the prototype of the process of globalization . . . [and] the motive force of universalization,"[18] for good or bad, intentionally or otherwise. Granted, for most college premed students on a summer mission trip to dig wells or put up mosquito netting in a developing nation, something this weighty may never cross their mind and may be wholly unrelated to why they felt called to participate. But it underscores the complexity and sensitivity of this subject that well-meaning young adults acting with honest conviction and a servant's heart may, through some eyes, be seen as unwitting agents of cultural imperialism.

A significant part of this story is the evolving professional role of clergy in hospital and healthcare settings over the past century. Delivery of spiritual care by healthcare chaplains, other clinical providers, and community clergy and religious leaders defines a vocational space in which religious professionals are employed by medical-sector organizations to minister to patients through services that cannot be offered by medical care practitioners. This is a mirror image of medical missions work, whereby medical professionals are employed by religious organizations to minister to health needs of client populations. Other new professional roles seem to overlap both categories, an important innovation being *faith community nursing*, originally known as parish nursing. As established by Rev. Granger E. Westberg in the 1980s,[19] faith community nursing is a specialty practice in which licensed registered nurses deliver healthcare in faith-based settings and, increasingly, provide spiritual care alongside or in lieu of pastoral care providers.[20]

Westberg's involvement here is significant. The most impactful and enduring twentieth-century figure whose labor lay at the intersection of religion and medicine, he is responsible for multiple firsts: the first academic center, medical school course, and faculty appointment focused on religion and medicine; the first wholistic health center; the concept of congregation-based health promotion programs; and, as mentioned, the field of parish nursing. He is also an important figure in healthcare chaplaincy and the development of bioethics. Westberg's story appears in several places in subsequent chapters. He was an innovator of many of the concepts and institutions defining the contemporary intersection of religion and medicine in North America and throughout the world.[21]

Medical Missions

The origins of Christian missionary activity can be dated to the earliest journeys of Paul and associates to spread the gospel in the first century CE. Inspired by words of Jesus, "Go therefore and make disciples of all nations,"[22] known as the Great Commission, for the past two millennia Christian missions have carried the message of Christ to every corner of the earth. In their comprehensive *To All Nations from All Nations*, Carlos F. Cardoza-Orlandi and Justo L. González document missions activity from antiquity to the present, across denominational groups (Roman Catholic, Orthodox, Protestant), and throughout the world, including the Middle East, Far East, South Pacific, sub-Saharan Africa, and Latin America.[23] They define missions as an "effort to expand the faith both within and beyond their borders of its own context,"[24] and in that sense Christian missions have been a monumental success.

But the history of missions also provides plenty of evidence that Christians "have used the words of Jesus as justification for lucre and for imperialistic purposes."[25] As well, historical works document resistance met by missionaries,[26] often resulting in violence from both sides and other evils, such as forced conversion of Jews.[27] The story of the Crusades and centuries-long conflict between the Christian and Muslim worlds is another troubling dimension of this subject, and scholars continue to contest historical evidence and debate the truth of what really happened and for what reasons.[28]

The work of Christian medical missionaries, beginning in the early nineteenth century, provided a different instrumentality and justification for efforts to spread the faith.[29] A largely evangelical movement at first, exemplified by the famed Scottish physician David Livingstone in South Africa,[30] captivating accounts of courageous journeys into godforsaken jungles for altruistic purposes "exercised a powerful hold on the Western imagination."[31] British historian David Hardiman elaborates on the public impact of these colonial missionary healers:

> These heroic figures were seen to carry on their different and dangerous work through a moral courage that was derived from strong religious faith. They provided a combination of Christian conviction, imperial mission, and science, a compelling amalgam for an age in which each value was held in high regard.[32]

Hardiman notes that evangelicals such as Livingstone "often depicted paganism as a sickness of both mind and body, requiring an all-round therapy administered by an evangelist."[33] This hints at a "harsh side to the medical mission,"[34] including use of coercion,[35] differing only in degree but not kind from the approach of centuries earlier during the Roman Catholic Inquisition in Europe.[36] Traditional indigenous worldviews were also subject to classification as madness or insanity, and social disruption caused by missionary activity was read as psychiatric illness requiring medical treatment and stepped up efforts at European socialization.[37]

In the twentieth century, imagery of "the mission 'jungle doctor' was depicted as fighting witchcraft, superstition, ignorance and degeneracy"[38] and accordingly, "walking in the path of Christ."[39] This patronizing view served as an excuse for medical missionaries to act as agents of "disciplinary control"[40] on the part of European powers seeking to preserve hegemony in the colonial world. This behavior in turn explains largesse dispensed to medical missionaries, suggesting motives not purely altruistic. A battle for the souls of so-called primitive people, in this view, was in part a cover for imposition of Western medical practices. Hardiman acknowledges this when he states, "A more lasting legacy of medical missionaries most probably lay not so much in the number of converts they won, but in their popularization of biomedicine. . . ."[41]

Notwithstanding these mixed motives, the second half of the nineteenth century was a seminal moment for Christian medical missions. Beginning in 1878, the next few years saw founding of the Medical Missionary Association in London, the New York Medical Missionary Society, and the American Medical Missionary Society.[42] The number of medical missionaries grew from only seven, combined, in India and China in 1858 to more than one thousand physicians and five hundred nurses worldwide by 1916.[43]

For the past two centuries,[44] Christian missionaries have provided medical, surgical, nursing, and dental care and shepherded environmental health infrastructure and health-impacting economic development projects in the developing world.[45] Medical missions in China, for example, date to the 1820s and the work of Robert Morrison and later Elijah Coleman Bridgman.[46] Since then, medical missions have been sponsored by almost every major Christian denomination on six continents, the scope of work evolving beyond establishing hospitals and clinics.[47] Today, extensive programs of global outreach have been established in partnership with nongovernmental organizations (NGOs), academic institutions, government agencies, secular foundations, and philanthropies, and serve as agents of social justice and change as well as means to address public health disparities.[48]

The phrase *medical mission* originally implied "one of the medical posts supported by a Christian congregation (dispensary for the poor, clinic, etc.),"[49] but later was broadened to imply the "medical branch of overseas mission."[50] In the latter context, medical missions continue to flourish throughout the world, sponsored by various institutions, such as private Christian organizations or NGOs, secular medical organizations, and student groups.

Compassion International is a nondenominational Christian NGO sponsoring missions addressing children's health, especially focusing on health and nutrition, water and sanitation, and child development.[51] Active in more than two dozen countries in Africa, South America, Asia, and Central America and the Caribbean, it works with over seven thousand indigenous church partners.

Compassion's mission is built on three foundations: it is Christ-centered, church-based, and child-focused. A fourth foundation is an expressed commitment to integrity.[52] A six-nation study published in the *Journal of Political Economy* determined that recipients of aid through its programs go on to complete more years of schooling, are more likely to finish their education, and experience a higher quality of employment opportunities.[53]

Use of the word *mission* does not imply that all medical missions are sponsored by faith-based groups. Non-faith-based organizations also operate health-related missions projects throughout the world. International Medical Relief, for example, which provides mobile medical and dental clinics, disaster relief, and community health education in fifty-seven nations, welcomes participants from all faith backgrounds. Student volunteers have come from 163 universities, including faith-based schools such as Baylor University.[54] Secular and faith-based humanitarian NGOs have a history of cooperation in "broad coalitions" to provide medical relief.[55]

Faith-based educational institutions are heavily invested in sponsoring missions activities for premedical and prehealth students. A case in point is Baylor, where I serve on the faculty. Baylor has a substantial missions presence, including multiple opportunities for medical missions experiences throughout the developing world, some projects ongoing for many years.[56]

Recent examples of medical missions for Baylor undergraduates include trips to provide medical services and public health outreach in Kampala, Uganda; to serve students and teachers of students with speech pathologies and other disabilities in Karen, Kenya; to prepare for the opening of a new medical clinic and conduct screenings in Collique, Peru; to shadow local doctors, assist the local pharmacy, and address barriers to healthcare in La Romana, Dominican Republic; and to offer maternal and child health education services in Hyderabad, India. Projects are conducted in partnership, variously, with local groups, established missionary organizations, and national student organizations. An example of the latter is a mission trip to provide basic healthcare, medical screening, and health education in Bogotá, Colombia, sponsored by the Baylor chapter of the American Medical Student Association.

Student participation in global medical missions makes an important contribution to premedical and medical education, but educators have a responsibility to ensure that projects are ethically above board.[57] Given the history of medical missions in the colonial era, noted above, this expectation is reasonable. Four principles have been proposed to guide implementation of educational experiences. Student missions projects must emphasize

- Skills building in cross-cultural effectiveness and cultural humility.
- Fostering bidirectional participatory relationships.

- Longitudinal engagement promoting sustainable local capacity building and health systems strengthening.
- Being embedded within established, community-led efforts focused on sustainable development and measurable community health gains.[58]

Many of these efforts, especially involving student volunteers, are short-term medical missions (STMMs). The STMM has been defined as a medical service trip sponsored by a faith-based organization (FBO) whereby "volunteer medical providers from [high-income countries] travel to [low- and middle-income countries] to provide health care over periods ranging from 1 day to 8 weeks."[59] The theological foundations for STMM trips, according to the Catholic Health Association, are grounded in several principles: respect for life and human dignity, the preferential option for the poor and vulnerable, solidarity with fellow human beings, and support for the virtues of charity, justice, and compassion.[60] This background places the STMM squarely in resonance with the ideals of Catholic social teaching,[61] which, according to Father Gustavo Gutiérrez, calls on Christians to begin "taking the road of the poor."[62]

In recent decades, a critique of the STMM's efficacy has appeared. Insightful and challenging analyses have originated from the missions field[63] and public health[64] and health services research,[65] and from Protestant[66] and Catholic[67] health professionals. Specific criticisms include lack of standards for selecting and training volunteers, as well as for implementation, safety, quality, and impact; absence of evaluative research to inform future efforts, as well as of standards for evaluation; minimal consideration for cultural differences that should inform design of missions projects; and poor coordination with the health infrastructure of host countries and local communities, inhibiting successful capacity-building efforts. Questions also have been raised about how well medical missions fit into missions work in general,[68] and medical missions have been criticized as potentially harmful expressions of "medical tourism"[69] and "humanitarian colonialism."[70]

Medical missions have received thoughtful attention within academic medical education.[71] Since the rise of global health as a field of study and practice, scholarly efforts have been made to examine the foundations of medical missions[72] and to suggest how they may contribute here.[73] Calls have been made for medical missiology to become an established scholarly discipline,[74] and an idealized future for medical missions has been envisioned.[75]

More recently, evaluative research studies,[76] reviews,[77] and quality-of-care analyses[78] have appeared in the medical and missiological literature. These include studies of missions experiences of medical and dental providers,[79] surgeons,[80] and residents participating in Operation Smile,[81] an international organization sponsoring volunteer surgical missions trips to repair cleft lips and palates.[82] Many challenges to missions work and its effective evaluation have been identified, including conflicts of interest[83] and ethical issues,[84] such as related to informed consent[85] and treating patients with dignity and sensitivity to cultural and religious norms.[86] In a provocative article titled "The Seven Sins of Humanitarian Medicine," the authors echo many of the concerns identified up to now, but at the top of their list is one that perhaps has not received enough attention: "Leaving a mess behind."[87]

It is an underreported fact that medical and public health missions are not solely sponsored by Christians or directed from the global West to the global East or South. For example, missions originating in Taiwan have sponsored medical outreach throughout the world, including forty-six missions to eleven countries in Central America and twenty-five missions to eight countries in the South Pacific.[88] These include the work of physicians, nurses, and pharmacists in hospitals and primary care centers and in the community, and entail health education and public health measures along with clinical services.

Another notable example is the Tobin Health Centre, which serves Abayudaya Jews and their Muslim and Christian neighbors in Mbale, Uganda.[89] Supported by Jewish philanthropy in the United States, its construction was motivated by religiously grounded principles of compassion and service and does not devote any efforts to religious proselytizing, which is not as actively pursued within Judaism as within other faiths.[90] The center was established in 2010 with support from the nonprofit Be'chol Lashon ("In Every Tongue"), a multiethnic research and community-building initiative based in San Francisco.[91] The center specializes in diagnostics and primary care and has made headway in addressing malaria, infant mortality, and other perinatal health concerns. Jewish philanthropy also supports Christian medical missions in Africa, such as through the annual Gerson L'Chaim Prize[92] sponsored by the African Mission Healthcare Foundation,[93] the world's largest prize supporting direct patient care.

Despite valid criticisms of features of STMMs, especially the perception of well-meaning but unprepared young Christian do-gooders helicoptering in for a brief stay then leaving, medical missions in the contemporary world are more likely than anytime previously to involve long-term established partnerships between reputable FBOs and host communities or nations. While there are troubling episodes to report, these do not originate exclusively from within the Christian missions community. Unfortunate incidents involving Hindu religious organizations in the United States, for example, have received public attention since the 1990s, including alleged sexual exploitation at the hands of Swami Rama[94] and Swami Satchidananda,[95] and an organized bioterror attack committed by followers of Bhagwan Shree Rajneesh.[96] Thankfully, these events are not representative of the outreach efforts of Hindus in the West, nor are they representative of the contemporary missions field.

Healthcare Chaplaincy

Just as physicians and nurses can minister to people, so can ministers and other clergy serve as agents of healing. As we saw in the previous chapter, religious institutions and pastoral professionals have had a formal role in hospitals and healthcare as long as there have been specialized sites for healing—for thousands of years. Since the 1920s, according to Wendy Cadge in *Paging God: Religion in the Halls of Medicine*, chaplains have become "the formal carriers of religion and spirituality in American hospitals."[97] *Paging God* documents evolution of the healthcare chaplaincy profession over the past century and is highly recommended to anyone seeking to understand the roots and antecedents of religion's presence within healthcare settings and academic medical institutions.

Prior to about a hundred years ago, according to Cadge, chaplains in secular hospitals were likely to be retired or volunteer clergy, without specialized training, who made the rounds of hospitals to minister to patients from their respective faith traditions.[98] After World War I, a series of developments established healthcare chaplaincy as a profession.[99]

Formal clinical training for clergy was proposed in 1925 by Harvard physician and divinity school lecturer Richard Cabot,[100] whose subsequent collaboration with Presbyterian minister Anton Boison led to creation of the first Clinical Pastoral Education (CPE) programs.[101] Boison went on to found the Council for the Clinical Training of Theological Students in 1930,[102] and over the next two decades hospital chaplaincy "began to organize as a distinct profession."[103] This was seen in establishment of training programs, certification bodies, and professional organizations,[104] as in other healthcare professions.

Subsequent decades saw further institutionalization of the profession through founding of professional and scholarly organizations. These included the HealthCare Chaplaincy Network, in 1961, a New York–based educational and research organization;[105] the Association for Clinical Pastoral Education (ACPE), in 1967, a multicultural and multifaith organization that accredits CPE programs and certifies healthcare chaplains;[106] and the Association of Professional Chaplains (APC), an interfaith membership society established in 1998, with roots dating to the 1940s, which publishes the *Journal of Health Care Chaplaincy*.[107] The APC issued a Code of Ethics in 2000, a set of Standards of Practice in 2015, and a statement of Common Qualifications and Competencies in 2016.[108] It also sponsors a Board of Chaplaincy Certification,[109] akin to the specialty boards that certify physicians and other health professionals.

Denominational communities of professional healthcare chaplains have coalesced, notably for Roman Catholic[110] and Jewish clergy,[111] with additional standards of practice. The Spiritual Care Association was founded in 2016 as an international membership society and professional certification organization "that establishes evidence-based quality indicators, scope of practice, and a knowledge base for spiritual care in health care."[112] Independent academic journals established for this field include the *Journal of Pastoral Care and Counseling*, founded in 1947, and *Pastoral Psychology*, founded in 1950. Noted religious scholars, including Princeton Theological Seminary's Seward Hiltner[113] and Southern Baptist Theological Seminary's Wayne E. Oates,[114] contributed to pastoral theology and the growth of pastoral counseling.

These institutional developments are signposts of healthcare chaplaincy's maturation into a formal occupational field, a well-established and full-fledged "companion profession,"[115] which Cadge describes as a profession that works "alongside another without seeking to challenge its jurisdiction."[116] While a unique, independent profession, healthcare chaplains nonetheless are engaged in an ongoing work of " 'translation' between the world of the patient and the world of hospital medicine."[117] Cadge describes this as something of a tightrope act, with chaplains "walking between the worlds of religion and medicine, pastor and clinician, and religious organizations and medical centers."[118]

Growth of the profession and expansion of its outreach and impact were facilitated by the American Hospital Association, which during the 1960s actively promoted healthcare chaplaincy as an integral part of the spectrum of patient care.[119] By the mid-1970s, most U.S. hospitals had a chaplaincy department or employed chaplains, whether CPE-trained or otherwise.[120] By the twenty-first century, national membership data suggest that the profession is religiously diverse,[121] although evangelicals and black Protestants remain somewhat underrepresented among professional chaplains.[122]

The institutionalization of CPE programs throughout the hospital sector has been most instrumental for professionalization of healthcare chaplaincy. At present, according to the ACPE, there are nearly three hundred accredited CPE centers, six hundred certified faculty, and twenty-three hundred active members. About nine thousand units of CPE are taken annually, and by now about seventy-five thousand people have undergone training.[123] At Texas Medical Center (TMC) in Houston, for example—the largest medical center in the world—there are five accredited CPE centers. These are at CHI St. Luke's Health–Baylor St. Luke's Medical Center, Houston Methodist Hospital, Memorial Hermann–Texas Medical Center, the University of Texas MD Anderson Cancer Center, and Harris Health System Ben Taub General Hospital. This must make the fourteen-hundred-acre TMC campus the healthcare CPE capital of the world, or close to it. Almost all major faith traditions and Christian denominations are represented among credentialed healthcare chaplains,[124] at TMC and nationally.

Despite these signs of professional success, significant challenges remain. According to George Handzo, a past president of APC and former director of chaplaincy services at Memorial Sloan-Kettering Cancer Center, "One of the major barriers to advancing the practice of spiritual care is a lack of definitional clarity among practitioners themselves."[125] A major figure in the healthcare chaplaincy field, Handzo has done much to provide the missing clarity through his research and writing. He makes the following conceptual distinctions among fields of practice whose descriptors are often, and wrongly, used interchangeably:

> In sum, *spiritual care* is the overarching category representing a domain of care comparable to "emotional care" that can and should be performed to a greater or lesser degree by all health care professionals. *Chaplaincy care* is the part of that care performed by professional chaplains. *Pastoral care* is performed by chaplains and other religious professionals, usually with persons of their own faith tradition.[126]

Chaplains in the healthcare setting perform many activities. Foremost among these are conducting spiritual assessments and creating spiritual care plans.[127] Spiritual assessment is itself multifaceted, and efforts have been made to further differentiate among spiritual screening, spiritual history-taking, and more in-depth and ongoing needs assessment through active listening.[128] The work of healthcare chaplains is typically conducted as a part of interdisciplinary and transdisciplinary teams,[129] in which chaplains serve in various roles, including facilitator, provider, caregiver, and adviser.[130]

Since the 1980s, healthcare chaplaincy has become increasingly introspective, which I believe is a healthy sign for the field. Efforts have been made to document its complicated history, identify how it can best meet anticipated professional challenges related to a rapidly changing healthcare environment, and set agendas comprising goals and objectives for guiding the profession into the future. Contemporary histories have made a point to emphasize clinical, educational, and scholarly developments,[131] as outlined above, that have shaped the field.

At the turn of the new century, Larry VandeCreek and Laurel Burton, two of the most important elder statesmen in the chaplaincy profession, edited the first joint statement on the role and significance of the profession signed onto by all the main healthcare chaplaincy organizations.[132] This consensus report included a section detailing benefits of spiritual care as provided by professional chaplains. These entail benefits to patients and families and to healthcare staff, healthcare organizations, and communities.[133] VandeCreek and Burton noted, especially, that healthcare chaplains "offers distinct benefits . . . [that] are increasingly demonstrated by empirical research studies."[134] Their evaluation carries weight: Burton was the first president of the APC, and was succeeded as editor of the APC's *Journal of Health Care Chaplaincy* by VandeCreek.

Over this same time period, the profession has continued to expand.[135] Data from annual surveys of the American Hospital Association show that between

1980 and 2003, just over half of hospitals had chaplaincy services.[136] These were mostly found in church-operated hospitals, not surprisingly, but such hospitals were also more likely to have eliminated these services than to have added them.[137] Greater prevalence of such programs in faith-based institutions "potentially indicat[es] different value commitments around religious/spiritual care and/or greater ease of finding and financially supporting chaplains."[138] Financial factors, however, may also play a role in their closing: more budgetary pressure on these hospitals may make them more inclined to drop chaplains in favor of retaining higher-priority services.

Accordingly, ongoing efforts to expand or rethink professional boundaries is apparent by a review of publications in major chaplaincy journals, as new roles continue to be identified for healthcare chaplains.[139] Creative innovations such as multicultural and multifaith practice models have appeared,[140] especially throughout the culturally diversifying Anglophone world.[141] All sorts of therapeutic approaches have been proposed, especially for working with psychologically distressed patients, such as Acceptance and Commitment Therapy (ACT).[142]

This is especially evident in ongoing research involving the U.S. Department of Veterans Affairs (VA) and Department of Defense, where a significant investment has been made to integrate mental health and chaplaincy services.[143] Such integration is requisite for veterans and service members to have "systems of care in place that can adequately address the complexity of their emotional, relational, spiritual, and mental health care needs."[144] Launched in 2010, this project has convened chaplains and academics in a series of needs assessments, task groups, invited conferences, training programs, and more, with an aim of meeting several strategic goals through more than two dozen specific actions.[145] I was honored to speak at one of their research events, in 2011, along with Ellen L. Idler, George Fitchett, Keith G. Meador, and other colleagues.[146]

Fitchett's lecture, titled "Envisioning a Research-informed Chaplaincy,"[147] resonated with my own experiences in teaching and consulting with the VA chaplaincy in the early 1990s. Whenever I was on campus to lecture at the National VA Chaplain Center in Hampton, Virginia, the leadership would ask me for ideas in ramping up a research agenda for the center and for the field. They recognized the importance of quantifiable endpoints in justifying their work, such as for reasons of demonstrating cost-effectiveness,[148] but, as in hospital environments outside the VA, multiple complexities made this a difficult task. Besides the challenging political realities of the healthcare sector, whether in public or private sectors, inhibiting factors also included issues related to availability of resources, time commitment, and lack of training in the sophisticated research methodologies required for publishable studies.[149] The movement to up the research game for healthcare chaplains dates to VandeCreek's research primer for pastoral care, published in 1988,[150] but it took several years for the research base of the field to visibly crystallize.

In the years since, healthcare chaplaincy and pastoral care in general have grown into a thriving research field. A major contributor to this effort has been Fitchett, director of research in the Department of Religion, Health, and Human Values at Rush University, in Chicago, and uniquely credentialed in both ministry and epidemiology. Since the 1990s his research and writing, alone and in collaboration with others, and his organizational contributions to the chaplaincy profession have helped to make for a more evidence-based field.[151] Fitchett's work as researcher and educator has been instrumental in strengthening the field's presence within academic medicine. Other contemporary leaders in this effort to solidify the field through outcomes research include Kevin J. Flannelly, George Handzo, and Andrew J. Weaver. This issue is contested, however, as some fear that greater emphasis on scientific validation may result in something important, and not capturable in numbers, being lost.[152] For the most part, this counterargument has not prevailed, and the field is moving rapidly in the direction of more systematic evaluative research.[153] The prevailing sense is that the potential value of research for securing the footings of the healthcare chaplaincy field, and directing its foci and efforts, has been acknowledged.[154]

Experts such as Handzo have noted that healthcare chaplaincy is finally "emerging from a marginalized role in the process of health care."[155] This is owed in large part to ramped-up efforts to provide recognized practice standards and mature as a research field. Accordingly, a culture of evidence-based care is taking root,[156] bolstered by innovative models of spiritual assessment[157] and spiritual processes[158] used in evaluative and outcomes research,[159] including studies of efficacy of care,[160] as well as research on patient satisfaction.[161] This change of culture has been reflected in the healthcare chaplaincy literature, with greater focus on research reports, theoretical papers, and review articles.[162] Since the start of the twenty-first century, the literature also includes reports of collaborative research among healthcare chaplains and other professional providers,[163] survey and qualitative data on integration of chaplaincy into mental healthcare within military and veterans' facilities,[164] and, not to be overlooked, basic demographics on patient contacts and staffing requirements.[165]

Significantly, there is the beginning of a scholarly literature of case studies in various patient populations and clinical settings—pediatric, psychiatric, and palliative care[166]—something not present in the chaplaincy literature prior to 2011, according to Fitchett.[167] This was an important lacuna to be filled, because "giving colleagues a published case study is an effective way to help them better understand the work that we do. Because case studies can be emotionally engaging, they are also an effective method for educating healthcare decision makers and the public about the work that chaplains do."[168] It would be hard to imagine physicians and nurses, for example, undergoing years of training without study or review of individual case reports, but to now this has not been a cornerstone of Clinical Pastoral Education. Accordingly, two volumes of such cases have been published.[169]

Currently, Fitchett and others are continuing to take an evidence-based, outcomes-focused approach to mapping out the future of the profession.[170] An important, and ongoing, frontier for the field is how to better integrate spiritual care and medical care.[171] To this end, the Transforming Chaplaincy project, funded by the John Templeton Foundation, was established as a partnership between Rush and Brandeis, under the direction of Fitchett and Cadge.[172] It sought to produce two cohorts of research-literate chaplains better equipped "to use research to guide, evaluate, and advocate for the daily spiritual care they provide patients, family members and colleagues."[173] In 2017 the project transitioned into a think tank focused on research-based chaplaincy practice and education. Other efforts to ensure a future for health-care chaplaincy have focused on reenvisioning how chaplains are trained in order to prepare for prospective challenges encountered as the healthcare system evolves.[174]

Faith-Based Psychotherapy

In 1988 psychiatrist David B. Larson and colleagues published results from an important study of clergy as mental health services providers for patients experiencing psychiatric symptoms.[175] Drawing on population data from the multi-site Epidemiologic Catchment Area study, findings showed that depending upon the particular diagnosis, patients were liable to seek care from mental health specialists only, clergy only, both mental health specialists and clergy, or neither. The most important finding was that "clergy are as likely as mental health professionals to be sought out by individuals from the community who have serious psychiatric disorders."[176] The study further noted that, methodologically, there was reason to believe that its prevalence estimate for clergy-only use was actually underestimated.[177]

The authors stated that "the conclusion is clear: the clergy are coping, with or without the assistance of mental health professionals, with parishioners who have a broad spectrum of psychiatric disorders."[178] Accordingly, the authors called on mental health providers "to make a concerted and diplomatic effort to reach out" to clergy,[179] offering two recommendations. First, clinicians might stand to gain significant insight on a respective patient by contacting the clergyperson initially consulted. He or she might have useful information on the patient's life history, ongoing mental health status, experience of stress, and means of coping. Second, national organizations of mental health professionals should reach out to clergy and theological seminaries so that each constituency may be involved in each other's respective training.[180] Larson and his associates noted, regretfully, that the need for such collaboration had been identified for twenty-five years at that point, without much progress.[181]

In the decades since, efforts to promote spiritually based mental health care, including psychotherapy, have arisen within the major faith traditions, practiced by psychologists and psychiatrists and grounded both in modern clinical practice and teachings of respective religions.[182] To be clear, this is a lay movement distinct from clergy-delivered pastoral counseling, as it involves efforts to integrate spirituality and faith concepts into mental health care by secular providers. Christian psychiatrists, psychologists, and marriage and family therapists, for example, treat patients presenting with a broad spectrum of challenges and symptoms and do so from a Christ-centered, Bible-based perspective complementing their professional training and informing their therapeutic approach.[183]

Christian psychotherapy is global movement,[184] not limited to North America. Professional societies such as the Christian Medical and Dental Associations' affiliated psychiatry section provide a safe space for fellowship, personal growth, and outreach to both the profession and the world, such as through sponsoring missions.[185] Members integrate modern therapeutic approaches with faith-based caring, including recommendations for prayer, into professional practice.[186] Well-known Christian clinics exist where patients receive medical and psychiatric treatment and psychotherapy from Christian providers in an environment that honors their faith commitment and does not intrinsically view it as an impediment to mental health or recovery.[187]

Significantly, efforts to integrate Christian beliefs into psychiatric and clinical psychological practice are not limited solely to evangelicals in the United States, as is often presumed.[188] There is, for example, a Catholic Psychotherapy Association, founded in 2002 and associated with the Institute of Psychological Sciences, offering doctoral training in Catholic psychology.[189] The association's stated mission is "to support mental health practitioners by promoting the development of psychological theory and mental health practice which encompasses a full understanding of the human person, family, and society in fidelity to the Magisterium of the Catholic Church."[190]

An especially close connection exists between Judaism and the mental health professions. Many pioneers of psychiatry and psychology were Jewish, although not necessarily observant of the Jewish religion, and psychoanalytic practice and psychodynamic theory would never have evolved as it did without seminal contributions from Jews. Important Jewish pioneers in the mental health professions included Sigmund Freud, Alfred Adler, Erich Fromm, Wilhelm Reich, Erik Erikson, Fritz Perls, and Viktor Frankl. The popular stereotype that psychiatrists are often Jewish is not entirely false. When the world-famous Menninger Clinic moved from Topeka, Kansas, where we were living at the time, to Houston in order to affiliate with the Baylor College of Medicine, our synagogue in Topeka lost several families.

The affinity between Jews and the mental health professions continues into the present. This manifests across the spectrum of Jewish affiliation and observance: from Abraham Twerksi,[191] scion of a famous lineage of Chasidic rabbis and expert on addictions, to Jon Kabat-Zinn,[192] a secular Jew responsible for popularization of mindfulness meditation as a contemporary therapy. There is a significant Jewish presence in clinical psychology, including important academic contributors from within Orthodox Judaism.[193] Ironically, this presence flourishes despite an observed stigma toward help-seeking for psychiatric problems among segments of the *charedi* (ultra-Orthodox) Jewish community.[194] Such individuals are more inclined to turn to prayer or rabbinic consultation.

Traditions of spiritually based psychiatric treatment, psychotherapy, and mental health counseling also flourish within other religions. Some associated theories and practice models are of putatively ancient origin. Others are contemporary expressions of body-mind-spirit thinking that emerged in psychology and other clinical disciplines with the human potential movement in the 1960s.[195] Published cases, reviews, and research studies appearing in English-language psychiatry journals in the current century have described features of psychiatric practice across faiths. This includes insightful writing on psychiatry within Islam,[196] including Sufism,[197] and in Hinduism,[198] Buddhism,[199] Sikhism,[200] Jainism,[201] Taoism,[202] and Confucianism.[203]

Buddhist psychology and the counseling tradition within Buddhism have been especially influential on contemporary psychotherapy on account of use of meditation and endorsement of mindfulness training.[204] *Mindfulness* has been defined by Kabat-Zinn as "the awareness that emerges through paying attention on purpose, in the present moment, and nonjudgmentally to the unfolding of experience moment by moment."[205] Hybrid forms of East-West spiritual psychology have emerged from synergies created between mindfulness and established religious therapies, such as in Islam[206] and Judaism,[207] as well as in nonreligious contexts for use as adjuncts to conventional and integrative medical practice.[208]

Closely associated with mindfulness has been the concept of transcendent experience,[209] which has been defined as an event or state that "typically evokes a perception that human reality extends beyond the physical body and its psychosocial boundaries."[210] Such experiences are termed *transcendent* because they entail "transcendence of one's personal identity and dissolution of a primary conscious focus on or grounding in one's ego."[211] Transcendence and related concepts, including mystical, unitive, transpersonal, and noetic experience,[212] have been the subject of research studies in psychology for the past few decades,[213] and therapeutic practices have incorporated these concepts for many years.[214] They also show some promise as foci of health research in the new field of study emerging around the concept of human flourishing.[215]

4

Congregations and Communities

When Granger Westberg relocated from Baylor to Wittenberg University, in Ohio, in the 1960s, he observed that "thousands of churches and synagogues were virtually empty most of the week and that . . . clinics could be located in the education or other space."[1] His pastoral work and seminary teaching led him to recognize an unmet need and that the pastoral care profession and field could be invigorated by shifting its base of operations from the "sterile" and "unreal" classroom to "on location where the people are."[2] As told by his daughters in his biography, *Gentle Rebel*, Westberg's vision was bold:

> Granger conceptualized the church clinic as "an action-research experiment to determine whether an ordinary congregation of people can assist physicians in providing health care to patients whose physical symptoms have been brought about chiefly by human problems, namely the stresses and strains of life."[3]

Westberg's first free clinic opened in 1970, sponsored by Good Shepherd Church, a middle-class Lutheran congregation in Springfield, Ohio, with substantial foundation and community support. Besides medical and pastoral care provided by a physician and clergy, respectively, the clinic expanded to include dental care, an eye clinic, immunizations and public health assistance, counseling, first aid, and other services.[4] Within a year, the facility "was swarming with people on clinic day."[5]

In 1972 Westberg returned to Chicago and expanded on his vision of pastoral ministry by establishing the first Wholistic Health Center.[6] In contrast to the original free clinic, this was a nurse-centric operation, creating a formal role for nurses as patient advocates. It favored a multidisciplinary team-based model, was whole-person-oriented in its approach to health needs assessment, and involved the patient in decision-making.[7] The model that Westberg pioneered eventually expanded beyond its base in the western suburbs of Chicago and was influential, directly or indirectly, in nearly every subsequent partnership between medical and public health institutions and agencies and religious denominations and congregations, whether respective contemporary religion-medicine alliances are aware of this or not. By now, half a century later, Westberg's work lives on in ways he may never have envisioned.

Religion and Medicine. Jeff Levin, Oxford University Press (2020) © Oxford University Press.
DOI: 10.1093/oso/9780190867355.001.0001

This chapter describes the progeny of Westberg's original clinic and center. His innovations were soon expanded on to include collaborations with academic public health professionals and religious denominations. This is best exemplified by the Health and Human Services Project of the General Baptist State Convention of North Carolina, established to focus on eliminating health disparities among African Americans.[8] Such programs, targeting underserved populations, have grown into a major feature of public health outreach in the United States, especially targeting risk reduction for serious chronic conditions among ethnically and socioeconomically diverse populations.

Another outgrowth of Westberg's early work is the numerous collaborative partnerships involving congregations and congregational networks working with local and state health departments and healthcare institutions, as well as with global organizations. Emory University has been a hub for programmatic work and scholarship in this area.[9] Medical care providers and public health agencies have come to recognize the advantages of reaching their target populations in local and regional communities through formal liaisons with faith-based institutions.

Yet another application of Westberg's ideas is organized outreach to special populations with substantial unmet needs—people disadvantaged, oppressed, or otherwise at heightened risk of deleterious health-related outcomes whose social status or living conditions may leave them invisible to established providers and formal systems of healthcare. In so many communities, faith-based organizations (FBOs) are the only institutions of the public or private sector with the available resources, connections, and commitment to reach out to these people and address their most pressing physical, material, and existential needs.

Churches as Clinics

Religious congregations have become familiar loci for community-based health promotion and disease prevention (HPDP) programs of various types.[10] Inspired and informed by Westberg's pioneering work, church-based health education interventions and healthcare delivery efforts throughout the United States and across the religious spectrum date back decades.[11] The most prominent and influential early such program was established in North Carolina in 1978.

The earliest major denomination-wide, congregation-based program was the Health and Human Services Project of the General Baptist State Convention (GBSC) of North Carolina,[12] a predominantly African-American denomination headquartered in Raleigh. A collaborative effort with the Department of Health Education (since renamed the Department of Health Behavior) at the University of North Carolina School of Public Health, its lead investigator was

John W. Hatch, currently William R. Kenan, Jr., Professor Emeritus. The project evolved from his earlier work as a community organizer with the Tufts-Delta Health Center in Mound Bayou, Mississippi,[13] the first rural community health center in the United States, and in leading the Community Health Education and Resources Utilization Project, described as "an effort to train lay people to be health resources in their local communities."[14] Influenced also by Westberg's idea of patient advocates, the churches project aimed to "mobilize natural helping systems within the churches and communities in order to provide appropriate counseling, screening, and social support to members at risk for selected health conditions . . . [through providing] support for lay advice seeking from family members or friends or others within the social system, leading eventually to increased self-care and health-seeking behavior."[15]

From the beginning, the project was oriented toward elimination of health disparities,[16] especially due in part to modifiable behavioral risk factors. Throughout its history, foci have included maternal and child health, chronic diseases (diabetes, hypertension, cancer, Alzheimer's disease), caregiving, and development of congregational health ministries. An important feature was identifying, recruiting, and training lay health advisers—community members relied upon to mediate between at-risk populations and health agencies and other community resources available for primary prevention and healthcare.[17] The challenge was to work with existing social support structures and networks, specifically operating within and among Baptist churches in African American communities in North Carolina, seeking ideally "to graft an intervention onto these existing roles and functions."[18] An extension of the health ministry of the GBSC, the project continues today under the auspices of the Center for Health and Healing, a nonprofit affiliate of the GBSC founded to provide organizational leadership for all of its health-related programs,[19] including its Faith and Health Initiative, which carries on its long-standing work in risk reduction and primary prevention.[20]

As a graduate student in public health at UNC from 1981 to 1983 I was an advisee of Hatch and one of many students who over the years interned in the project.[21] My assignment was to conduct a process evaluation of the project's hypertension screening activities in rural churches throughout the state. Traveling to these churches in a state car, often driving many hours to a destination, was an eye-opening experience. I learned so much about the promise of religious congregations for reaching communities with health education and healthcare, but also about challenges and barriers that may render these good intentions inert. Naively, I would arrive armed with a list of precise questions to be answered in formal interviews with respective congregational leaders, usually following church services on Sunday mornings, but in some instances found this to be pointless. While many churches were quite large and had modern, well-staffed clinics with nurse volunteers who were members of the congregation, others had no space, no resources, no supplies, and hardly any personnel.

I especially recall driving hours to one small home back in the woods, down miles of dirt road, without an address ("turn left at the old tree"), in an unincorporated part of the state. The resident, an elderly woman, was the contact person for the project in her small, one-room church. She kindly welcomed me into her home and offered me some tea. Then without any prompting, this dear person began telling me how wonderful the project was, how many people it had helped, and all the great things it was doing to combat "high blood." At the end she added, "Oh, one more thing, do you know when they'll send us one of those sphygmomanometers?"

An essay in the inaugural issue of the *American Journal of Health Promotion* in 1986 penned by the journal's founding editor, Larry S. Chapman, identified "spiritual health" as "a component missing from health promotion."[22] At the time, this was a mostly accurate assessment, although one-off health programs in particular churches, such as those affiliated with the Westberg and Hatch projects, do have a history dating to the 1970s, as noted. Have things evolved in the subsequent three decades? Yes, they have, but this does not mean that these efforts are always well planned, successfully implemented, and competently evaluated. As a result, while much has been learned, much is left to learn in order to more effectively develop faith-health partnerships to fill lacunae in health services delivery and address population-health disparities within so many communities. This may sound like a clichéd response, but it is accurate here. An especially understudied issue relates to what health educators term *outcome evaluation*.

Among priorities for researchers, Chapman noted, "We need to correlate health promotion interventions with discernible effects on human health and well-being. Do [they], in fact, have a direct and measurable effect on human health?"[23] This may seem like an obvious point, but most HPDP program evaluation, when it even occurs, is focused on impacts—change in quantifiables, such as particular health-related behaviors, as a result of an intervention—not on outcomes, on whether there is a lasting effect on health status. This may require substantial longitudinal monitoring, typically beyond the scope of most projects. It is much easier to focus on near-term changes in whatever discrete behavior or institutional parameter the program targeted—less cigarette smoking, better medication compliance, healthier snacking, shorter hospital stays, and so on—than to determine whether this eventually impacts on population rates of morbidity or mortality in a given community. To be fair, such evaluation may not be feasible given the operational and funding parameters of most programs.

Almost thirty years after Chapman's commentary, I published my own commentary in the same journal on the same theme, taking stock of whether we had made any progress in the intervening years.[24] I concluded that we indeed have, as far as the content breadth of programs. Congregational interventions and other health programs involving FBOs have been implemented successfully across the domain areas of public health, including health education (e.g., HPDP programs), health management (e.g., establishment of church-based clinics), and environmental health (e.g., community advocacy to clean up polluted neighborhoods).[25] Based on these successes, I called on the Obama administration to take the lead "in institutionalizing faith-based partnerships as an integral component of national health promotion efforts."[26] In my opinion, this was a solid recommendation, but to date not much action has been taken at the federal level to move this idea forward.

Common emphases of congregational public health interventions include risk reduction (via screening, referral, and primary care delivery), chronic diseases (including primary prevention of hypertension, diabetes, HIV/AIDS, mental illness, and adverse perinatal outcomes), and underserved populations (especially rural, urban, older adults, single mothers, and ethnic minorities).[27] The ubiquity of church service participation and other faith group involvement in communities across the United States makes religious congregations "essential partners" in HPDP programs and other health-related outreach.[28] For communities and populations with limited access to healthcare for financial or other reasons, such partnerships may be a godsend. Health educators have long recognized this, and accordingly, such "non-traditional channels are often employed to deliver health-based interventions to populations that are sometimes considered hard to reach or who view traditional health care channels with distrust."[29]

Programs in the most historically underserved locales also draw on long-standing traditions of self-help and mutual aid, such as within African-American communities and centered in local churches.[30] The Black Church since its origins has been the primary autonomous and independently run organization functioning in rural and urban African American communities with a history of being ignored by government and denied access to needed resources.[31] It has been identified as a "therapeutic community,"[32] a system of social or formal organizations that can provide physical and psychological support to African Americans and contribute to mental health promotion.[33] Potential government support, such as through faith-health partnerships underwritten by the federal faith-based initiative, raises complex and concerning challenges pitting the historic autonomy of African-American churches against the organizational benefits of public funding for faith-based health ministries.[34]

African-American churches have been popular sites for intervention programs since the earliest days of congregational HPDP,[35] exemplified by the North Carolina churches project. Such programs have existed for decades, addressing rural and urban populations with limited access to primary care and community mental health services, focusing on issues from health-behavior change to health-policy advocacy.[36] Black pastors as well have served as agents of social and behavioral change within their communities and church networks, laboring to improve the health and well-being of their constituencies.[37] Again dating back decades, they have served in numerous health-directed roles at the primary, secondary, and tertiary levels of prevention: public health educator, counselor and community psychologist, liaison with community health programs, community health activist, program development consultant, medical history-taker and mental health diagnostician, referral agent, hypertension detection specialist, family liaison to local hospitals, support group organizer, and more.

The success of the North Carolina program encouraged other ethnic-minority churches and state and national denominational bodies to follow suit. Contemporary examples of established HPDP programs can be found throughout the United States within minority churches or congregations or within statewide or regional offices of minority denominations, as with the North Carolina Baptists. Such programs have addressed cardiovascular disease risk,[38] HIV/AIDS,[39] diabetes,[40] mammography,[41] exercise and physical activity,[42] and mental health.[43] Evidence exists that African-American church congregations can successfully "create and collaborate in the birthing of a strong faith-based health education program focused on health prevention strategies."[44] Still, an important review, published in 2002, noted that "very little research has empirically examined church-level and pastor-level factors that may aid or impede the successful implementation of such programs" in Black churches.[45] Only recently have sustained efforts been made to systematically evaluate such programs and investigate factors that bear on their successful implementation.[46]

Other programs exist that are thematically linked but organizationally independent across congregations and draw on broader faith-based communities, including minority and nonminority racial and ethnic groups and churches.[47] Still other thematic programs involve unique faith-based coalitions among religious congregations, community organizations, and educators.[48] Since the North Carolina project began, variations of this work have proliferated across the country, especially in medically underserved communities.

The most prominent and influential exemplar of local faith-health collaborations is the Congregational Health Network (CHN), in Memphis, Tennessee, a program widely known as the Memphis Model. Founded in 2004, it benefited greatly from the expertise of Gary R. Gunderson, who came to Memphis the following year from Emory University's celebrated Interfaith Health Program (more on that in Chapter 6).[49] Gunderson drew on successes elsewhere, from the North Carolina churches project to global health initiatives in Africa,[50] in developing a model that recognizes that "strengths of the *social infrastructure of congregations* inherently provide strong social 'interventions' to support health and healing."[51] In operational terms, this means "allowing the clergy and congregational leadership and intelligence to define what they want and need and meeting those named training needs,"[52] resulting in a grassroots network of empowered partners sealed in a covenantal relationship that respects the autonomy of congregations and innate wisdom and insight of the faith sector to identify health needs and pathways to meet those needs.

The CHN is currently a network of over six hundred congregations in partnership with Methodist Le Bonheur Healthcare, serving over twenty thousand congregants and supported by over seven hundred congregational and community laypeople.[53] The CHN evolved out of earlier local efforts, including the Church Health Center (CHC), a local program providing health education, wellness promotion, and healthcare and other human services to over sixty thousand patients. Established in 1987 the CHC is the largest faith-based healthcare organization of its type in the United States.[54] Evaluative research of hospitalized CHN participants through 2011 revealed significantly longer time-to-readmission, lower overall mortality rates, and greater likelihood to be discharged from the hospital into home health.[55]

Today, the CHN is influential far beyond Memphis. Other programs in other locales are patterned after the Memphis Model.[56] A briefing by Gunderson to senior staff of the Obama administration in Washington in 2011, following a government delegation's site visit to Memphis, was significant in giving the federal imprimatur to the work of the CHN.[57] The important role of Gunderson in all of these developments cannot be overstated. He has had a hand in so many of the significant developments in this field, either directly through his leadership or through his scholarship and ideas. Especially influential for the Memphis Model was the African Religious Health Assets Program,[58] itself based on an earlier model known as assets-based community development.[59] Originating in faith-based activism during apartheid-era South Africa, insights gleaned from this work piloted, in essence, the concepts and best practices later applied in Memphis and elsewhere.

The South African connection here is significant. Much of the modern fields of social and community medicine, social epidemiology, and public health education derived from the work of a group of South African expats who settled at UNC many decades ago.[60] These included John Cassel and Sidney L. Kark of the Department of Epidemiology and Guy W. Steuart, chair of the Department of Health Education during my time as an M.P.H. student. Based on their work in South Africa at the Pholela Health Centre in Natal[61] in the 1940s and 1950s, Dr. Kark laid the groundwork for what became known as *community-oriented primary care*,[62] Dr. Cassel conducted the first programmatic research in social epidemiology,[63] and Dr. Steuart formulated a vision of health education far more expansive than the patient-education-oriented model then in vogue.[64]

Steuart envisioned HPDP as ideally focused on bottom-up community organization and community development for purposes of planned and natural (unplanned) health-related and health-directed social change. Change agency, for Steuart, was an organic process best facilitated—but not directed—by public health professionals working as consultants through and with the endorsement of existing networks of people, who retained control of the parameters and goals of their participation.[65] One of his initial hires at UNC was John Hatch, who had been applying Steuart's model in rural Mississippi[66] and who then built on this work to establish the North Carolina churches project. Incidentally, one of Cassel's first hires upon becoming chair of the Department of Epidemiology was Berton H. Kaplan, a pioneering social epidemiologist and one of the earliest figures in the field to write seriously about religion. My own research and indeed career's work on this subject date to my mentoring from both Hatch and Kaplan as their student at UNC.

The story of the many interconnections among work in South Africa, North Carolina, and Memphis has come full circle. After establishing both Emory's Interfaith Health Program and the CHN in Memphis, Gunderson was recruited to North Carolina in 2012, joining the faculty at Wake Forest University.[67] The Wake Forest Baptist Medical Center, in partnership with philanthropies and the hospital sector, had decided to replicate the Memphis Model statewide in North Carolina, through a program named FaithHealthNC, and set their sights on hiring Gunderson. The program was rebranded as the North Carolina Way, and it too has met with success, although there have been unique challenges due to substantial differences between the two settings.[68]

A couple of denominational efforts also deserve mention. The United Methodist Church's Health Ministry Fund, for decades under the direction of attorney Kim Moore, is a Kansas-based initiative focused on improving the health of rural and underserved communities in the state.[69] Established in 1986 the fund has provided more than $70 million in grants to support over twenty-four hundred programs seeking to increase access to healthcare, improve early childhood development, and build healthy congregations.[70] The Kalsman Institute on Judaism and Health was established in 2001 as a unit of Hebrew Union College–Jewish Institute of Religion, the rabbinical seminary and graduate institution of Reform Judaism. In 2010 the institute issued a comprehensive review of health and healing programming within Reform congregations and elsewhere sponsored by Reform and other Jewish institutions.[71] This document nicely complemented a best-practices report prepared in 2008 by the National Center for Jewish Healing that summarized existing programming on Jewish healing.[72] Earlier in the 2000s I was privileged to have a small role in both programs, consulting on the fund's Healthy Congregations project and serving as a scientific consultant to the Kalsman Institute.

Closer to home for me in Central Texas are a couple of faith-based programs, one ongoing and directed by a single medical institution and the other in the planning stages (at the time of writing) and involving a community-wide network coordinated by a regional denominational group. The Office of Mission and Ministry is an executive office of Baylor Scott & White Health System with a charge to promote "the spiritual aspect of patient care."[73] It operates four projects: Second Life Resource Center, which donates used medical equipment and supplies to medical missionaries in thirty-five countries; the Sacred Vocation Program, focused on the spiritual growth of employees; Faith Community Health, which recruits individuals to serve as liaisons with patients discharged back into the community, based on the Memphis Model; and Direct Pastoral Care: Hospital Chaplaincy, the traditional mission of a hospital spiritual care department and also the most labor-intensive and difficult to evaluate.[74]

Faith Health Waco, also based on the Memphis Model, is a project of the Church Health Ministry of the Waco Regional Baptist Association.[75] Its goal is to establish "a partnership between churches/faith communities and hospitals, clinics and the health district to provide a network of support to improve the health of the Waco community."[76] The project team seeks to train laypeople within the local faith community to serve as "faith health liaisons" for their respective congregations. They intend to focus their efforts on healthy lifestyle behavior change, improving healthcare access, and achieving better community health outcomes, such as a lower rate of hospital readmission, fewer billable costs, heightened access to primary care, and even lower mortality rates. Their plan has been to build a large congregational network since launching their pilot program in 2018.

These two programs, operating in a single community, exemplify the kinds of faith-health partnerships that exist throughout the United States. They include programs and interventions directed by individual congregations or denominational groups, as in Faith Health Waco, as well as medical-center-based programs that liaise with institutions and people in the local faith community, as in aspects of the Baylor Scott & White program. The latter program also exemplifies partnerships originating in medical or healthcare institutions or agencies, rather than in local congregations, and these expand the universe of faith-health partnerships beyond the types of interventions characterized by church-based HPDP programs. More detail on these healthcare-sector partnerships appears in the next section of this chapter.

With notable exceptions, program evaluations and evaluative research of faith-health collaborations have been slow in coming, which has been identified for decades as a substantial gap in this work. I can remember as a graduate student in public health in the early 1980s speaking with experts, hearing talks, and reading articles in which better evaluation of congregational HPDP programs was being "called for" repeatedly; it still is today. Far less of a systematic nature is known about the success of such programs than one would hope.[77] Further, according to a recent nationwide review, "There is little empirical data informing public health professionals of factors influencing the translation of faith-based health promotion research into practice."[78] According to a 2004 review, only a small proportion of published reports of congregation-based health programs or interventions (about 7%) presented data on outcome measures,[79] but what data were presented "nonetheless demonstrate that faith-based health programs can produce positive effects. . . ."[80] So we do have more than an inkling that these programs can be effective, but systematic evaluation is required for us to understand what makes for successful and unsuccessful ventures.

Competent evaluation, moreover, can and should serve a formative as well as summative function.[81] That is, results of program evaluations can and should be used not just to summarize whether a project has met its objectives but also to be fed back into the design and implementation of the intervention or project. This may be done on an ongoing basis or for purposes of improving subsequent rounds of intervention. Program evaluation for a respective project may comprise both summative and formative elements; they are not mutually exclusive. Each type can additionally involve evaluation of processes and impacts, whether quantified or qualitative. All these approaches to evaluation, as well as use of meta-evaluations, have been applied to faith-based HPDP programs of one sort or another, but until recently they were not widely applied, concomitant to the general neglect of evaluation, as noted.

Since the start of the new century, conditions have improved somewhat, and programs are by now more likely to have built-in evaluation components; funding agencies require them as a condition of support. Broader meta-evaluations are fewer, but the lens has been zoomed out enough to enable valuable feedback for program planners and public health policymakers.[82]

A helpful study from researchers at the University of Nebraska identified critical factors in the success of congregational HPDP programs. Among the most important is cultivation of "positive health values," best facilitated when clergy and congregational leaders "value and demonstrate commitment to health promotion projects."[83] This may seem obvious—programs fail without leadership and a shared set of aims—but FBOs provide a unique "model of caring"[84] specially influential and necessary to promulgate lasting behavioral change. Committed congregational leadership can provide tangible benefits as well: access to facilities, a denominational network of fellow congregations, and socially supportive relationships that can reinforce positive change.[85]

To date, according to a major review, HPDP programs have achieved success in effecting change in intrapersonal characteristics such as health-related knowledge, attitudes, beliefs, and feelings; interpersonal influences such as social networks of family and friends that support healthy behaviors; organizational policies, facilities, and structures within congregations, such as health ministries; and policies related to the physical and economic environment, such as advocacy for farmers' markets, urban victory gardens, and hiking trails.[86] Moreover, the "potential for reach and long-term sustainability of health programs is perhaps the most compelling rationale for partnering with FBOs for health promotion."[87]

One should not take away from this the notion that faith-based programs, interventions, and behavior-change research in health are only found in Christian churches and perhaps a few Jewish congregations and community centers. Such programs and projects exist across faith traditions, although the readiness or amenability to sponsor HPDP programs for particularly sensitive diagnoses (e.g., HIV/AIDS) may be culturally and religiously constructed.[88] Still, health-related programs—educational, clinical, and research-focused— have been sponsored by congregations and organizations representing Asian religions in the United States, and this is not a recent phenomenon, as a personal example shows.

In the summer of 1979, while in college, I spent a couple months at the Himalayan Institute of Yoga Science and Philosophy, a residential retreat center and Hindu ashram located on four hundred acres in rural Pennsylvania. Founded by Swami Rama, the Institute was established to promote *Rāja yoga*, meditation, and holistic health in the West.[89] I volunteered in the medical department while staying in living quarters among the resident-renunciants. My job, under the supervision of a Harvard-trained internist, was to take precise measurements, by hand, of the wave components on EKG strips collected from medical patients undergoing stress tests while participating in studies of the effects of yogic practice on cardiovascular health. This was a terrific, if unusual, summer experience for a young religion major planning a career in the health sciences: besides participating as a lab grunt in some fascinating medical research, I spent two months practicing *Haṭha yoga*, eating organic vegetarian food, and even learning a bit of Sanskrit.

Collaboration with the Healthcare Sector

So far, we have examined health-related programs operating within congregational or other religious settings. As noted, there is another side to this issue: partnerships with local congregations in programs operating within or directed by healthcare organizations or public health departments. Healthcare systems and state and local governments have partnered with religious denominations and congregations for HPDP programs or, more broadly, for community health development. This can encompass working collaboratively to foster social, environmental, and health policy change, besides the sorts of be-havior change programs that have been a staple of health education efforts for decades.

Partnerships between local health departments and FBOs are present in every region of the United States, offering a collaborative means to provide for vulner-able populations using shared resources. This is not a fringe activity: a national survey of a representative sample of over five hundred local health departments reported that 83.1 percent of them had partnership activities with FBOs.[90] These activities included exchanging information through networks of community or-ganizations, working together in planning health fairs and screening programs, and health-sector funding or leadership of joint programs. This may be the most underpublicized and unrecognized success story in public health management in the twenty-first century.

Existing models outline how such partnerships can coalesce and function more harmoniously. Summative and formative evaluation efforts have been made to review these collaborations and, ideally, learn from the experience to create more effective models for future partnerships.[91] Creative solutions have been proposed as well for navigating complex data management issues involved in evaluating such programs, such as pertaining to healthcare data and medical records.[92]

Other types of collaborations exist, such as among congregations, the public health sector, and academic institutions, as in the North Carolina churches pro-gram. Much has been learned here, too, as far as strategic organizational lessons that can be applied to ensure successful programs that meet their impact and outcome objectives.[93] These sorts of partnerships, assisted by input from in-formed academic scholars and scientists, are vitally important in formulating strategies to meet public health goals and objectives, according to a discerning review, because they provide "a plausible solution to overcoming obstacles to engaging hard-to-reach populations in efforts to eliminate health disparities."[94] Especially important if these efforts are to succeed is for government agencies, such as public health departments, to be willing to transfer some of their power and decision-making authority to local congregations and community leaders,[95] who, after all, know their people and most pressing needs better than govern-ment bureaucrats, no matter how earnest and well meaning. Local ownership of programs is also essential for ensuring long-term sustainability of programs and continuity of efforts to achieve program aims.

This theme was reinforced in a review of successful faith-health partnerships undertaken by researchers at Emory's Interfaith Health Program.[96] Factors most associated with successful collaborations were passion and commitment, sup-port from community and faith leaders, and mutual trust and respect.[97] A top-down, rule-by-edict approach only serves to engender distrust of health-sector partners such as public health agencies, which can be as serious a barrier to program success as lack of resources and internal team conflicts. Private-sector FBOs and public-sector government health agencies not only have distinct worldviews; they may also have different agendas.[98] These may differ, too, across congregations or faith-based groups within a particular partnership or program. Some churches or ministers may be very otherworldly in their outlook and see prayer and reliance on God as the only acceptable approach to dealing with community health challenges. Others may view collaboration with public health professionals as essential to achieving health equity and social justice, which may be seen as authentic extensions or expressions of Christian ministry.

Progress in reducing population-wide health disparities requires addressing systemic issues—it is not all about implementing individual-level behavior change programs in selected congregations. Accordingly, successful partnerships require participation across sectors: government, philanthropies, the faith community, and local organizations and advocacy groups. Team-building among all players is requisite for evolving and sustaining both a truly collaborative structure and a healthy pool of leaders.[99] Faith-based interventions and partnerships do not occur in a vacuum. FBOs and institutions may be embedded into networks of other organizations, formal and informal, whose leaders and constituents may have involvements in multiple groups and sectors that are stakeholders in the issues being addressed.

Another factor to consider is the diversity of meanings of *faith-based*. This phrase covers a lot of ground, and not every partnership between a congregation or FBO and a public health department or healthcare provider or agency is the same in all respects. Another Emory researcher, Ellen Idler, the Samuel Candler Dobbs Professor of Sociology and director of Emory's Religion and Public Health Collaborative, along with her coauthor Allan Kellehear, proposed a continuum of faith-based collaborations with healthcare institutions and agencies.[100] These range from partnerships defined by merged identities to relationships in which the institutions remain entirely separate.

Drawing on existing programs in both the United States and the United Kingdom, Idler and Kellehear developed a model of six categories of faith-health institutional relationships. From the most independent to the most connected, they are as follows:

- *Faith-secular partnerships*: religious congregations or groups that join together informally with clinics, hospitals, or government agencies to provide services.
- *Informal faith role*: the presence of religious themes occurring, for example, in nonpastoral interactions with patients in medical care settings.

- *Formal faith role*: secular healthcare institutions that provide a formal role for spiritual care, such as through chaplaincy.
- *Faith-background institutions*: religiously founded healthcare institutions that are now mostly secular in orientation but that maintain a religious affiliation or identity along with selected religious traditions.
- *Faith-centered institutions*: healthcare institutions with a strong public religious identity, but open to public (secular) funding and participation.
- *Faith-saturated institutions*: healthcare institutions that are run and staffed exclusively by a religious institution and require a specific profession of faith for employment and/or service.[101]

This taxonomy was developed to categorize relationships between religious institutions and medical care providers and organizations, but can be applied to healthcare and public health agencies just as easily. The authors anticipate that their conceptual model will be "particularly valuable for identifying those health-care institutions where the religious influence was an important part of their history, but of which only vestiges remain."[102] Partnerships with such institutions may present opportunities for more direct and collegial collaboration than with faith-centered or faith-saturated institutions, but challenges that are considerably more complex and multifaceted may also arise. Faith-secular or informal-faith-role healthcare partnerships may require leaders to negotiate a tricky terrain in which competing forces within the religious institution alternately welcome and encourage secular collaboration and resist such efforts as overly secularizing.

This work is ongoing throughout the United States. It is not without challenges, but existing partnerships are successfully negotiating this terrain, which is heartening given the reality of limited healthcare access, rising costs of medical care, increases in the incidence and prevalence of degenerative chronic disease, and resultant population-health disparities that plague so many communities. Establishing partnerships with FBOs has been a solution, in part, and the decision to explore this option can be considered prescient. In *Building Healthy Communities through Medical-Religious Partnerships*,[103] Johns Hopkins physician Richard G. Bennett and psychologist W. Daniel Hale succinctly explain the motivation underlying such collaborative efforts:

> There is a way for health care organizations, large and small, to address these challenges. But they cannot do it by themselves. To reach and maintain contact with people, providing them with the information and resources they need to make good decisions about their health and medical care, health care organizations need partners. They need to work closely with institutions that are deeply rooted in the community and are trusted by people in the community.

Health care organizations need to develop alliances with institutions that have a strong tradition of caring for others and that attract people who identify with this tradition.

Religious congregations—churches, synagogues, mosques, and temples—clearly fit this description.[104]

Hospitals, medical centers, healthcare systems, public health departments, social services agencies, and community organizations and support groups across the United States are participating in such partnerships, and the numbers continue to expand. *Building Healthy Communities* is a compendium of such programs and projects, as well as a source of guidance and tangible resources for developing new programs. Examples include faith-health collaborations addressing serious illnesses, as well as associated risk factors, including coronary heart disease, hypertension, cancer, diabetes, depression, dementia, and respiratory diseases. Additional examples include faith-health programs focused on advanced directives, patient-provider communication, risk factor modification, medication compliance, and accidents and falls.[105] Note how many of these efforts pertain to issues of relevance to geriatric populations.

In their insightful book *Religion and the Health of the Public*, Gary Gunderson and James R. Cochrane, a South African religious scholar, summarize what religion brings to the table—ideally, in partnerships seeking to contribute to the health of public.[106] They define and develop the concept of *religious health assets* (RHAs), which runs counter to the thinking of many health professionals who see religion as a liability.[107] The authors believe that it is "both disrespectful and strategically irresponsible to ignore those religious assets that can be discerned, built upon, and supported."[108] While the tacit view within medical and public health circles may be that faith does more harm than good, the authors remind us that "if faith can be toxic, it can also be generative."[109]

In their book, Gunderson and Cochrane provide a matrix of RHAs, distinguishing between tangible and intangible assets, and proximate and distal assets.[110] Forty such assets are identified. *Proximate tangible assets* include faith-based hospitals and clinics, hospital chaplains, hospices, faith healers, and volunteer-sector projects. *Distal tangible assets* include healing sacraments and rituals, funeral and rites of passage, and various fellowships and networks that address health issues. *Proximate intangible assets* are healing prayer, resilience (i.e., religious coping), healing relationships with caregivers, and health-directed advocacy from pastors, congregations, and FBOs. *Distal intangible assets* include cultivation of faith and hope, creation of sacred spaces, and the sense of meaning and belonging that come through faith and fellowship.

These RHAs, according to Gunderson and Cochrane, supply "spiritual cap-ital" and are animated by "spiritual capacity,"[111] which is "embodied in human persons and their communities as a dynamic life force,"[112] making them more akin to "living organisms than material objects."[113] This understanding of faith and religion is provocative and probably counterintuitive for many people in the health sector, but the authors are boldly optimistic:

> RHAs generally are increasingly recognized as potentially crucial components of a comprehensive, sustainable strategy for advancing health. To mobilize them, however, requires new, sophisticated understandings of the interwoven logic of faith and health, new ways of linking social and scientific approaches, and a new set of leadership capacities to make it work.[114]

Outreach to Outsiders

Alongside partnerships occurring within or under the aegis of local congregations or local healthcare providers, HPDP alliances between religious and medical institutions may be diffused across larger networks of organizations that serve identified constituencies in local communities. This type of community-based outreach to special populations marshals participation of healthcare and human services professionals in conjunction with, or under the direction of, pastors, congregations, interfaith organizations, and other community groups sponsored or staffed by people of faith.

This substantial domain of the volunteer sector comprises faith-based commu-nity programs and activities that welcome participation by medical, healthcare, and human services professionals and target specialized populations of outsiders. By this I refer to identity groups located outside of population norms—according, for example, to race, ethnicity, nationality, religion, social class, or disability status, or who are otherwise disadvantaged, oppressed, excluded, underserved, or func-tionally disenfranchised. In numerous communities throughout the United States, collaborative efforts to reach such groups have organized and staffed primary care clinics, faith community nursing programs located in congregational buildings, patient education efforts sponsored by individual church congregations or denom-inational districts, hospices and other services to the terminally ill, and specialized programs operated by and/or within religious bodies: food banks, clothing banks, job programs, shelters (for the homeless, for abused women and their children), re-covery programs for substance abusers, assistance for the physically or cognitively challenged, and more. A special focus has been the proportionally growing popu-lation of underserved older adults, especially those who are infirm or homebound or who have limited financial, tangible, social, or personal resources.

A representative example was the Partnerships for Healthy Aging (PHA) Project, an interfaith community-based program established in Houston in the early 1990s.[115] The PHA was initiated by faculty at the University of Texas School of Public Health, under the leadership of health educator Vilma T. Falck, and assisted by my wife, Lea Steele, who participated while a graduate student. The PHA sought to address ongoing problems of ill health and dependence among the elderly through a multipartner citywide HPDP effort that brought together multiple stakeholders—religious and secular, public and private. These included Protestant, Catholic, and Jewish congregations, along with health agencies and community health centers and representatives from the University of Texas Health Sciences Center and even the mayor's office. This kind of cross-sector buy-in, along with an ability to obtain seed funding, is instrumental in the sustained success of such programs. Nonetheless, despite demonstrable benefits of the kind of collective-governance approach exemplified by the PHA, a write-up of the project noted that "'turf' issues continue to present challenges."[116] Such conflicts are probably unavoidable when bringing together so many diverse partners, but they can be minimized by thoughtfully involving as many parties as possible from the outset of the vision-making and planning stages.

Throughout this domain of community-based HPDP programming, interfaith efforts are becoming commonplace, by design or necessity, and such cooperative service activities represent a significant force for cross-cultural and interclass cohesion in many communities. Such programs also may serve as a radix for mobilizing constituents for other projects involving community organizing for social or political change. When people come together for one purpose—altruistic service to "outsider" groups, for example—they may discover other shared interests that lead them to making common cause in addressing systemic issues in their community or in a broader setting. Interfaith collaboration is especially valuable in this regard as it brings together people and assets from across the spectrum of religions, cultures, and nations of origin in a shared covenantal relationship for purposes of public service. Such groups exist in most medium- to large-sized communities throughout the United States, coordinating activities among local congregations and across faith traditions, and targeting myriad special populations.

In Topeka, Kansas, for example, where my wife and I lived for many years, the local Roman Catholic parish founded an initiative called Let's Help, which sought to address concerns of those living in poverty.[117] One of their ongoing projects is a food bank and lunchroom that serves a free lunch each weekday to anyone who is hungry. Each day, a different local religious congregation takes responsibility for purchasing, preparing, and serving the meal, and staffs the kitchen and handles clean-up duties. Our synagogue was one of those participating, once a month, and I was part of the crew. This was one of the most rewarding (and labor-intensive) activities that I have ever participated in. Throughout the country, in communities large and small, the work of interfaith organizations also extends beyond provision of services to participation in coalitions involved in community organizing and health-directed social and political change agency,[118] such as combating poverty or safeguarding the environment.

National networks have expanded on this idea. An example of the latter is the Shepherd's Centers of America, a national network of nearly sixty local, interfaith community-based centers serving older adults.[119] Founded in 1972 by Rev. Elbert Cole, a United Methodist minister in Kansas City, Missouri, the Shepherd's Centers provide meaning and purpose for adults throughout their mature years, through health, learning, and various assistance programs. From 2000 to 2002 I was honored to serve on their national board, and I chaired the research committee, preparing a major report and encouraging ongoing impact evaluation.[120]

Each local Shepherd's Center is uniquely focused around the interests and needs of respective communities, with an emphasis on providing opportunities for learning and volunteering. A third emphasis is a program titled "Adventures in Wellness." Across the network of centers this entails numerous classes and activities on various topics and skills: exercise, nutrition, health screening, health literacy, healthy lifestyles, *tai chi, yoga*, water aerobics, line dancing, and more. Most centers also provide support programs to enhance caregiver wellness.[121]

Local missions in many urban communities serve as multifaceted, holistic coordinating centers addressing myriad issues and challenges among the neediest of the needy, often out of sight of the rest of the community. Foremost among such types of outreach is the operation of free health clinics.

One of the most successful and celebrated local missions in the United States is Mission Waco. Since its founding in 1992 by Rev. Jimmy Dorrell, it has developed into an influential player in delivering human services within Central Texas and a model for other local missions. Its mission statement declares, "Provide Christian-based, holistic, relationship-based programs that empower the poor and marginalized. Mobilize middle-class Americans to become more compassionately involved among the poor. Seek ways to overcome the systemic issues of social injustice which oppress the poor and marginalized."[122] Baylor students and faculty have been involved in the work of the mission since its founding.

Located on a multibuilding campus site in a low-income neighborhood in Waco, the mission accomplishes its work through a remarkable range of donor-supported and volunteer-staffed family and adult programs, youth programs, and children's programs, as well as multiple facilities, including retail. Programs and activities include meals, legal services, job training, recovery groups, transitional housing, social services, shelters, after-school programs, camps, a grocery store and fair trade market, a toy store, a theater, a neighborhood park, a chapel, a coffee shop, and too many other programs and demonstration projects to list here.[123] Foremost among these is the Meyer Center Community Clinic, offering free medical care and dental screening and referrals two afternoons a week to residents without insurance. Mission Waco, like other local missions, is steadfast in its commitment to "[stand] firmly in the biblical affirmation that 'faith without works is dead' and the widow, orphan, poor, naked, hungry, homeless, stranger, and voiceless people are the 'least of these' we are all called to serve."[124] While our family is Jewish, my wife and I are honored to provide financial support to the mission each year.

What the Future Holds

In 1998 I was invited to coedit a special issue of the peer-reviewed journal *Health Education and Behavior*, along with University of Michigan psychologist Linda M. Chatters (the lead editor) and University of Texas sociologist Christopher G. Ellison.[125] This is the leading journal in the HPDP field and flagship publication of the Society for Public Health Education. The issue was put together to summarize and broadly examine "the interconnections among public health, health education, and faith-based communities."[126] Contributions elaborated on many points identified here, exemplifying them with ongoing health education projects or studies in the United States and overseas. Topics included behavioral risk reduction among a national sample of adolescents,[127] breast cancer screening among a multiethnic sample from Los Angeles,[128] mental health help-seeking from black clergy among a national sample of African Americans,[129] and roles for faith community nursing practitioners in Australia.[130]

From what has been said up to now, one might imagine that the most daunting barrier to the success of faith-health partnerships is resistance to working alongside the faith community on the part of medical or public health officials skeptical about or antagonistic toward the institution of religion. This has been true to a point, but according to real-world experiences and observations of public health professionals in the field, this resistance goes both ways. In our introduction to the special issue we noted,

> Efforts to conduct research and practice in the area of religion and health are often met with skepticism on the part of religious institutions and their representatives regarding the motivations of public health professionals and/ or outright rejection of the idea that religious matters are appropriate topics for scientific inquiry. Anyone who has attempted to conduct church-based health interventions is aware of the difficulties often encountered in initiating

such efforts and the pivotal role that clergy play in their acceptance and implementation.[131]

Two decades later I was privileged to be invited to coedit another special issue on this subject in another prestigious peer-reviewed publication, the *American Journal of Public Health*.[132] The lead editor for the issue was Ellen Idler, and the other coeditors were Tyler J. VanderWeele, the John L. Loeb and Frances Lehman Loeb Professor of Epidemiology at the Harvard T.H. Chan School of Public Health, and Anwar Khan, president of Islamic Relief USA. This generous invitation provided an opportunity to revisit this subject over twenty years downstream. The papers and associated commentaries published in the issue highlight how faith-based healthcare and public health partnerships have flourished in local communities, statewide settings, nationally, and globally. Featured in the issue were deep descriptions of a diversity of programs and projects in the United States and overseas, along with expert commentaries by William Foege, Howard Koh, David Williams, and Gary Gunderson and Teresa Cutts.

Summarizing this work, we concluded,

We recognize that some observers in both communities may be skeptical about the utility of such partnerships, or will call to mind undeniable examples of stances taken by some religious groups that often seem harmful to public health. . . . [W]e provide examples, perhaps less publicized, that show the history and potential of collaboration between public health and faith-based organizations. Professionals in these two domains have a deep understanding of the nature and power of organizations and how to get things done on a large scale when the actors share common commitments and responsibilities and participate together across sectors.[133]

Besides the partnerships described in the journal, other major programs exist or have been supported in recent years by philanthropies and private foundations. The highest-profile example was the Faith in Action program sponsored by the Robert Wood Johnson Foundation (RWJF).[134] From its inception in 1983 as a demonstration project (known at the time as the Interfaith Volunteer Caregivers Program) through the turn of the century, it awarded over one thousand grants, making it the largest funding program in RWJF's history. These grants underwrote respective local interfaith coalitions of volunteer caregivers from a diversity of religious congregations who united with other healthcare and social services providers to offer "informal care and support to the community's homebound chronically ill and disabled residents."[135] The program expanded further, ultimately supporting 1,715 projects, involving over nine thousand individual congregations, with over $77 million of funding by the time it closed in

2008.[136] Projects focused on chronic conditions, geriatric issues, AIDS, mental illness, dementia, children with disabilities, substance abuse, and other health-care concerns.[137]

It should be clear by now that religious congregations and FBOs are contributing players in efforts to address the health needs of local communities and help meet national population-health goals and objectives. The faith sector provides primary sites for HPDP programs and interventions, partners with public health departments and medical centers, and operates community social service agencies. Religious institutions and their pastoral and lay leadership foster health-related change in a variety of contexts: from reinforcing healthy behavior to organizing constituents for social and environmental activism and to working for more just social policies. In short, there are few limits to what churches and other places of worship—and their denominational bodies and affiliated institutions—can accomplish in the way of improving the health of people and populations.

Faith-based institutions are thus vital components of a multilevel empowerment process that entails "individual involvement, organizational development, and community change" familiar to community organizers.[138] The faith sector incorporates and bridges these multiple levels of action and influence. This has direct relevance to the promotion of health and prevention of disease.

A sole focus on promoting lifestyle and behavior change may be of limited effectiveness in improving health because it overlooks "the systemic issues that limit health equity, such as unequal access, limited economic opportunity, racial discrimination, and cultural incompetency."[139] As the determinants of population health encompass a multiplicity of personal and environmental factors—from the biological, psychological, and behavioral to the physical, social, and political[140]—any strategy for population-wide prevention "that omits or deemphasizes one or two of these foci will necessarily be compromising its effectiveness."[141] Without addressing the more macro-level, social-structural, or systemic influences on physical or mental health, lasting impact on the health status of populations is unlikely,[142] and effecting any enduring change in reducing population-health disparities is probably doomed.[143] Because of its centrality and influence within communities, especially those that are underserved and less advantaged, the faith sector can play a lead role here.

A renewed emphasis on partnerships between local congregations and FBOs, on the one hand, and healthcare institutions and public health agencies, on the other, remains a promising if challenging undertaking. Yet this is consistent with principles that would be familiar to early leaders of public health in the nineteenth century. For these pioneers, according to Gunderson, the public health profession was rooted "in the understanding that the environmental factors in disease could be engaged through rational social change."[144] Accordingly, "strong alliances with the religious community were common."[145]

In subsequent decades, things changed, perhaps reflecting the secular optimism of scientific advances and biomedically driven conquest of killer diseases. But as the threat of poverty-driven infectious diseases reemerges, socially mediated health disparities widen, and medical care becomes more expensive and out of reach to larger segments of our diversifying population, public health and medical leaders have come back around to recognizing that they need all the allies they can muster, and that the faith sector can serve a valuable function.[146] According to Gunderson, there is much common ground and shared purpose between the religious and public health sectors—"sacred ground," he called it— and thus reason for making common cause.[147]

5

Scientists and Scholars

In 1988 an unusual study appeared in the *Southern Medical Journal*. San Francisco cardiologist Randolph C. Byrd published results of a prospective, double-blind, randomized controlled trial (RCT) of distant intercessory prayer for hospitalized patients in the coronary care unit at San Francisco General Hospital.[1] Between 1982 and 1983, 393 cardiac patients were randomly assigned by computer-generated list to either a treatment or control group, the former receiving prayer from Christian groups outside the hospital. Each patient received prayer from three to seven intercessors. Blinding meant that neither doctors and nurses nor patients, nor even Byrd, knew what group each patient was assigned to, and intercessors received only the first name of a respective patient and his or her diagnosis. Pray-ers included born-again Christians and religious Roman Catholics active in a church or fellowship. What was the result?

According to Byrd's analyses, prayer worked. At follow-up, analyses showed that prayed-for patients had significantly less congestive heart failure, pneumonia, and cardiopulmonary arrest; required fewer antibiotics and diuretics and less intubation/ventilator assistance; and received a lower severity score based on a measure of the course of their postentry hospital stay.[2] In the acknowledgments at the end of his paper, Byrd humbly added the following: "In addition, I thank God for responding to the many prayers made on behalf of the patients."[3]

Publication of Byrd's study created a firestorm of comment and critique.[4] Fallout included denunciations from secular skeptics[5] and devout Christians[6] alike. But there was also an emerging apologetics from secular physicians and proponents of a more welcoming role for spirituality in healthcare.[7] Notably, the response from readers of the *SMJ* was mostly positive, with one exception—a letter to the editor accusing the journal of an "attempt to return medicine to the Dark Ages" by publishing a study that sought "to undermine reason."[8] The writer demanded that the journal "no longer publish articles of that kind."[9] The editor was unapologetic: the paper was methodologically sound, well executed, and passed peer review, and he pledged not to cater to any agitated reader's definition of what does or does not count as rational.[10]

To critics, the mere idea of having done such a study, regardless of its results or soundness, was galling. This reaction does not take into account that scholarly discussion on nonconventional healing, including as a result of faith or prayer, goes back to the earliest days of Western biomedicine. This includes a

Religion and Medicine. Jeff Levin, Oxford University Press (2020) © Oxford University Press.
DOI: 10.1093/oso/9780190867355.001.0001

famous essay on "the faith that heals" by William Osler, a father of modern scientific medicine, published in the *British Medical Journal* in 1910,[11] and a three-part essay on religious healing published in the *Journal of the American Medical Association* in 1926.[12] Desire to attribute interest in this topic solely to cranks and quacks may still be powerful in some quarters but does not map onto the reality of the Byrd study's long-standing antecedents in reasoned speculation dating back over a century.

A countercritique soon emerged, supporting the value of medical research on outside-the-box topics, even including unusual topics such as the possible healing effects of prayer.[13] Yes, results of research such as the Byrd study may cause consternation for some, but his execution of the RCT was methodologically sound. There may be reasons for caution about overinterpreting results from such studies, and I share these concerns. For example, a study using methods for testing natural phenomena in the physical world cannot possibly prove or disprove actions of a presumably supernatural being that may exist in part outside of the physical universe. That is, even the best-designed RCT of distant intercessory prayer cannot decisively reveal whether results were due to something that God did. All it can show is that distant prayer anteceded healing and that results cannot easily be attributed to something "naturalistic," at least according to currently mainstream understandings of science and the natural universe. They remain a mystery. Nonetheless, the trial was well designed and well executed, produced statistically significant results, and successfully passed through peer review at a major medical journal. By itself, that makes the Byrd study worthy of notice.

In the years since, I have spoken about this study with many colleagues, including epidemiologists, experts in conducting clinical trials, and social scientists known as skilled methodologists. Some were not religious nor familiar with or invested in research on religion and health. But, to a person, they agreed with the editor of *SMJ* that the Byrd study was well done and did not make any egregious methodological errors that would invalidate its findings—other than seemingly broaching a mechanism of action that appeared physically impossible. Despite the contentiousness of the topic, this was pretty much a garden-variety RCT. According to Larry Dossey, well-known internist and author, the Byrd study and those that followed in the same vein have been "one of the best-kept secrets in modern medicine."[14]

While the Byrd study was the first of its type to reach wide public awareness, as well as the attention of physicians and scientists, it was not the first healing prayer study conducted, nor the last. In the 1970s Bruce and John Klingbeil, a father-and-son team of Christian Science practitioners, designed a series of experimental tests of prayer directed at various organic systems, including germinating seeds, beans, sprouts, and yeast.[15] They tested whether prayer could cause these biological organisms to grow or flourish, and many of the experiments succeeded.

They believed their experiments "reflect the Christian viewpoint that there is in consciousness a pattern-developing, pattern-mending . . . power. Such a power is reflected in prayer and is, by definition, a healing power."[16] The Klingbeils founded an organization called Spindrift to support their investigations and issued a research report circulated among other prayer researchers but otherwise not well known.[17]

The Spindrift studies met with heated opposition not just from skeptics but also from the Christian Science Board of Directors, which forbade them to conduct their experiments and then, when they continued, expelled Bruce from the healing ministry of the church.[18] The rejection of the Klingbeils' work by their church led them to become despondent, and in 1993 they committed double suicide. The history of the Klingbeils and their tragic story is told in Bill Sweet's *A Journey into Prayer*.[19]

For the twenty years following the Byrd study, new research was published as well as thoughtful (and sometimes not so thoughtful) reviews and critiques of this literature. Other experimental clinical trials of prayer were conducted in various settings, some providing significant evidence of a distant healing effect. Notable among these was an RCT of Christian prayer for coronary care unit patients in Kansas City, modeled after the Byrd study and published in the *Archives of Internal Medicine*;[20] and an RCT of prayer and other distant healing techniques applied by healers from several diverse spiritual traditions to advanced AIDS patients in San Francisco, published in the *Western Journal of Medicine*.[21] Both studies produced positive, statistically significant results indicative of a successful trial. In the latter study, healers included Christians, Jews, Buddhists, Native Americans, practitioners of shamanism, and secular practitioners of bioenergy or meditative healing. Apparently, if there is indeed a healing power of prayer, it is no respecter of religion.

These studies, and many more, were most famously reviewed by Dossey in his bestselling *Healing Words*.[22] Although published in 1993 this book remains essential reading for anyone interested in exploring this topic, and offers a fascinating take on the scientific issues this research raised and the fallout and controversy these studies elicited. Dossey did more than anyone else to bring this research and its startling implications to the attention of the public, medical profession, and scientific community. This made him something of a lightning rod for skeptics and debunkers seeking to disparage this research and shut it down. For many years, Dossey was unfairly targeted by people unhappy with the existence of the Byrd study and the research that followed, as if Dossey himself had conducted these studies. It was a perfect example of "shoot the messenger," but Dossey held up admirably and remains an outspoken voice encouraging rigorous scholarship on themes at the interface of spirituality, consciousness, and healing.

The earliest and still most comprehensive review of this research was conducted by Daniel J. Benor, an American-born psychiatrist who spent much of his career in the United Kingdom and founded the Doctor-Healer Network.[23] Through careful bibliographic collation of existing studies, first published a few years following the Byrd study, Benor discovered that the research literature of prayer and distant healing studies was far more vast than anyone could have imagined. By the time of his most recent update, in 2001, his list of studies included 191 experimental or quasi-experimental trials addressing various medical outcomes. More surprisingly, these were not just human trials. Besides the Spindrift studies, Benor uncovered studies of all sorts involving biological organisms, including animals, plants, single-celled organisms, bacteria, yeasts, in vitro cells, enzymes and chemicals, and DNA.[24]

Benor helpfully graded each study into one of five categories on the basis of methodological quality. As skeptics often note, most studies were not up to par for one reason or another—whether it was flaws in study design, sampling of subjects, assessment of variables, or data analysis. But more than a quarter of the studies passed muster, and what Benor found regarding those studies has been mostly ignored by people with a stake in declaring all of this research worthless. While most of the poorly designed studies did not reveal statistically significant results indicative of a healing effect of prayer, about three quarters of the well-designed studies *did* find such an effect.[25]

I am convinced that this finding is responsible for Benor's work being largely disregarded by academic medicine, especially by critics of the prayer studies. It is much easier to attack Dossey, who bravely put himself forward in public forums and debates for many years as a proponent and face of this research. But Benor's comprehensive bibliography and systematic review of studies, careful and even-handed assessment of methodological quality, and cumulation of results leave little to criticize. About all that disconcerted critics can honestly say about this research is that the study results are mysterious. Perhaps pretending that they do not exist is an easier approach.

As it turns out, some experimental studies have been even more provocative than these prayer trials. All sorts of strange phenomena have been observed:

- *Experimenter effects*, whereby results of a blind trial of a seemingly "para-normal" phenomenon depend upon the perspective of the person directing the study. In one study, when a skeptic conducted the experiment, it failed, but when someone open to positive findings conducted the identical experiment, it succeeded.[26]
- *Retroactive prayer*, whereby a double-blind RCT methodology is applied to test the healing power of prayer backward in time. When intercessors were

randomly assigned, after the fact, to patients hospitalized with sepsis four to ten years previously, the prayed-for patients were found to have had shorter hospital stays and shorter duration of fever.[27]

- *Cardiac energy exchange between people,* whereby the electromagnetic energy field produced by the heart is detectable in another person's field. When two people were in proximity, but not touching, the signal generated by one person's electrocardiogram registered in the other person's electro-encephalogram and elsewhere in their body.[28]

- *Direct mental interaction with living systems (DMILS),* whereby there is a measurable mental connection or interaction between two people spatially separated. A review of two dozen published laboratory experiments validated the presence of physical or physiological changes in a "receiver" as a result of projected mental intentions of an "agent."[29]

- *"Spooky actions at a distance,"* Einstein's phrase for phenomena whereby physical objects or people appear to exert measurable effects on each other nonlocally, or across space and time. When Yale-trained physician and philosopher Drew Leder examined the studies of distant healing he concluded that results could be accommodated by existing theories in physics, which he termed *energetic transmission, path facilitation, nonlocal entanglement,* and *actualization of potentials.*[30]

As with Benor's contribution, rather than attempting to debunk or discredit this work, which would bring it to wider attention, Western medicine and biomedical science have tended to look the other way and simply ignore it.

None of this research has succeeded (yet!) in altering the practice of medicine, but as evidence for the nonlocal characteristics of human consciousness, the prayer studies and its cousins remain influential.[31] Considerable attention has been paid to these studies by intrepid physicists, philosophers, psychologists, and biomedical scientists[32]—just not many academic physicians up to now. Careful and dispassionate literature reviews and commentaries have been published,[33] and efforts have been made to identify explanatory mechanisms that can account for the results of the trials.[34] These include taxonomies proposing all sorts of naturalistic, transpersonal, nonlocal, and other hypothetical explanations for the strange and persistent fact that nonmedical interventions involving distant prayer, intentionality, and related phenomena seem to antecede healing.[35]

In the new century, ongoing controversy over the prayer studies has not abated, although the studies themselves have, in large part due to research conducted by Harvard Medical School and funded by the John Templeton Foundation. In 2006 the *American Heart Journal* published results of a multicenter clinical trial of intercessory Christian prayer for patients undergoing coronary bypass surgery.[36]

Directed by Harvard physician Herbert Benson, analyses found that prayed-for patients actually had more postoperative complications than controls; for all other outcomes there were no statistically significant findings. Because of the gravitas conveyed by the Harvard brand and by a finding that contradicted previous studies, results were received enthusiastically by skeptics and the media, which found this story to be newsworthy.

Overlooked in such reports was the strongly negative reception to this study from other researchers, including in the pages of the *American Heart Journal*,[37] who pointed out several disqualifying methodological flaws. To be blunt, this RCT was not well-designed, either conceptually or methodologically. Especially egregious, from my perspective, is that the intervention—intercessory prayer— did not resemble the way that anyone that I know prays, whether for themselves or another person, including for anybody's healing. Intercessors were given a prescripted passage to insert into their regular prayers ("for a successful surgery with a quick, healthy recovery and no complications"), imposing on them a "prayer" with which they may have been unfamiliar, with which they may have had no experience or success in offering up for healing, and which may have gone against their religious beliefs about how to pray to or petition God. The pray-ers were also instructed when, how long, and how often to pray. Akin to a drug trial, this seemed to be an effort to create some sort of standardized unit of intercessory prayer. According to Dossey, "The most important criticism of the Harvard prayer study is that prayer was employed in ways that simply do not occur in ordinary life."[38]

The aftermath of the Benson study coupled with another well-publicized null finding from a large-scale funded research study at Duke[39] have served to mostly kill off this line of research. The abrupt halt in these investigations is not without good reason: many studies were half-baked, methodologically and conceptually speaking, as Benor's review found.[40] Some were solid, but most were not. On this point, skeptics and proponents agree.[41] Nonetheless, systematic reviews and meta-analyses, taking a cue from Benor's bibliography, suggest that, on the whole and across this body of studies, there is indeed a modest, statistically significant, and observable effect,[42] even if little momentum encourages exploration of this subject at present. About the best advice came from Dossey, who called for a "time out" on these studies:

> I would like to see a *temporary* moratorium, because currently the protocols in healing experiments wander all over the place. People don't benefit from scrutinizing prior studies to see what worked and what didn't. Amazingly, they even duplicate the methods that failed in prior studies. This is nuts. It also reveals laziness on the part of experimenters. Perhaps we need a healing summit that would bring together researchers who are interested in this field. We could put

all of these studies under the microscope and examine what works and what doesn't.[43]

When physicians and other health professionals, as well as the media and general public, hear of research on religion and health, these prayer studies are still generally the first thing that comes to mind. Public and professional reaction to the idea of empirical research on the impact of religion and health invariably refers back to these studies, and the same arguments, pro and con, that have been made for the past thirty years keep getting rehashed. Yet these studies are only a fraction of all the research on religion and health, which dates back over a century. Indeed, they are such a small fraction that in the larger scheme of religion and health research, these unusual RCTs barely register. Most of my colleagues who conduct research on religion and health show little interest in clinical trials of prayer, nor do they consider them relevant to what they do. All of them by now have heard of the Byrd study, but it is generally thought of as a curiosity, one example of a more substantial (if flawed) research literature on prayer and healing and not an exemplar of the larger body of religion and health studies.

What is not widely recognized by the many voices commenting on this literature—from the media, from organized skeptic groups, from strident physicians taking pro or con stances toward these studies—is that these prayer RCTs are but a drop in the bucket of a much larger research literature addressing religious and spiritual influences on health, healing, and well-being. This broader research subject is, for the most part, not particularly controversial, either methodologically or conceptually—that is, it does not seem to presuppose or imply forces or mechanisms that conflict with consensus laws of nature nor require physicists or philosophers to make sense of it. Most studies are simply standard-issue investigations by psychologists, sociologists, health services researchers, physician and nurse researchers, epidemiologists, and biomedical scientists working in various fields.

Population-based studies of religion and health, such as those conducted by epidemiologists and social scientists, are what I am most associated with since the mid-1980s. By *population-based* I mean studies using a sample of people drawn from a defined population, rather than a hospital or patient cohort,[44] and that express results in terms of morbidity or mortality rates or associations between exposure variables ("causes") and disease outcomes ("effects"). For about four decades, at the time of this writing, epidemiologists, social scientists, and other investigators have been employing methods of population-health research to explore the impact of religion, faith, and spirituality on physical and mental health—the functioning and well-being of the human body and mind.

The Epidemiology of Religion

Among the most misconstrued intersections of the religious and medical domains is the surprising number of studies identifying religious or spiritual predictors of health and medical outcomes in the general population. Research on this subject dates to the nineteenth century and by now encompasses thousands of published studies and reviews, according to the two editions of Oxford University Press's authoritative *Handbook of Religion and Health*. These include clinical, epidemiologic, biomedical, social, and behavioral research studies on almost every imaginable medical or health-related outcome, conducted among respondents, subjects, or patients in almost every one of the world's major religious traditions and denominations.[45] Results are mostly positive, depending upon the respective disease or health condition under study, and have been found regardless of sociodemographic characteristics or religious affiliation.[46] Discovery of these studies makes for an interesting story, in which my own efforts were front and center.

In 1982, as a young graduate student in public health at UNC, I was taking a class called Culture and Health in the Department of Epidemiology, taught by Bert Kaplan. One of the assigned readings was an analysis of data from a large population study in Evans County, Georgia.[47] The authors found significantly lower systolic and diastolic blood pressure and less hypertension among men who attended church services regularly (one or more times per week) compared to men who attended church less frequently (less than once per week). I thought this was one of the oddest epidemiologic studies I had ever seen. Another article in the course pack was by Kaplan himself, an essay in which he reviewed findings from several other studies in which religious differences were found in a variety of cardiovascular outcomes.[48] Apparently there was more than one such study. As someone with an undergraduate degree in religion, I was mightily intrigued.

Kaplan's essay closed with a summary statement that, though written in the dry academic style typical of medical journals, electrified me: "So we are left with a challenge to refine our concepts, and perfect our methodologies to see if, in fact, specific religious processes are related to the etiology, precipitation, recovery, or prevention of heart disease."[49] Little did I know that this sentence would set the stage for what ultimately became my life's work—research on how religion influences health.

With Kaplan's encouragement I chose as a term paper project a review of published research on this subject and headed off to the library. I found about a dozen more studies, made my presentation to the class, and Kaplan suggested that I write up my results as a review article for submission to a medical journal. So back to the library I went to ensure that I found every study and had not missed anything. As weeks and months went by, I kept uncovering more and more studies from all over the world. By the end of my search, more than four years had passed and I was now finishing my doctoral work at the University of Texas Medical Branch. Upon final tally I had located over two hundred published studies dating to the nineteenth century that reported religious differences in cardiovascular disease, hypertension and stroke, overall and cause-specific cancer, mortality rates, morbidity and health status, and more.

Although these studies had been done and their results published, apparently almost no one knew they existed. This includes most of the authors of these studies themselves: the reference sections of their respective articles rarely cited more than one or two prior studies, and most cited none. I felt like an explorer who had made a startling discovery—an epidemiologic Roald Amundsen.

Again with Kaplan's encouragement, from afar, I wrote up my review with the help of Preston L. Schiller, another UNC public health professor, as coauthor. Titled "Is There a Religious Factor in Health?," the paper was published in the *Journal of Religion and Health*, a peer-reviewed pastoral care journal, in 1987.[50] That same year, a pair of Canadian sociologists also published a review of some of these same studies, categorized by religious denomination.[51] In 1987 as well, Ellen Idler published her first important study of religion and health, including a helpful effort to interpret findings in light of existing theories of health.[52] There must have been something in the water that year.

Lack of attention to these studies before 1987 is especially unusual because they had been published in the world's most venerable and prestigious medical journals. Studies reporting statistically significant religious differences in morbidity or mortality rates, or significant associations between religious measures (such as attendance at worship services) and scales or indices of health, had appeared in the *New England Journal of Medicine*, the *American Journal of Public Health*, the *Journal of the American Medical Association, The Lancet*, the *Archives of Internal Medicine*, the *American Heart Journal*, the *American Journal of Epidemiology, Cancer*, the *Milbank Quarterly*, and other top-tier journals. Yet until the late 1980s, this research seems to have been mostly invisible—a kind of "collective amnesia" on the part of Western medicine.[53]

This is even more surprising in that research on religion and health goes back a long way. For example, in 1891, pioneering surgeon John Shaw Billings, founder of both the National Library of Medicine and the Johns Hopkins University School of Medicine, published a study of differences in morbidity and mortality rates by religious affiliation.[54] He noted the relative absence of reproductive-related cancers in Jewish men and women, an observation first made in the European medical literature half a century earlier.[55] Following the Billings study, this particular topic was subject to about two dozen research studies published throughout the first few decades of the twentieth century,[56] followed by a detailed literature review in 1948.[57]

Over the past half century, more sophisticated population-based research has been conducted using state-of-the-art epidemiologic methods. Many of these studies of religious differences in overall and cause-specific morbidity and mortality rates were conducted by prominent investigators. Most notable throughout the 1970s was the work of George W. Comstock, dean of American epidemiologists, and his colleagues at Johns Hopkins using data from the Washington County, Maryland, epidemiologic census.[58]

After publication of the Levin and Schiller review, I worked on a follow-up review with one of my Texas professors, religious and medical historian Harold Y. Vanderpool. We focused on that subset of the religion and health studies that had presented data on religious attendance. Out of twenty-seven studies that we identified, twenty-two reported positive and statistically significant results—that is, more frequent attendance at religious services was associated with better health or lower rates of illness. We published the review in the British journal *Social Science and Medicine*, also in 1987.[59] We subtitled the article "Toward an Epidemiology of Religion," a phrase I have come to regret, as it has caused some confusion and I suspect is likely to be carved as an epitaph on my gravestone.

A semifunny anecdote: We initially submitted the paper to a leading epidemiology journal and received very positive reviews. The editor, however, rejected the paper, and his cover letter went on for nearly two single-spaced pages, specifying in painstaking detail how unacceptable, even misguided, our paper was, and why we should just give up the idea altogether and not pursue it any further. Most rejection letters contain nothing but a couple paragraphs of boilerplate, so for this editor to take the time to go on and on about a paper that he was not even inviting to be revised and resubmitted, and to be somewhat unfriendly about it, was unsettling. But that was not all. He made sure to let us know that not only was our paper unacceptable, but the very concept, the very idea, of an epidemiology of religion was, in his words, "execrable."

For several years I was under the impression that the word derived from the same root as excretion or excrement, and concluded that the editor was using a scatological term to tell us that our ideas were full of you-know-what. One day in the early 1990s, as I related this story to a group of VA chaplains-in-training, one member of the class, a Catholic priest knowledgeable in Latin, mentioned that he thought the word derived not from excretion but from execration. There was a dictionary in the classroom, so all of us walked over to it and looked up *execration*. According to the dictionary, it means "worthy of being detested, abominated, or abhorred." Well, that's a whole lot better, I said, and we all laughed.

In the years since 1987, growth of population research on religion and health has accelerated. In 1990 I received the first research grant from the U.S. National

Institutes of Health (NIH),[60] followed by successful funding of my research collaborators Robert Joseph Taylor and Linda Chatters, from the University of Michigan.[61] Major research conferences and comprehensive bibliographies were sponsored by the private-sector National Institute of Healthcare Research,[62] the NIH,[63] and a joint NIH/Fetzer Institute committee,[64] resulting in funding of a national study in conjunction with the National Opinion Research Center at the University of Chicago.[65] Also appearing were important review articles,[66] academic handbook chapters,[67] and significant field-mapping summaries.[68] By the twenty-first century it could be truthfully said that religion and health research had consolidated into a genuine *field*.

The most significant marker of the arrival of this field was publication in 2001 of the first edition of the *Handbook of Religion and Health*. Edited by Harold G. Koenig, Duke professor and psychiatrist, the encyclopedic *Handbook* is the most important work of scholarship on religion and health and widely considered the bible of the field. Koenig is by far the most published investigator in this area and universally acknowledged as the medical world's leading expert on the role of faith and spirituality in clinical practice and research. I was honored to pen the foreword to the first edition of the *Handbook* and the preface to the second edition in 2012.

For physicians, scientists, and laypeople unfamiliar with this subject, publication of the *Handbook* came as a shock. The first edition of the *Handbook* identified about twelve hundred published studies, far more than the two hundred or so that I found in 1987. The second edition identified another three thousand studies just in the intervening decade. At the back of each book is a summary table listing details of each study in a spreadsheet format. In the first edition, the table is about 75 pages long; in the second edition, the table goes on for more than 350 pages. Little wonder that a review published in the *Journal of the American Medical Association* stated, "This is an unparalleled resource not only for physicians with an interest in the relationship between religion and health but perhaps even more for those who doubt its significance."[69]

The *Handbook* is such a prodigious work of scholarship that it is not easy to summarize its contents in a small space. But focusing on the number of studies that Koenig and colleagues uncovered, by health- and disease-related categories, can provide a synopsis of the scope of published research and consistency of findings. In a recent published summary of studies in the epidemiology of religion, I used the *Handbook* editions as a kind of database and extracted information that provided a good indication of where things stood in this field as of 2011.[70]

Cumulating the bibliographies from both editions of the *Handbook*, and focusing on several selected categories, I came up with the following totals for the number of population studies and proportion of those reporting at least some positive findings—that is, indicative of a salutary or health-promoting influence of religion:

- *Heart disease morbidity and mortality*: 64 studies, 47 (73.4%) with positive findings.
- *Hypertension and cerebrovascular disease*: 87 studies, 55 (63.2%) with positive findings.
- *Cancer morbidity and mortality*: 84 studies, 64 (76.2%) with positive findings.
- *All-causes mortality*: 116 studies, 92 (79.3%) with positive findings.
- *Self-rated health*: 70 studies, 44 (62.9%) with positive findings.
- *Pain and somatic symptoms*: 118 studies, 50 (42.4%) with positive findings.
- *Physical disability*: 64 studies, 30 (46.9%) with positive findings.
- *Depression*: 459 studies, 317 (69.1%) with positive findings.
- *Anxiety*: 314 studies, 170 (54.1%) with positive findings.

The grand totals for these selected disease- or health-related categories are 1,376 studies, with 869 (63.2%) reporting positive findings. As noted, this research literature is not solely the product of one-off studies in small samples with results published in obscure journals. The best of this research has been conducted by important scientists at top universities—Duke, Johns Hopkins, Michigan, Harvard, Yale, Rutgers, Emory, Berkeley, Texas, Baylor, North Carolina, and elsewhere—many with funding from the NIH or major foundations, and findings were published in top-tier journals. The best of this work involves analyses of data from well-regarded community-based epidemiologic studies, such as the Alameda County (California), Washington County (Maryland), Evans County (Georgia), and Tecumseh (Michigan) studies.[71]

Many of the initial cohort of investigators who began their research in the 1980s are sociologists.[72] They have ensured that research in this field focuses on variables typically studied by medical sociologists: indices of physical health status, scales of somatic symptoms, self-ratings of overall health, and checklists of functional health or disability status. They also have set a high bar, methodologically speaking, ensuring that studies utilize the best designs and population sampling procedures and apply the most sophisticated statistical analyses. Idler, notably, is the world's leading authority on self-assessment measures of health.[73] Her presence in the religion and health field since the beginning has been beneficial in providing leadership and lending methodological credibility to population-health research on religion.

As unusual as this work may seem to nonspecialists, it is consonant with the mainstream of social and population research on health. It is just that the subject of research—the combination of the predictor variable (religion) and outcome variable (health)—is out of the ordinary. But social scientists conduct studies of determinants of health all the time, including research by medical sociologists, social demographers, and social and psychosocial epidemiologists. Many also study patterns of religious identity and participation, independent of health, such as in relation to matters like fertility rates, and have done so for decades. So both of these categories of variables—religion and health—have been much researched by nonmedical scientists for a long time. What is distinctive about the work considered here is that these variables have been looked at in relation to each other.

Critics who would never say boo at the thought of research on, say, the impact of poverty on rates of cancer mortality or depressive symptoms or on the impact of church participation on political affiliation or voting behavior—standard fare for medical sociologists and sociologists of religion, respectively—nonetheless react dismissively or angrily at studies in which these variables are combined differently: such as studying the impact of church participation on physical or psychological illness. At times the criticism is strident—that these studies are somehow an affront to the laws of science, whatever that means. This criticism is off-base and, in my opinion, simply a way for critics to signal that they do not ap-prove of the implications of such studies, perhaps because findings suggest that religion is not a reflexively malign force.

Criticism often comes from partisan organizations opposed on principle to religious faith or the existence of God, such as the Freedom from Religion Foundation, or from gatekeeper groups protecting the sanctity of science from heresies and apostasies, an example being the Committee for Scientific Investigation of Claims of the Paranormal. For many years, when a new religion and health study was published, reporters would commonly solicit comments from representatives of one of these groups in order to offer an "opposing view," even though the individuals presenting such comments were usually not re-search scientists. I even experienced this response after publication of my early literature review referencing a couple of hundred studies of religion and health. What in the world is the "opposing view" to a literature review calling atten-tion to hundreds of studies? The studies are not really there? After many years of reading angry denunciations of this research, I still have not figured out how a study identifying, say, lower morbidity rates of depressive symptoms among older adults participating in church groups somehow represents a claim of para-normal forces.

In contrast to the healing prayer studies, which are typically experimental trials using RCT methods and indeed seem to result in findings that challenge conventional understandings of physics and of healing, these population-based studies, as noted, draw on research methods from epidemiology, medical sociology, and demography and on well-accepted theories of social and behavioral determinants of health. Their results do not mean what many skeptics think they imply. Perhaps because of confusion with prayer RCTs and the notion that all medical research involves study of treatments that cure disease, misinterpretations are commonplace—for example, that these studies claim or prove that religious involvement promotes healing, religious people do not get sick, religion is the most important factor in health, and evidence exists of a supernatural influence on health.[74] These studies prove no such thing and, anyway, were not designed to do so.

Another large body of studies has investigated the impact of religion on psychiatric diagnoses and mental health. These studies, too, go back further in time than most physicians and scientists may be aware. A bibliography published by the National Institute of Mental Health in 1980, long before my colleagues and I began conducting our own research, already contained 1,836 entries, including research studies, review essays, chapters, books, monographs, practice guidelines, and other scholarly works.[75]

Focused research on religion within the field of psychiatric epidemiology originated in the 1950s. The best-known early example is from the Midtown Manhattan Study, a landmark community-based study of urban mental health.[76] Throughout the 1990s, data from major multisite epidemiologic studies of mental health were also used to examine the effects of religious identity and practice. These included the authoritative Established Populations for Epidemiologic Studies of the Elderly (EPESE)[77] and Epidemiologic Catchment Area (ECA) research programs.[78] Studies of the impact of religious participation on measures of psychological well-being have for decades been a regular subject of research in gerontology and geriatrics.[79] These are not formal psychiatric diagnoses but rather things like life satisfaction, happiness, affect balance, mood tone, and distress. This category of religious research is of longer standing than most people may realize,[80] dating to a series of studies by sociologist David O. Moberg beginning in the early 1950s.[81]

However, unlike for the physical health studies, reviews of the religion and mental health literature have reached conflicting conclusions. Early reviews found mixed evidence of a salutary association[82] or no significant empirical evidence at all.[83] More positive evidence was provided in a series of case studies,[84] but these were not based on systematic samples. In the 1980s modest evidence of a positive effect of religion was found in a meta-analysis[85] and in a series of systematic reviews.[86] Koenig published a comprehensive annotated bibliography in the 1990s[87] and, under contract from the NIH, I published a systematic review of studies published in leading gerontology journals.[88] Both of these reviews found that most studies had produced at least some positive findings.

A subsequent review acknowledged what is by now plain: that research "has found both negative and positive associations between religious involvement and mental health."[89] But the authors suggested an explanation:

Although early research seemed to confirm the widespread clinical lore that religion impaired mental health, many more recent studies utilizing better methodologies within the past two decades appear to reveal quite the opposite, i.e. that religious involvement is generally associated with greater well-being, less depression and anxiety, greater social support, and less substance abuse.[90]

Since the 1990s, the standard for research on religion and mental health or well-being has become population-based epidemiologic studies or large-scale social surveys characteristic of studies of religion and physical health. Recent studies are less likely to rely on nonrandom convenience samples and simplistic correlational analyses. They are more likely to lay out the impact of religiousness on rates of morbidity due to specific psychiatric diagnoses or in relation to validated indices of well-being, in the United States or globally, and across religious and sociodemographic categories. This research is also more likely to include patients or subjects from racial and ethnic minority groups.[91]

Clearly, the studies described here are not the same type of studies as RCTs of intercessory prayer. This nuance is typically glossed over or not grasped by media accounts, laypeople, physicians and clergy, skeptics hoping to debunk all religion and health research, and even some contemporary researchers doing these population studies. Most published studies on religion and health are population-based or community studies designed to identify religious predictors of health or well-being in general populations, at one point in time or followed prospectively. These trials are not experimental nor do they test any type of therapy (e.g., prayer) seeking to cure disease. These are dramatically different types of studies with different aims and methodologies.[92] As I explained several years ago, "This body of research has *nothing* to do with medicine, with physicians, with patients, with illness, with the clinical setting, with medical therapies, or with healing."[93]

Rather, these reports are observational studies of mostly healthy populations conducted by social scientists, epidemiologists, and physician-researchers investigating how measures of religious identity, practice, or belief are associated with increases or decreases in risk of subsequent medical or psychiatric outcomes, often expressed in terms of population-wide rates of morbidity, mortality, or disability.[94] Moreover, research findings on this subject are generally consistent with current understandings of how other social institutions, psychological processes, and lifestyle behaviors influence the health of people and populations.[95]

Nonetheless, these facts remain stubbornly difficult to convey, and confusion persists even after a quarter century of researchers like me parsing distinctions among these types of studies.[96] I recently noted, with considerable frustration, that "literature reviews by physicians and social scientists alike still sometimes mix together the controversial results from randomized clinical trials of distant prayer as a therapeutic intervention with the abundantly replicated findings of standard population surveys on prayer and associated religious correlates of physical and mental health, even though these are plainly different research topics."[97]

While I believe that making these distinctions is helpful, continually bemoaning the fact that such confusion exists serves little purpose. After all, the two categories of studies—clinical trials of praying to cure disease and population-based studies of religiousness as a preventive resource in healthy people—are not unrelated. Each provides a different type of evidence suggesting that human spirituality has a role to play in human well-being, whether through mobilizing internal resources that help to ameliorate symptoms of disease or through providing access to social or psychological resources that keep us well and enable us to prosper. It may be constructive to explain that valid criticisms of clinical trials of prayer do not invalidate epidemiologic studies of religion, but in the court of public opinion, as in the halls of medicine, these two types of studies will sink or swim together.

Religion as Healthcare

RCTs of healing prayer and population studies of religiousness and physical and mental health are not the only types of medical research studies to have been conducted on the impact of religion. Clinical investigations conducted by physicians and psychologists, as well as health services research, experimental and laboratory studies, and scientific inquiries even further afield—these, too, are important provinces of the world of empirical religion and health research.

The prominence of the prayer trials has drawn attention away from other types of clinical research on religion conducted since the 1980s. Some of this work is quite interesting and directly relevant to patient care or the daily lives of people with physical or emotional challenges. It deserves better than to be obscured by the controversy elicited by the RCT literature.

Most clinical studies of religion are not experimental in design: they include, for example, community- or hospital-based studies of patient outcomes, or case series of recruited subjects drawn from medical practices. Koenig and his collaborators at Duke and throughout the country have published many such studies.[98] For example, medical in-patient studies showed that a lower level of religiousness was associated with a greater severity of depression[99] and a lengthier time to remission of depressive symptoms.[100]

This important work is underrepresented among research studies on religion, which are more likely to involve comparing religious and nonreligious people among general populations and following them forward to see who becomes ill and who remains well. Studies using clinical samples—people already sick or being seen within the medical care system—can provide different and more immediately relevant information about how people get better. This is a subtle distinction for nonresearchers but has major implications for understanding the relevance of religion to the healing of illness, not just the maintenance of health or prevention of disease.[101]

All sorts of research questions come to mind: Do religious people do better or worse than the nonreligious when facing illness? Does an active spiritual life contribute to a more successful course of treatment? Do people who are able to maintain continuity in their religious life when ill, such as participating in the life of their congregation, adjust better to physical or psychological challenges? Can faith in God enable people to remain cognitively and emotionally well, even in the face of permanent disability or impending death? These questions may not be as provocative and newsworthy as, "Does distant prayer heal?," but in my opinion they are more directly relevant to patients' recovery and well-being.

Much interesting and high-quality research and writing on the impact of religion have been undertaken by psychologists—clinical psychologists and researchers with specialties in social, health, or developmental psychology, as well as in the psychology of religion.[102] Many leading academic psychologists of religion have focused their research on physical and mental health, whether specific psychiatric diagnoses or dimensions of psychological well-being. Psychological research on religion and health has become a much bigger enterprise than sociological and epidemiologic research, which remain the work of a smaller niche of investigators. Within psychology, studies of religion have entered the mainstream of the field,[103] even if many academic psychologists do not themselves profess or value religious beliefs.[104]

Important studies and review essays by psychologists have identified features or dimensions of religious expression as significant factors for physical health,[105] mental health diagnoses such as depression,[106] and overall well-being.[107] Specialized studies also focus on the concept of spiritual well-being,[108] and other studies have found neuroanatomical[109] and neurophysiological correlates of spirituality.[110] These studies are from major figures in academic psychology and published in top-tier peer-reviewed psychological or medical journals or as chapters in important books or texts.

The most prominent clinical psychologist among religion and health researchers is Kenneth I. Pargament, Professor Emeritus at Bowling Green State

University. One of the original cohort of investigators in the religion and health field, his research in the psychology of religion dates to the 1970s. His most visible and important contributions to religion and health research, in my opinion, are his studies of religious coping[111] and his having trained a couple of generations of psychologists to conduct research on the impact of religion on mental health and well-being. Foremost among these is David H. Rosmarin, Harvard psychologist and clinician at McLean Hospital, whose own prolific research has pioneered the study of mental health among Orthodox Jews.[112]

Pargament, Rosmarin, and colleagues also have conducted fascinating studies of spiritual therapy for mental health problems. For example, a randomized controlled trial of a spiritually integrated treatment in religious Jews confirmed its efficacy for treating subclinical anxiety symptoms.[113] In another study, conducted among patients in a day-treatment program in a psychiatric hospital, simply believing in God, regardless of religious affiliation, was associated with better outcomes in response to treatment.[114] Rosmarin's latest book documents his success in integrating spiritual and religious content through using cognitive-behavioral therapy to alleviate emotional distress and improve psychological functioning.[115]

Pargament's revered stature was signified by his selection to serve as editor-in-chief of the American Psychological Association's multivolume *APA Handbook of Psychology, Religion, and Spirituality*,[116] the most authoritative resource in the psychology of religion. Many chapters focus on health-related issues, such as depression, anxiety, mental illness, and addictions.

The field of health services research is another unexpected place to find large-scale studies of religion. Since the 1920s, researchers have drawn on data from health surveys to map patterns and determinants of medical care use.[117] Endpoints include physician and hospital utilization rates and other parameters of the use of and satisfaction with medical care, as well as its organization, delivery, and financing. Research typically uses data from large general population surveys or patient samples drawn from defined clinical populations or medical catchment areas. Ongoing national surveys are also sources of data for health services research, including the National Health Interview Survey, National Health and Nutrition Examination Survey, and various Medicare, Medicaid, and VA databases containing information on patient encounters.

In 1981 the former U.S. National Center for Health Services Research (NCHSR) published a comprehensive annotated bibliography of studies of the utilization of medical care and health-related services.[118] For many years prior to the birth of the internet and online searching capabilities this was a valuable resource for health services researchers seeking to review specific topics. It was a great tool for answering questions such as: How many studies have looked at the effect of educational level on vaccine utilization, and what are the references? Surprisingly, when I first saw the bibliography while in graduate school, I found that among the hundreds of published studies and dozens of sociodemographic and other variables used throughout analyses to predict utilization were a group of studies examining religious affiliation.

Following up on our review of the epidemiologic studies of religion, I again collaborated with my former UNC professor Preston Schiller to conduct a literature review of health services research studies of religion. Starting with the NCHSR bibliography and supplemented with an additional search, we identified thirty-one published studies.[119] Of these, twenty-four reported statistically significant religious differences in the utilization of physicians and dentists; maternal and child health, pediatric, psychiatric, ambulatory, extended, and primary care; family planning, hospital, and preventive services, and health care systems; and medications and vaccines. The earliest study was an investigation of oral polio vaccine acceptance in Florida, from 1962.[120]

Despite the presence of these studies, many indexed in the NCHSR bibliography, the authors of the bibliography nonetheless asserted, "Religious preference does not predict the use of health services."[121] When I first read that comment it reminded me of the response to my own then-current efforts to cumulate the largely unknown literature of epidemiologic studies of religion. These health services studies of religion were there in plain sight—indeed the bibliography cited ten of them,[122] half reporting statistically significant findings[123]—but apparently it was easy to dismiss the results because they did not match with expectations.

That explanation, though, never sat well with me. Other researchers in health services had already acknowledged the possibility that one's religious background was an important factor that could influence healthcare use. Since the 1970s, experts had noted there was good reason to believe that religious identity, beliefs, or practices could predispose people to use or not use certain types of healthcare,[124] influence patterns of illness behavior,[125] or create barriers to appropriate utilization.[126] Accordingly, questions about religion had been included in national health services research surveys since the 1970s, as the bibliography made clear. Yet despite a history of research on this topic and the presence of statistically significant findings, awareness of this work was limited. Or perhaps it was another example of collective amnesia.

Following publication of our review article in 1988, more systematic studies documenting the influence of religion on healthcare use began to appear in the medical literature. This included research on use of religious resources, such as clergy, for treatment of mental health issues.[127] In the first edition of Koenig's *Handbook*, an entire section was devoted to reviewing religion and health services studies through the turn of the century.[128] By the time of publication, there had been more than fifty studies of medical and mental healthcare use and related topics, such as treatment compliance and preventive health behavior.[129] Koenig's own studies of hospitalized inpatients at Duke, conducted in the 1990s and 2000s, found that religiousness was associated with fewer long-term care days[130] and fewer hospital admissions and shorter length of stay.[131]

For the past several years I have revisited this issue in my own research, with special focus on the utilization of prayer and spiritual healing in lieu of or in conjunction with other forms of medical care. This offers a different take on the prayer and healing angle, one unfortunately overlooked in favor of the controversial RCTs. The question here is not of efficacy—whether healing prayer works—with all its attendant controversies, but rather a more basic line of inquiry: Who does this, how often do they do this, and why? Addressing these issues does not require broaching unconventional theories about space-time, consciousness, or nonlocal connections among people or with God. Moreover, it promises to provide insight about a practice that, for better or worse, may be more prevalent than physicians and healthcare planners realize.

Along with Taylor and Chatters, using data on 6,082 adults from the National Survey of American Life, we explored the lifetime prevalence and sociodemographic predictors of use of faith healers.[132] Our results exploded some persistent myths about the practice. Contrary to presumptions found in the medical literature, we concluded that

> Use [of] a spiritual healer is not due, on average, to poor education, marginal racial/ethnic or socioeconomic status, dire health straits, or lack of other healthcare options. To some extent, the opposite appears to be true. Use of a spiritual healer is not associated with fewer social and personal resources or limitations in health or healthcare.[133]

These results, we noted, should encourage "a rethinking of tacit assumptions about the determinants of the use of healers, and CAM generally, that have driven much of the research in this field."[134]

More recently I analyzed data from the third round of the nationally representative Baylor Religion Survey in order to map the prevalence and predictors of healing prayer use. In a nationally representative sample of 1,714 adults,[135] I found that nearly nine of ten adult Americans have used healing prayer at some point in their lives, praying for themselves or others, with nearly a third having prayed often for their own healing and over half having prayed often for the healing of others. More surprisingly, over a quarter of Americans have performed laying on of hands, nearly one in five having done so on multiple occasions. Over half of Americans reported participating in a prayer group, prayer circle, or prayer chain.

The most provocative finding, in my opinion, was that the most consistent predictor of use of healing prayer was reporting a loving relationship with God. "People who feel a close connection to God, who love God and feel loved by God," I remarked, "are the very people most likely to pray for healing: for themselves or others, alone or in a group, and verbally or through laying on of hands."[136]

Besides clinical and health services research on religion, additional studies have begun to take faith into the lab, in a manner of speaking. These types of studies, known as *basic science* or *bench research*, include investigations of the physiological, psychophysiological, and pathophysiological features and correlates of meditation and spiritual states of consciousness. The earliest example that I found, from 1957, was an experimental study of stress in college students.[137] Subjects whose parents were regular religious service attenders were more likely to have a norepinephrine-like cardiovascular response, indicating a propensity to express emotions such as anger; those whose parents did not attend services regularly were more likely to react to stress with an epinephrine-like response, indicative of greater anxiety and holding in anger.

Another early study, from the field of neuroscience in 1978, examined brain-wave patterns of Christians during prayer.[138] Findings revealed that electrocortical rhythms in a sample of adult Protestants, as measured by electroencephalogram readings, sped up during prayer, contrary to expectations. The investigator noted that this matched brain-wave patterns of "highly experienced Yoga meditators and advanced Transcendental Meditators capable of advanced meditative states."[139]

The highest-profile research from the 1970s was the work of Benson and colleagues on the relaxation response.[140] He described this as "an integrated hypothalamic response which results in generalized decreased sympathetic nervous system activity, and perhaps also increased parasympathetic activity."[141] Significantly, he added, this is the opposite of the famous fight-or-flight response, and can be elicited through relaxation techniques, meditation, prayer, mystical experiences, autogenic training, Zen or *yoga*, or quiet contemplation, with eyes closed, in a place of worship.[142] This research was highly formative for mind-body medicine, leading to decades of research on mindfulness and efforts to incorporate meditation into Western clinical settings.[143]

Substantial bodies of health and healing research investigate the effects of states of consciousness characteristic of, or engendered by, religious practices. These include practices associated with Eastern and non-Judeo-Christian faith traditions. It is likely, I suspect, that most Western physicians and biomedical scientists are unaware that such research exists in such quantity. A few examples:

- *Meditation.* According to a bibliography compiled by the Institute of Noetic Sciences (IONS) in 1997, over fifteen hundred studies had been published on the physical and psychological effects of meditation,[144] dating to 1931. From 1997 through 2013 the bibliography was maintained and updated as an online resource, at its peak comprising over six thousand references.[145] Still, the physiological and health impact of meditation remains contested territory for academic psychology, including denial that evidence supports such effects.[146]
- *Yoga.* Parallel to the meditation literature, a large body of studies has investigated the physiological and health impact of *yoga*, in its many variants. The first substantial review of this research that I encountered was in a book by James Funderburk titled *Science Studies Yoga*, published in 1977 by the Himalayan Institute.[147] Funderburk detailed studies of muscular-articular, circulatory, respiratory, and endocrine and nervous system responses to the practice of *Haṭha yoga*. In the forty-plus years since, research on *yoga* has flourished. A search of PubMed, at the time of this writing, turned up over five thousand hits on "yoga," with hundreds of new studies and reviews published every year of the past decade.
- *Spontaneous remission.* Another project sponsored by IONS, published in 1993, was a remarkable annotated bibliography of published case series and reports of spontaneous remission.[148] This was defined as "the disappearance, complete or incomplete, of a disease or cancer without medical treatment or treatment that is considered inadequate to produce the resulting disappearance of disease symptoms or tumor."[149] The authors cited 1,385 published reports of spontaneous remission throughout the peer-reviewed medical literature, including remission of neoplasms (cancer) of almost every imaginable site, infectious and parasitic diseases, diseases of every imaginable bodily system and organ, diseases of the skin and tissues, and injury-related disorders. Some remissions seemed "miraculous" or the result of "spiritual cures"; others were examples of "pure remission."[150] That is, they "followed periods of doing precisely nothing."[151]

For many years I have tried to make the case that for scientific knowledge in this field to progress and better inform medical practice, several changes need to occur in how religion and health research is conducted. Most importantly, investigators need to incorporate harder measures of health and healing into their studies, such as indicators of physiological, psychophysiological, and pathophysiological functioning.[152] The aim here would be to investigate whether religious participation is associated with reductions in biological risk.[153] As noted, most research to date has come from social, behavioral, and population scientists, and has helped make the case that faith and spirituality matter for health. But what remains, as with other psychosocial research on health, is to connect these observations to "inside the body" functions—physiological and biochemical processes and functions that involve anatomical features and systems and that are coherent with our biological knowledge of how the body works. Short of that, it is difficult to envision the medical field ever fully accepting the validity of these studies, no matter how many thousands continue to accumulate.

One promising area of research involves a possible connection between religious beliefs, practices, and experiences and psychoneuroimmunology (PNI).[154] This field of medical research, dating to the mid-1970s, focuses on interactions between psychological processes and the human nervous, immune, and endocrine systems. In a 1993 article in the *New England Journal of Medicine*, Tufts neuroendocrinologist Seymour Reichlin suggested that research on this subject, still in its early stages at the time, showed great translational promise—that is, potential for laboratory findings to affect clinical practice.[155] Since publication, this article has been cited over seven hundred times, and the NIH established a lab to conduct intramural research on the subject.

There appears to be a sound basis for a connection between PNI and religion.[156] For example, Esther M. Sternberg, former section chief of Neuroendocrine Immunology and Behavior at the U.S. National Institute of Mental Health and director of its Integrative Neural Immune Program, has stated that faith and prayer may exhibit therapeutic effects by "act[ing] through well-defined nerve pathways and molecules—molecules that can have profound effects on how immune cells function. A part of prayer's effect might come from removing stress—reversing that burst of hormones that can suppress immune function."[157]

Published findings bear this out. Over both editions of Koenig's *Handbook*, more than ninety studies were identified and nearly two-thirds of them found statistically significant associations between indicators of religiousness and respective markers of immune system and neuroendocrine function.[158] This includes examples from Koenig's own research, notably a study using EPESE data that found a modest but statistically significant effect whereby frequent religious attendance was associated with higher levels of plasma Interleukin-6, a marker of immune system function.[159] These results withstood adjusting for effects of depression, stress, medical history, and physical functioning. In *The Link between Religion and Health: Psychoneuroimmunology and the Faith Factor*, Koenig and his Duke medical school colleague Harvey Jay Cohen[160] lay out a detailed agenda for this new area of research, focused especially on identifying mechanisms of effect.

Faith Matters

If a reasonable conclusion can be drawn, it is simply this: for people of faith, religion can serve as a vital resource for coping with life's challenges, thus enhancing one's well-being. For sure, the healing prayer studies are an ongoing source of contention, but as noted, they are a fraction of the medical and health-related research published on the impact of religion. The takeaway from the thousands of social, behavioral, biomedical, epidemiologic, and other clinical and population-health research studies is really quite straightforward and ought not be a lightning rod for controversy: namely, that "religious participation, on average, exhibits primary-preventive effects in well populations by an association with lower morbidity. No more, no less."[161]

The implications tend to be overstated by advocates who look to these studies to validate beliefs about God, the universe, and reality. This is troubling for two reasons. For one, it is disconcerting that these studies, especially on healing prayer, have tended to reinforce some very unhealthy and unrealistic expectations about God and healing, leading some folks to attribute their illness or failure to be cured or to recover to their own lack of faith. No medical study can possibly suggest such a thing, and shame on any investigators who attempt to do so. But there is another troubling undercurrent to this field of research:

> Science and biomedicine have become lenses through which religion—something seemingly ephemeral, subjective, mysterious, and transcendent, perhaps even intractable—can be rationalized and made reducible to something amenable to systematic inquiry by observational or experimental science. This adaptation presents problems for the discourse, as it asks scientific methodologies and theories to do work that they may not be equipped to do. Questions related to the existence of God or supernatural realities and the nature of their putative influence on the manifested universe and on the course of human affairs have challenged the greatest minds for thousands of years. *It requires great hubris to presume that the sorts of studies conducted by medical scientists are the ideal way to obtain answers.*[162]

If we are looking to religion and health studies to provide insights into psychosocial and behavioral determinants of population health and personal well-being, then their cumulative findings have something substantial to offer. But if we are looking for this research to give us insight about existential questions, the actions of God, divine justice, or the meaning of life, then we might want to reconsider. Several years ago I made this same point as succinctly as I could: "If folks are looking to scientific research (on health, of all things) to validate the existence or motives of God, then they are looking in the wrong place."[163]

For religion and health research, much remains to be learned. Many of us in this field have been proposing agendas for future research for many years,[164] hopeful that the next generation of scientists will chart a new course and not keep rehashing the same questions. Thankfully, our suggestions are bearing fruit, as new research frontiers emerge. Many studies of the past few years are especially fascinating and creative:

- *Religion and mortality rates.* Epidemiologic studies of religion and mortality go back to the earliest days of religion and health research. At least 60 studies appeared through the mid-1980s, mostly comparing rates of death between categories of religious affiliation.[165] More recently, sophisticated methods of analysis have been used to calculate precisely the longevity or survival benefit attributable to religious participation.[166] A meta-analysis of studies through the 1990s found that religious participation was associated with about a 29 percent reduction in all-causes morality.[167] By the second edition of Koenig's *Handbook* there had been 116 religion-mortality studies, of which 92 (79.3%) reported higher levels of religious participation associated with lower mortality.[168]

- *Religion and leukocyte telomere length.* Within the past few years, studies suggest that higher levels of religious involvement, including church attendance, prayer, and strong self-assessments of religiousness, are associated with longer white blood cell telomeres.[169] These are DNA-protein complexes located at the end of our chromosomes, and their shortening is a marker of cellular aging associated with reduced life span.[170] Results of these religion studies, although promising, have been called into question on methodological grounds.[171] Researchers are encouraged to continue investigating this issue, provided they can make use of large prospective cohort studies and longitudinal designs.[172]

- *Tefillin and cardiovascular function.* A controlled study of twenty Jewish men, conducted at the University of Cincinnati, found that use of tefillin (nonocclusive leather straps attached to the arm during morning prayer, also known as *phylacteries*) appeared to have an ischemic preconditioning effect.[173] Long-term daily use among Orthodox Jews was associated with an anti-inflammatory response (decreased levels of circulating cytokines and attenuated monocyte chemotaxis and adhesion), while acute use in both religious and nonreligious Jews was associated with improved vascular function (greater brachial artery diameter and flow volume) after thirty minutes of use. I must admit that I am not sure what to make of these results, but as a practicing Jew I find the possible implications fascinating and encouraging.

- *Energy healers and healing.* A long-standing interest of mine,[174] the work of individuals purporting to heal through access to a subtle bioenergy is a provocative and underinvestigated subject even within the field of integrative medicine. It is difficult to study, due in part to conceptual fuzziness that makes it hard to distinguish between prayer, distant intention, and energy healing. Fewer methodologically sound studies thus exist than even for healing prayer, so there is a pressing need for scientists to begin a focused discussion around the concept of healing and its possible dimensions and determinants.[175] In the meantime, evidence from a systematic review of healing studies suggests the possibility of efficacy,[176] but as noted, there remains a need for better conceptual work[177] and theory-building.[178] One important question: Does what is being called *energy healing* even involve "energy"?[179] There is also a pressing need to consider the possibility of research fraud in this highly charged area of study.[180]

The most important unanswered question left to address is how and why, specifically, religion, spirituality, and faith exert measurable effects on health and healing among individual people and population-wide. Does this idea even make sense? Sure, by now reams of studies have been conducted and most report statistically significant results of one sort or another, but what does this all mean? Another way to state it: What is it about religion that is or should be health-promoting? What are the characteristics, functions, expressions, or manifestations of being religious or spiritual or practicing one's faith that decrease the risk of illness or help us to recover or heal from a medical challenge?[181]

For social scientists and epidemiologists, this question is defined as a search for what are termed *mechanisms*, or mediating factors that lie between religion and health in a sort of causal chain or pathway. That is, being religious or doing religion leads to *something* that in turn leads to physical health or emotional well-being or lower mortality rates or whatever. The issue here is to identify that *something*. This has also been referred to as a search for the "active ingredients" in faith or spirituality that contribute to health or healing.[182]

Since as far back as the 1970s, efforts have been made to answer this how or why question for religion and health. This is a decade before publication of the first major literature reviews documenting the scope of published research. The earliest systematic take on this issue was from Presbyterian theologian and ethicist Kenneth Vaux.[183] He outlined three dozen health-related activities, grounded in religious belief or behavior, that may account for observed associations linking religion and health. These included preventive health behaviors (e.g., involving diet, vaccination, hygiene) and health-promoting attitudes regarding ethical decision-making, such as related to medical compliance, substance abuse, and reproductive issues. Each is an outgrowth of being religious or doing religion that in turn may affect our health.

Other notable takes on this issue—efforts to list health-impacting mechanisms or active ingredients in religion—have come from sociologists,[184] psychologists,[185] and interdisciplinary teams of scientists and social scientists.[186] My own research, beginning in the 1980s, proposed a comprehensive model of hypothetical ways that dimensions of religious expression affect health. Each respective form of being religious or practicing religion was linked to disease prevention, health promotion, or healing by way of known scientific mechanisms,[187] including

- *Healthy behavior.* Religious commitment encourages avoidance of smoking, alcohol and drug abuse, unprotected sex, and other destructive behaviors, thus lowering disease risk and enhancing well-being.
- *Social support.* Religious participation and fellowship embed us in networks of supportive social relationships that provide emotional and tangible resources that alleviate effects of stress and enable coping with health challenges.
- *Positive emotions.* Religious worship and prayer involve rituals through which we experience feelings of peace, love, acceptance, grace, and other emotions that activate psychophysiological, neuroendocrine, and psychoimmunologic processes associated with health and healing.
- *Healthy beliefs.* Religious theologies and worldviews (e.g., Calvinism) are consonant with certain health-related beliefs, personality styles, or behavioral patterns (e.g., Type A) that may elevate or decrease risk of respective disease outcomes (e.g., myocardial infarction).
- *Salutary thoughts.* Religious faith involves psychodynamics that stimulate hope, optimism, and positive expectations, cognitions that in turn may activate something akin to a placebo effect that can heal or cure disease.
- *Healing states of consciousness.* Religious, spiritual, and mystical experiences may invoke a state of consciousness or activate a healing force associated with remission of disease and elevated states of psychological well-being.

Each possible active ingredient in religion or faith is proposed as a mechanism for explaining how and why faith matters, for making sense of the religion-health associations observed in studies. Have all of these mechanisms been validated as explanations for results of published studies? No, not yet; they are merely hypotheses. Further, they were put forward to help us account for findings from clinical and population-based studies of religion. The healing prayer RCTs likely require a different set of explanatory mechanisms—including, perhaps, "God did it"—that are highly speculative, at best, and probably not the sort of thing that observational science is capable of addressing.

In the final analysis, the mechanisms question is yet to be answered completely.[188] Many or all of these factors may likely come into play in certain situations, among certain populations, and for certain health conditions. The reality of human health is not always neatly captured by simple equations that link a single variable (e.g., religiousness) to a single mechanism (e.g., healthy behavior) to a health-related outcome (e.g., less heart disease). How the body holds off disease and maintains or recovers health is much more complicated. But thinking through the how and why of religion's putative effects on health, proposing hypotheses, and then testing them as best we can is essential if we are ever to advance beyond the stage of cumulating interesting one-off studies of this or that measure of religion correlated with this or that rate of disease in this or that study sample.

In order to advance, any scientific field needs both good research studies and development of reasonable theories to test.[189] For this field, lack of theoretical development up to now, save for the few efforts to formulate takes on the how-and-why issue, is a stumbling block needing to be overcome for this to become a mature and respected area of medical research. It is not there yet.

One way to help achieve this is for researchers to extend their search into other areas of scholarship outside the comfort zones provided by one's home discipline, whether medicine, epidemiology, sociology, or psychology. As noted, valuable insights have already emerged from studies done by physicians and biomedical researchers and those social scientists and epidemiologists for whom research means statistical analysis of quantitative data. But that does not exhaust the possible ways to investigate this issue.

There is much to learn, for example, from historical, ethnographic, phenomenological, and other types of qualitative research at the interface of medicine and religion, including from the humanities, history, anthropology, and religious studies. Recent examples include an interdisciplinary roundtable discussion of cross-cultural perspectives on faith and mortality;[190] an edited collection of over two dozen essays on religious healing in North America, written from a diversity of religious and cultural perspectives;[191] and an analysis of the concept of transcendence and how it contributes to healing in the lives of individuals and is engaged by investigators working outside the mainstream of medical science.[192] Each contribution provides insights into how and why religion, spirituality, and faith matter for health and healing, for better or worse.

Important works of humanistic scholarship have appeared that focus on spirituality in the life experience of older adults.[193] The best includes creative ethnographic studies by University of Connecticut gerontologist L. Eugene Thomas.[194] My favorite was an observational study of Hindu *sannyāsis* (renunciates) living in Varanasi and Pondicherry, in India.[195] Thomas's dialogues with these *sādhus* (mystical ascetics) convinced him of their spiritual maturity and depth of wisdom. His conversations also convinced him of the irrelevancy of most current research on the determinants of mental health and well-being.

> By any standard, these men were socially disengaged—the number of roles they occupied had shrunk dramatically. Their economic level would place them below the poverty level. Their health ranged from fair to quite poor. They had no support from their families, and they had no personal friends. Despite these and other negative correlates of life satisfaction (at least, as derived from research with Western respondents), *these men would have bumped the top of any scale of life satisfaction.*[196]

Clearly, something important is going on here that has not been captured in the number-crunching statistical studies to which I and my colleagues gravitate in our research.

Nursing research is an overlooked domain of high-quality work on spirituality and health and healing, including both empirical studies and trenchant conceptual and theoretical analyses. The work of Joan C. Engebretson and Diane W. Wardell, for example, distinguished nursing professors at the University of Texas Health Science Center at Houston, has been instrumental in documenting the efficacy of touch healing and the historical, psychological, and cultural contexts where it occurs.[197] They know as much as anyone about how and why healing happens, yet their insights are not as widely circulated and cited among religion and health researchers as other streams of research noted in this chapter. My sense is that this is due to a troubling silo effect in contemporary medical research that marginalizes contributions of nurses, females, and qualitative researchers, especially those who focus on spirituality, energy healing, and integrative medicine. Their excellent work deserves a wider airing.

Theologians, too, are underrepresented in scholarly work on religion and health, to the detriment of the field. Or, rather, their niched writing on the topic, which is prolific, insightful, and extends back centuries, is mostly invisible to the medical and social scientists who conduct most research, if patterns of citing references are any indication. In an excellent critique of the religion and health field, theologian Joel James Shuman and Vanderbilt physician Keith G. Meador made the case that research studies, on the whole, are guilty of assessing religiousness in simplistic ways inconsistent with normative religious belief and practice within Christianity and the great faith traditions.[198] These studies, moreover, seem to reinforce existence of "a generic spirituality and an instrumentalized deity" that can be marketed as a commodity to improve health.[199]

Religious faith and spiritual involvement may indeed be capable of promoting health and well-being and even healing, for reasons that involve still somewhat speculative or mysterious mechanisms of effect. This is a hopeful observation, for sure. But we must be careful lest we trivialize religion and faith in ways that diminish its majesty and holiness and reduce it to a discrete commodity. More specifically, as I have noted, religion

> ought not be viewed in the way that we regrettably have come to view diet and exercise and meditation and routine preventive checkups. Faith is not some discrete "thing" that we can "do," something to "plug in" to our "life style," and thus attain some sort of amorphous state of "wellness." Such a notion, such a misconstrued notion of faith, is, if anything, the therapeutic version of martyred Pastor Dietrich Bonhoeffer's famous theological concept of "cheap grace."[200]

It seems misguided that despite the thousands of studies of religion and health conducted by physicians and scientists, those professionals and academic scholars with content expertise on religion are mostly excluded and not even consulted when it comes to formulating hypotheses, asking questions, and interpreting results in ways that make sense. As a result, much of this work—no matter its methodological sophistication—does not make much sense religiously speaking. It does not seem to adequately capture or represent religion or spirituality or faith as lived out in the lives of real people. One prominent researcher, sociologist Neal Krause, referred to this entire research enterprise as "a disheveled literature" in part for these very reasons.[201]

Such exclusion of content experts would never happen for any other topic of medical or epidemiologic research. Could you imagine planning a study of the health effects of, say, toxic exposures, personality disorders, or abusive relationships in which an environmental toxicologist, a clinical psychologist, or a social worker or family therapist were not consulted? But because religion—the subject and even the word—carries so much emotional and ideological baggage for so many people in the scientific world, it may be that prospective investigators assume that good scholarly work does not exist on the subject or that one's own tacit presumptions constitute full and accurate knowledge of the topic and will suffice for designing a study. Thus there is little reason to run one's ideas by a professional scholar knowledgeable about religion before designing or conducting a study. The result? The wrong questions are asked of the wrong people, analyses are conducted that may not make sense, and findings are misinterpreted and result in misleading messages about religion reaching the general public. This is unfortunate no matter the reasons.

To address this lacuna, I collaborated with Meador on an edited book soliciting perspectives of leading Jewish and Christian theological scholars as to why we should expect (or not expect) spirituality, in its broadest sense, to be impactful for health.[202] Entitled *Healing to All Their Flesh*, from a verse in Proverbs (4:22, ESV), we gave our contributors carte blanche to reflect on what their respective faith tradition—its canon, theology, ethics, and pastoral writing—have to say about health, healing, medicine, and healthcare. We wanted to know whether it even makes sense to expect that the human body, its physiology, and its state of health are in any way a function of the well-being of the human spirit, and if so, how and why—and especially, what questions researchers should ask so as to make sense within the context of these religions.

Although religion and health research remains controversial in the medical and scientific communities, this response is no longer warranted. As described, most studies fall squarely within the mainstream of social, behavioral, or population-based research on health, and most do not broach concepts that challenge the limits of current scientific and biomedical knowledge. My own opinion about the implications of this work mirror the famous words of psychiatrist and Holocaust survivor Victor Frankl, who stated that "when a patient stands on the firm ground of religious belief, there can be no objection to making use of the therapeutic effect of his religious conviction and thereby drawing on his spiritual resources."[203]

As for the deservedly more contentious clinical trials of distant prayer, even here I am hopeful and defer to the opinion of Larry Dossey:

> There is evidence that the scientific and medical community may be slowly opening to the cumulative evidence.... Those who believe in prayer might pray for this process to continue.[204]

6

Teaching and Training

In the 1940s a diverse group of Texas physicians, philanthropists, educators, and politically connected private citizens laid the groundwork for what became Texas Medical Center (TMC) in Houston.[1] A joint project of multiple public and private health sciences schools, hospitals, specialty clinics, academic research centers, and other member institutions, TMC evolved into what today is the largest medical center in the world.[2] Alongside the medical schools and other health sciences programs of Baylor University and the University of Texas; M.D. Anderson cancer hospital; the Methodist, Hermann, St. Luke's, Shrine Children's, and naval hospitals; and the library of the Houston Academy of Medicine—and other institutions soon to come—a most unusual member was added to the original TMC roster. On May 9, 1956, the building housing the Institute of Religion was dedicated, the first of its type founded at a U.S. medical center.[3]

Established the year before, the institute's mission encompassed research and education of physicians, nurses, other healthcare professionals, and ministers, especially training of hospital chaplains. A founder of TMC described the importance of the institute: "It rounds out the total purpose for our Medical Center. That is, for the care of all phases of man—religious, mental, and physical."[4]

Just as TMC was the product of a collaborative vision and many years of planning, so too was the institute. Its founders benefited from consultation and sage advice from leading figures in pastoral theology and ministry, including Granger Westberg,[5] and had support from an ecumenical and interfaith group of Houston clergy and theological leaders.[6] From the beginning, the institute was affiliated with five mainline theological seminaries and academically connected to Baylor. In 1965 it hired Westberg away from the University of Chicago, where he had served for eleven years with joint appointments in the medical and divinity schools,[7] to become dean of the institute.[8] He was also was appointed as Professor of Religion and Medicine in the Department of Psychiatry at Baylor,[9] the first such titled academic appointment in a U.S. medical school.

The institute sought to become a center for promoting integration of religion and medicine, including through joint programs for research and training of medical and ministerial students.[10] This covers a lot of ground, something recognized at the time. Accordingly, the institute has gone through a few distinct epochs in its history, with specific foci waxing and then waning. For its first two decades, it was a major player in pastoral care and healthcare chaplaincy, and

Religion and Medicine. Jeff Levin, Oxford University Press (2020) © Oxford University Press.
DOI: 10.1093/oso/9780190867355.001.0001

instrumental in pioneering and coordinating CPE at TMC.[11] Westberg was influential here, and developed and implemented ideas he would build on when he left to go to Ohio and then back to Chicago.[12]

While at Baylor and the institute, Westberg added another first to his résumé: he offered the first formal coursework on religion and medicine at a U.S. medical school. He taught seminars to medical students and chaplaincy trainees on the interrelation of medicine and religion and on preventive medicine, and offered supervised clinical experiences. He also developed a series of Interdisciplinary Religion-Medicine Case Conferences, based on a clinical education model he had implemented at Chicago.[13]

By the 1970s, after Westberg left Houston, the institute changed focus. It was no longer TMC's center for CPE; individual programs had diffused out into the medical center's member institutions. Institute leadership was candid in acknowledging that "it was searching for a new mission."[14] In 1972 the institute asked Kenneth Vaux, already on staff for the past few years, to become acting director. Like Westberg, he had an appointment at Baylor, where he taught medical ethics. Also like Westberg, he left after a couple years, settling in Chicago where he joined the faculty of Garrett-Evangelical Theological Seminary and Northwestern University.[15] Vaux's tenure at the institute and Baylor was as instrumental for academic bioethics as Westberg's time there was for pastoral care. The first edition of the *Encyclopedia of Bioethics*, published in 1978, acknowledged the institute as "the first major institution devoted to medical ethics in the United States."[16]

In the 1980s the institute's focus shifted again. Since that time it has undergone multiple changes in leadership and a couple of name changes—first to the Institute for Religion and Health in 2003, and then to the Institute for Spirituality and Health in 2008. It has strived to become a center for congregational health ministries, psychotherapy and religion, and research on spirituality and health, and has initiated various programs on various topics, including meditation and *yoga*, but in my opinion has not yet recovered the traction it had during its time as a pioneer in pastoral care and bioethics. It is financially secure, however, thanks to a generous arrangement with Houston Methodist Hospital, which agreed to provide substantial funding for one hundred years in exchange for the space it was occupying. In 2002, when Methodist needed to expand its footprint into the small grove where the institute building stood, the institute moved off campus to its current home, a suite just south of TMC.[17]

The institute is no longer formally partnered with Baylor, although collegial relationships exist with many TMC institutions. Two downstream descendants of the institute's collaboration with Baylor continue aspects of its earlier work, one with direct lineage back to Vaux and his efforts in medical ethics, the other with only an indirect connection to the institute's early days.

In 1982 Baylor (by then known as Baylor College of Medicine [BCM]) entered into a partnership with the Institute and Rice University to establish the Center for Medical Ethics. They hired Baruch Brody, chairman of Rice's Department of Philosophy, to become the first director.[18] Under the leadership of Brody, among the world's preeminent bioethical scholars,[19] the center became the top program of its type in the country, as well as one of the earliest academic centers focused on non-biomedical content—e.g., medical humanities, philosophy, religious studies, law, clinical ethics, history of medicine, and health policy— that now exist at most leading medical schools. Today known as the Center for Medical Ethics and Health Policy, it continues under the leadership of Amy Lynn McGuire, attorney and Leon Jaworski Professor of Biomedical Ethics at BCM.

The other Baylor-branded academic center is the Program on Religion and Population Health (PRPH), which I direct at Baylor University's Institute for Studies of Religion. Founded in 2009, when I was recruited to Baylor, the mission of PRPH is "to conduct and promote research on the impact of religion on healthcare and indicators of population health."[20] Over the past decade, the program has had three foci: population-health research on religion and physical and mental health and well-being, study of faith-based partnerships in health policy and public health, and documentation of theories of healing and the work of healers. The program has been successful in publishing dozens of scholarly works, including several books, and sponsoring visiting speakers and my own lectures and teaching.

To be clear, no formal relation exists between the two programs—PRPH and the BCM center—nor between PRPH and Westberg's efforts at Baylor in the 1960s. This work is separated by decades, and, since a contentious divorce in 1969, Baylor University and BCM have been officially independent institutions.[21] But I am nonetheless proud to claim a "genealogical" connection for PRPH with this earlier work. Baylor University's historic faith-based mission provides a welcoming home for my research, as does the Institute for Studies of Religion, an interdisciplinary academic think tank that specializes in social research and public policy analysis on religion. I feel a personal obligation to ensure that the pioneering work of Westberg and Vaux and their colleagues is remembered and that Baylor remains a place where scholarship on faith and medicine continues to flourish.

For the record, the Institute for Spirituality and Health, BCM's Center for Medical Ethics and Health Policy, and Baylor University's PRPH are not the only loci in Baylor's long and multifaceted history where religion and medicine have come together. Founded in 1963, through combined efforts of the Houston Jewish community and over one thousand local Jewish donors, the Jewish Institute for Medical Research was established as a site for medical research on land belonging to BCM and adjacent to the medical school's main basic sciences building.[22] It does not operate as a separate academic unit, but rather as a location housing labs and research programs, including Nobel Prize–winning research.[23] Its scientists have been instrumental in bringing BCM to the forefront of American medical schools in funded biomedical research.

The original Jewish Institute building remains a centerpiece of the BCM campus—with a prominent *Magen David* (Shield of David) carved into the main entrance wall. As well, every year at Chanukah a large *menorah* is stationed in front of the building. These evidences of Jewish provenance must cause cognitive dissonance for visitors from the main Baylor campus in Waco who believe that the university's history is exclusively Baptist. The true narrative, especially as it concerns the medical school, is more complex, as it was a product in part of local Jewish philanthropy[24] and continues to benefit from Jewish administrative leadership. Since Baylor University and Baylor College of Medicine split half a century ago, the institutions continue to share some regents/trustees, so this history rightly belongs to both schools, as well as to the Baylor University Medical Center in Dallas, original home of the medical school, and Baylor Scott & White Health, one of the largest not-for-profit healthcare systems in the United States.

I do not wish to give the impression that the Baylor brand is the center of the academic universe when it comes to religion and medicine. Decades ago, this was so, but no longer—although Baylor does count as ground zero for development of this field in the United States. The leadership role for academic research, teaching, practice, and service has been supplanted by other institutions—notably Duke, Harvard, and George Washington—and by a growing presence in undergraduate and postgraduate medical education at several other universities. At most of these schools, this work flourished due in large part to a small group of visionaries who came together, at great odds, to establish a safe space to explore religion. These efforts, in turn, owe a great debt to two men who were devoted to making inroads for research and education on religion and faith within academic medicine.

Sir John and David

For many years following establishment of the Institute of Religion and its partnership with BCM, formal institutional linkages between religion and medicine for educational purposes were scarce. Outside of academic medicine, the most visible efforts were the American Medical Association's creation of a Department of Medicine and Religion in 1961, and an associated board-level Committee on Medicine and Religion in 1962.[25] A recent history has documented how the department and committee met with considerable success, as together they fostered collaborations with medical and theological schools to establish courses in medicine and religion. These groups also established state- and county-level committees on medicine and religion, which, in turn, organized events designed to bring physicians and clergy together around issues of mutual interest.[26]

By 1965, committees had been established in forty-nine states, and programming on religion and medicine was organized in over seven hundred county-level medical societies.[27] The AMA's goal was to create a healthy climate of cooperation "to enable physicians and clergypersons to better care for individual patients in their actual practices and local communities."[28] As one might anticipate, Westberg had an active role on the Committee.[29] Soon, though, the AMA called it quits. For a variety of complicated reasons—some political, some ideological, some perhaps a result of antireligious bigotry from secularists among the association's membership, some perhaps due to fallout over internal AMA conflict regarding abortion laws[30]—the committee was disbanded in 1972, and the department followed suit in 1974.[31]

In the years following, activities at the Institute of Religion were still the focal center of the religion and medicine field. Throughout the United States, individual physicians continued to write insightful papers on religious aspects of patient care, medical specialists continued to collaborate with clergy, and one-off educational experiences were developed for health sciences students in selected schools. But, for the most part, academic medical centers shied away from formal recognition of this subject as worthy of institutional investment.

Toward the end of the 1980s, this began to change. Emboldened by publication of several medical review articles, two men took up the mantel of leadership in incorporating religious content within academic medicine. These were billionaire Sir John Marks Templeton, investor and philanthropist, and David B. Larson, psychiatrist and epidemiologist.

In the 1980s, as noted in the previous chapter, publication of several comprehensive literature reviews brought attention to the substantial body of existing research findings pointing to a salutary role for religion in physical and mental health. This included my own reviews and original research, as well as those of Harold Koenig, Ellen Idler, Ken Pargament, Robert Taylor, Linda Chatters, and several others, including sociologists Chris Ellison, David R. Williams, and Linda K. George. Of all of us cataloguing results of these studies, no one took to the task more enthusiastically than Dave Larson. Nobody around at that time who participated in this groundswell of research and writing would possibly debate this point. A biography of Dave described him as the tireless captain of a team of beleaguered sociologists, psychologists, epidemiologists, gerontologists, and physicians who shared not much else but a desire to do scholarly work, sometimes in collaboration and sometimes alone, in an area that most everyone else in academic medicine, public health, and the medical, social, and behavioral sciences, it seemed, derided or ignored.[32]

Dave was educated at the Temple University School of Medicine, followed by a psychiatry residency and geriatrics fellowship at Duke. He then received a graduate degree in epidemiology from UNC, funded by a fellowship from the NIH. While at Duke, he was mentored in psychiatry by William P. Wilson, well-known leader in Christian psychiatry who gathered around him a team of resident trainees that came to be referred to, not always approvingly, as the "God squad."[33] Dave was chief resident.

In the first half of the 1980s, unbeknownst to me since I had never met Dave nor heard of him, we had been bit by the same bug: cataloguing the many studies of religion existing throughout the medical literature but, to that point, largely undiscovered. Whereas my focus was on studies of physical health, morbidity, and mortality, Dave focused on the psychiatric literature and on mental health. His important reviews were cited in the last chapter.

In 1985, after completing a fellowship at the National Institute of Mental Health (NIMH), Dave accepted a commission as an officer in the U.S. Public Health Service, eventually rising to the Naval-equivalent rank of captain. He served in assignments at NIMH, NIH, and the Department of Health and Human Services, including as a senior analyst in the Office of the Director of NIH. He later had adjunct appointments as professor of psychiatry at Duke, Northwestern University, and the Uniformed Services University.[34]

All the while, Dave continued to write literature reviews of religious research. Unlike the rest of us also doing this work, Dave was responsible for innovations in how research summaries were conducted and literature reviews written. He was a pioneer in the *systematic review* (SR), a methodology that, like its name suggests, offers a more systematic way of defining a topic, identifying journals to search, critically assessing the content of articles, making judgments about the quality of the research design and methods, and then numerically summarizing results.[35] SRs represent a midpoint between old-school narrative literature reviews and more sophisticated meta-analyses, which involve quantifying effects from numerous studies using statistical techniques. Besides his reviews of religion and mental health, Dave and colleagues published SRs on the impact of religion in fields as diverse as pastoral counseling, gerontology, criminology, child development, psychology, health services research, medical education, and primary care.[36]

Dave did not invent the SR—systematic reviews within medicine were conducted since the 1970s.[37] He did, however, popularize the method within medicine and the social and behavioral sciences, especially for reviewers seeking to summarize the impact of particular predictor variables not subject to previous reviews.[38] Dave's adoption of the SR was timely, as it paralleled emergence of an evidence-based culture within academic medicine and biomedical science that valued reproducible metrics to gauge the efficacy of medical outcomes and salience of proposed determinants of health.[39]

Dave's work upped the game for all of us actively collating and summarizing the unmined troves of research studies on religion and health discovered in the medical literature at the time. Over the past thirty years, because of Dave, the SR has become the norm for summaries of religion and health research. Many of his early reviews were written in collaboration with John S. Lyons, at the time a psychologist at Northwestern's School of Medicine, who shared his interest in documenting effects of religious participation on physical and mental health and other social, psychological, and quality-of-life indicators.[40] Dave's reviews, with Lyons and others, were instrumental in documenting the mostly positive contribution of religious participation and faith, in contrast to the tacit presumption at the time that religion was detrimental for personal well-being.[41]

I first met Dave in 1989, while in Chicago attending the annual meeting of the American Public Health Association. He was moderating a panel on religion and mental health, featuring some people I knew, and I was in the audience.[42] After the session was over, I introduced myself. Dave's eyes got big: every presenter had cited my work and most had mentioned my name, including Dave, who did not know that I was present. He invited me to go out to eat with the panel and we remained good friends and in close touch, on occasion collaborating on research papers, until his untimely passing in 2002.

Of greatest significance in the Dave Larson story, for both his career and the historic rapprochement between religion and medicine that he expedited, was his fated meeting with John Templeton.[43] Sir John, as he was known, was one of the world's most famous and successful investors, incorporating the John Templeton Foundation (JTF) in 1987 to serve as a philanthropic organization promoting character and virtue development, individual freedom, exceptional cognitive talent, and exploration of big questions in science. JTF sponsors the Templeton Prize, a de facto Nobel Prize in religion, whose recipients have included the Dalai Lama, Mother Teresa, Rev. Billy Graham, Rabbi Jonathan Sacks, and Bishop Desmond Tutu, and also supports academic research on a variety of subjects, including the contributions of religion and spirituality to physical and mental health. JTF also hosts the Templeton Press, which publishes books on all these subjects. Sir John's own insightful writing was far-ranging, and he had a special interest in what he called "unlimited love," which he believed had the power to transform lives and to heal body and mind.

Sir John was taken by Dave's rigorous and methodical reviews and commissioned him to devote more time to these and to conduct other scholarly activities.[44] In 1991 Dave took a leap of faith, and with JTF support he founded the National Institute for Healthcare Research (NIHR), a Washington beltway think tank devoted to research and education on issues of common interest to Dave and Sir John. After three years, in another leap of faith, Dave resigned his officer's commission and went to work full-time directing NIHR out of an office suite just outside the beltway in Rockville, Maryland.

Together, Dave and Sir John made a remarkable team, and products and projects flowed from NIHR in a steady stream. The SRs kept coming, as did a series of major conferences[45] and published reports.[46] Typical of Washington think tanks, NIHR had a list of affiliated senior fellows, and I was honored to serve in that capacity from the beginning. When I left academic medicine in 1997 Dave was even gracious enough to let me use this professional affiliation as my academic title for the next couple years.

The most lasting contribution of NIHR, in my opinion, was its administrative leadership of Faith and Medicine, a JTF-funded educational program for medical schools beginning in 1995. Directed by Dale A. Matthews, Georgetown internist and author,[47] Faith and Medicine consisted of a lecture program in which Matthews spoke at many leading medical schools, as well as a course competition soliciting submissions from medical educators to develop learning experiences for medical students. Matthews described the project as an opportunity "to encourage the development of exciting new educational programs by medical schools seeking to train the next generation of doctors to be sensitive to this domain."[48]

The competitive grant program for medical school courses requested proposals "for the development of a curriculum that integrates religious components with medical care."[49] More than forty inquiries were received, from about one-third of U.S. medical schools. A panel of judges made awards of five grants at ten thousand dollars apiece.[50] In the second year of competition, an additional six grants were made. In the first three years, nineteen schools received funding, including the medical schools at Johns Hopkins, Georgetown, Wake Forest, Case Western Reserve, Emory, George Washington, Rochester, Brown, West Virginia, and Washington University. At most of these schools, the courses were required for all students.[51]

In 1997, the awards were worth twenty-five thousand dollars. Among awardees were Morehouse University, the first historically Black institution to win one of the curriculum awards. The content of the course, which began that fall, ranged "from African religious beliefs [and] death and dying to taking religious and spiritual histories."[52]

Leadership of the program transferred in 1998 to Christina M. Puchalski, George Washington University palliative care physician, and a new course competition was initiated for psychiatry residency programs. These awards were for fifteen thousand dollars each, and recipients were Baylor, Harvard, Yeshiva, University of California–San Francisco, Loma Linda, Thomas Jefferson, and Pittsburgh.[53]

Faith and Medicine was a transformational moment for medical education in North America. Before the program, only three medical schools had any course content on religion or spirituality, even a single lecture. Within the first six years of the program, this number had increased to more than sixty, approximately half of all medical schools. Sir John was well aware of this success,[54] grateful that his investment in Dave resulted in a tremendous dividend. He was not exaggerating when he noted, "Worldwide, the health of people will benefit for generations to come by the dedicated work of Dr. David Larson and his wife, Susan."[55]

Medical school deans were initially skeptical,[56] but by now religious content is well institutionalized throughout North American medical schools. By 2010, fifteen years after the first courses were funded and nearly a decade since Dave's passing and the shuttering of NIHR, a review showed that 90 percent of all medical schools had instituted required or elective courses or course content on religion or spirituality.[57] It is likely that few of the professors and teachers overseeing this coursework have any idea that its presence in the contemporary American medical curriculum is owed mostly to the vision and labor of one person. Along with his coworkers and colleagues, and with JTF's largesse, Larson influenced the mainstreaming of spirituality and spiritual content into Western medical practice more than anyone else, including those of us like Harold Koenig and our colleagues who have conducted so much of the research on religion and health and physician-authors like Larry Dossey, whose writing brought widespread public attention to this subject.

In contrast to a generation ago, religion is no longer considered so off-putting a topic for medical education. No matter one's own religious beliefs or practices, it has become tacitly recognized that understanding how and why faith may matter in the lives of patients, for better or worse, makes for a more effective and compassionate clinician. Since the passing of Larson and the demise of NIHR, the most significant means by which religious content has taken its place within medical education has been through establishment of dedicated academic units within major medical and health sciences schools and universities.

Religion in Academic Medical Centers

By the 1990s programmatic research on religion, faith, and spirituality in health, healthcare, and healing from established investigators had begun to supplant a literature of one-off small studies. The success of NIHR in raising the profile of this research and promoting its medical school course competition was instrumental in the founding of formal academic institutes, centers, and programs that began popping up at universities and medical centers by the turn of the century. The oldest and still most prominent were established at Duke and Emory.

The Duke Center for Spirituality, Theology and Health was founded in 1998[58] with financial support from JTF. Administratively, it is a unit within the Center for the Study of Aging and Human Development at the Duke University School of Medicine. Directed by Harold Koenig, the spirituality center describes its mission as

conducting research, training others to conduct research, and promoting scholarly field-building activities related to religion, spirituality, and health. The Center serves as a clearinghouse for information on this topic, and seeks to support and encourage dialogue between researchers, clinicians, theologians, clergy, and others interested in the intersection.[59]

Since the beginning, the Duke center has been the most research-intensive of all academic centers of religion and health, due to the prolific research program directed by Koenig in collaboration with numerous colleagues at that university.[60] There are many facets to the center's work. It sponsors an annual summer workshop in clinical research methods;[61] is home to numerous ongoing clinical, community-centered, and population-based research projects;[62] hosts a monthly seminar series featuring visiting lecturers from across the country; and presents the annual David B. Larson Memorial Lecture in Religion and Health, which I cohost along with Koenig.

The first Larson Lecture was held in 2003, a year after Dave's passing. It was created to honor his memory and to recognize leading scholars, scientists, and medical and pastoral figures whose work lies at the intersection of religion and medicine. It is supported in part by proceeds from a *festschrift* volume that we coedited to honor Dave[63] and by private donations. The Larson Lecture was the first on this subject in academic medicine, and many esteemed figures in religion and medicine have received the honor of delivering one. Besides several individuals associated with Duke University, honorees have included Stephen G. Post, Daniel P. Sulmasy, Ken Pargament, George Fitchett, Gary Gunderson, Tracy A. Balboni, David Williams, John R. Peteet, Gail Ironson, and Ellen Idler. At the time of this book's publication, we are looking forward to the nineteenth annual lecture, held each year in March, around the date of Dave's passing.

The center has a lengthy list of resident and nonresident faculty scholars, whom it draws on for lectures and research collaboration. As both a Duke alumnus and adjunct faculty member I am privileged to serve as one of these scholars. It is a curiosity that so many key figures in the religion and health field were connected with Duke, whether as a student, resident, fellow, or faculty member, including Larson, Koenig, Matthews, George, Ellison, and many others, such as Keith Meador, Harvey Cohen, Kimberly A. Sherrill, Farr A. Curlin, and Warren A. Kinghorn.[64] The latter two also codirect the Duke Divinity School's Theology, Medicine, and Culture initiative, which sponsors fellowship and graduate certificate programs, a seminar series, and various research projects and partnerships on themes at the intersection of the health professions and church community.[65]

Along with the Duke center, the other largest and most successful religion and health center in the United States is located at Emory University. The Interfaith Health Program (IHP) has a much different focus than Duke— global public health, rather than clinical medicine—and a much different mission, organizational structure, and program of activities.[66] The IHP was established at the Carter Center in Atlanta in 1992, a few years prior to the Duke center, and even before the existence of the Rollins School of Public Health at Emory, where the program has been housed since 1999, currently within the Hubert Department of Global Health.[67] It was founded by former CDC director William Foege, with assistance from President Jimmy Carter, and its first director was Gary Gunderson, who remained there until leaving for Memphis in 2005. Its associate director was Lutheran theologian Thomas A. Droege, former student of Westberg at Chicago and author of important works on faith-health partnerships.[68]

From the IHP's mission statement, its distinctives come into focus, especially a characteristically public health orientation that distinguishes its work from that of Duke:

> Established to actively promote the health and well-being of individuals and communities who face health disparities, the Interfaith Health Program (IHP) brings together a diverse community of scholars and public health practitioners to assure access to health programs and services. Through alliances with national and global partners, IHP facilitates collaboration, provides training, builds networks, conducts research, and implements programs that improve the health and wellness of communities around the world. IHP's work is rooted in respect for diverse religious beliefs and practices, justice, and human rights for all people.[69]

The institute sponsors and participates in numerous projects, in the United States and globally, especially in Africa. These include programs establishing faith-based community partnerships, conducting community mapping and mobilization, and fostering public health development efforts. The IHP has a long history of hosting conferences, conducting basic and evaluative research, teaching both in the classroom and the field, and creating collaborative networks among public- and private-sector partners and NGOs. Its course offerings at Emory include Health and Social Justice and Understanding Religion's Role in Global Health and Development Practice. The institute has an accomplished and devoted staff, led by John Blevins and Mimi Kiser, and a tremendous website presence that archives two decades of scholarly work and publications, including its series of IHP Reports.[70]

An important subproject has been the Institute for Public Health and Faith Collaborations, founded in 2002 as an initiative of the IHP and also located at Emory. It has become a global leader in mobilizing institutional faith-based and healthcare resources to create partnerships for addressing health disparities.[71] It describes its mission as training collaborative teams of faith and health leaders to address health disparities within their communities. Since its establishment, hundreds of individuals have been trained throughout the United States and have successfully focused on mental health, HIV/AIDS, teen pregnancy, and so-cial, behavioral, and environmental determinants of population health.[72]

Also located at Emory is the Religion and Public Health Collaborative, directed by Ellen Idler. The collaborative is an interdisciplinary program with links to the IHP and Emory's schools of public health, nursing, and theology, as well as Emory's religion department.[73] Founded in 2006 the collaborative is involved in research, teaching, and service across intellectual disciplines and fields, with special emphasis on ethics; oversees one of the only M.Div./ M.P.H. dual-degree programs in the world; and sponsors research studies, vis-iting lectures, and conference events. The most notable was "Religion as a Social Determinant of Health," held in 2010, whose proceedings were later published by Oxford.[74]

In the decades since Baylor, Duke, and Emory established their respective centers and institutes, multifaceted programs dedicated to medical and public health research and education have flourished at prominent universities. These include units located within major academic medical centers. Each has devel-oped a special focus tailored to a respective institutional culture and to the exper-tise, interests, and professional and religious background of respective faculty.

The George Washington Institute for Spirituality and Health (GWish), founded in 2001 by Christina Puchalski, has led the way in thoughtfully integrating spirituality into the clinical setting and patient care.[75] Located within the George Washington University School of Medicine, GWish is preeminent among religion and health centers when it comes to curriculum development and evaluative research of initiatives in undergraduate and postgraduate medical education.[76] It has staked out a leadership role here as pronounced as Duke's in clinical research and research training and Emory's in global public health. GWish has been instrumental in initiatives outside of the United States, including founding the Global Network for Spirituality and Health[77] and the Interprofessional Spiritual Care Education Curriculum,[78] and ongoing research throughout North America. Puchalski has written prolifically on incorporating religious content in academic medical education and training, including an article coauthored with Larson and me, solicited by *JAMA* in 1998.[79] She also coedited the landmark *Oxford Textbook of Spirituality in Healthcare.*[80]

The Center for Spirituality and Health at the University of Florida was founded in 1998 as an interdisciplinary, university-wide center for teaching and research.[81] Its mission statement acknowledges a commitment to "academic exploration of the wider contexts of spirituality, religion and sciences as a whole, using the interface of spirituality and health sciences to bring Humanities, Natural and Social Sciences into relationship."[82] Founding codirectors were Allen H. Neims, former dean of the medical school, and Shaya R. Isenberg, at the time chair of the religion department—a synergy providing a secure footing within the university much different than other religion and health centers. Its affiliated faculty members are positioned throughout the various colleges at Florida, and offer courses in many departments, including classes for undergraduates. The center sponsors a lecture series, and I was honored to speak there in 2003.[83] In contrast to other religion and health centers, Florida's perspective focuses on human consciousness, integrative healing, spiritual self-actualization, and mindfulness meditation, and many faculty have personal and professional interests in Eastern religions and metaphysical spirituality. Its current director is neuroscientist Louis A. Ritz.

Another important institution is the Program on Medicine and Religion at the University of Chicago.[84] Cofounded with JTF support in 2009 by physicians Farr Curlin (currently at Duke) and Dan Sulmasy (currently at Georgetown), the program is one of the younger religion and health centers. Uniquely among such centers, the emphasis at Chicago is on bioethics and the practice of medicine. It identifies its mission as conducting "empirical, historical, theological, ethical, and legal scholarship to enrich our understanding of the meaning of illness and the myriad ways that religion and medicine each respond to the human predicaments of illness, injury, disability, suffering, and death."[85] The current director is Muslim physician and bioethicist Aasim I. Padela,[86] under whose leadership the program has established an Initiative on Islam and Medicine. It aims to become the foremost academic center "for study and dialogue at the intersection of the Islamic tradition and biomedicine."[87] Other projects focus on spiritual and ethical issues in medical practice, coursework is offered in both the medical and divinity schools, and, like Duke, a monthly seminar series hosts experts from throughout the world.

The Initiative on Health, Religion, and Spirituality at Harvard hosts multiple research and educational programs, a deep roster of distinguished faculty and senior fellows, and a guest lecture series featuring experts from throughout the academic world.[88] Codirected by radiation oncologist Tracy Balboni, theologian Michael J. Balboni, and epidemiologist and biostatistician Tyler VanderWeele, the initiative has defined for itself a conceptual space at the intersection of medicine, theology, pastoral care, and public health.[89] Faculty direct ongoing research programs in chaplaincy and medicine, religion and public health, religious communities and health, spirituality and mental health, and other subjects,[90] producing a steady stream of important scholarly articles published in high-profile medical journals.[91]

Besides the initiative, Harvard also is home to the Religion, Health and Medicine Program, an interdisciplinary collaboration among the divinity school, medical school, and school of public health. It is a part of the divinity school's Science, Religion and Culture Program, and has a set of faculty, fellows, research foci, and educational activities distinct from the initiative.[92] Current project themes include spiritual care in medicine; race, religion, and health; religion, medicine, and sexuality; and religion, culture, and global health.

This does not exhaust the roll call of academic religion and health or religion and medicine programs, centers, or institutes. Many such academic units have existed over the years, coming and going as funds dry up or faculty move on or retire.[93]

The University of Minnesota's Earl E. Bakken Center for Spirituality and Healing, founded in 1995, is a strong and thriving interdisciplinary center focused on teaching, research, and clinical care from an integrative medical perspective.[94] Its director is Mary Jo Kreitzer, a prominent figure in academic nursing,[95] and the center is a major international leader in research on complementary and integrative medicine.

The Spirituality and Health Interest Group at the Medical University of South Carolina was a successful multidisciplinary group of faculty and students interested in promoting research and education on "the spiritual concerns of patients and the spiritual context of medical illness and compassionate health care."[96] It existed for several years beginning in 2003, led by family physician Dana E. King,[97] a longtime collaborator with Koenig,[98] until King left for West Virginia.

Indiana State University's Center for the Study of Health, Religion and Spirituality, in operation from 2002 through 2013, for many years hosted an annual interdisciplinary research conference featuring presentations from important figures in the field.[99] The center was directed by Harvard-trained pastoral counselor Christine Kennedy,[100] until she moved to Jefferson University.

Other centers exist or existed outside of medical schools or health sciences centers, but as units within faith-based universities. One example is the former Center for Catholic Health Care and Sponsorship, founded in 1994 as a project of the Beazley Institute for Health Law and Policy located in the law school at Loyola University Chicago.[101] Another example is the Kalsman Institute on Judaism and Health, established in 2000 at the Los Angeles campus of Hebrew Union College–Jewish Institute of Religion.[102]

Religion and health centers have also been established outside the United States. One notable example is the University of Aberdeen's Centre for Spirituality, Health and Disability,[103] directed by theologian John Swinton.[104] Membership organizations exist as well, unaffiliated with a particular university but sponsoring scholarly programs and conferences. Examples include the Scientific and Medical Network, headquartered in London,[105] and the United States Spiritist Medical Association[106] and its affiliated International Spiritist Medical Association.[107] I have been honored to receive invitations to speak before all three of these organizations, at conferences in Canterbury, Washington, and Paris, respectively.

Since the events sponsored by NIHR in the 1990s, other centers or organizations have sponsored scholarly conferences on religion and health for professors, students, and medical and pastoral professionals. Beginning in 1995 Harvard Medical School, under the leadership of Herbert Benson, sponsored a conference on the theme of Spirituality and Healing in Medicine that was held at least annually for over a decade.[108] Subsequently, beginning in 2008, the Duke center sponsored with JTF support an annual conference on Spirituality, Theology, and Health that ran for three years.[109] Since that time, staring in 2012, an annual Conference on Religion and Medicine has been held, with multiple current sponsors including Harvard, Duke, Baylor, TMC's Institute for Spirituality and Health, and other academic institutions.[110] Initially supported by seed funding from JTF and sponsored by the University of Chicago, the Conference on Religion and Medicine has become the premier annual event in the field. The conference's mission is

> to enable health professionals and scholars to gain a deeper and more practical understanding of how religion relates to the practice of medicine, with particular attention to the traditions of Judaism, Christianity, and Islam. The forum

is intended in a spirit that builds bridges between theory and practice, science and theology, the academy and lay communities, the various health professions, and the Abrahamic religious traditions.[111]

Two other scholarly organizations, both now shuttered, played an important role in academic research on religion within medicine and healthcare.

The Academy of Religion and Mental Health, founded in 1954 in New York with the support of the Josiah Macy Jr. Foundation, sponsored a series of annual symposia in the 1950s and 1960s on themes at the intersection of religion, medicine, and the behavioral sciences.[112] The published proceedings, featuring contributions from world-famous scholars, are among the most essential documents ever produced in this field.[113] The academy also founded the influential peer-reviewed *Journal of Religion and Health* in 1961, still publishing after nearly sixty volumes. In 1968 the academy and journal merged with other institutions to become the Institutes of Religion and Health, and in 1972 was renamed the Blanton-Peale Institute.[114]

The Park Ridge Center for Health, Faith, and Ethics, founded in 1985 by University of Chicago professor Martin Marty, filled an important role into the early 2000s.[115] Its mission was as an interfaith, interdisciplinary organization that "explores and enhances the interaction of health, faith, and ethics through research, education and consultation to improve the lives of individuals and communities."[116] The center published a magazine titled *Second Opinion*, hosted research fellows, and produced many scholarly works, including an important book series called Health/Medicine and the Faith Traditions.[117] This project was designed "to deal systematically with the contributions of the various faith traditions to . . . core themes in life confronted by the sick and those who care for them." In all, fourteen monographs were published, mostly by Crossroad, covering the world's major religions and Christian denominations.[118]

Religion in Medical Education

A primary function of these centers and organizations, alongside research and service, has been the education of medical and premedical students and continuing education of healthcare professionals. This reason, above all, is why most were established within or in conjunction with educational institutions. Religious content is delivered in many ways, some quite creatively, not solely through lecture-based classroom teaching.

If there is an underlying motive for incorporating learning about religion into medical education it is simply this, according to Puchalski and Larson: medical educators have begun to recognize "the need to bring the art of compassionate caregiving back into the medical school curriculum."[119] This statement suggests that something was lost that once was present in the education of physicians before modern laboratory-based, specialty-organized, technology-driven medical education was introduced at the turn of the twentieth century. Perhaps the implied critique of how doctors train since then is responsible in part for the animosity from secular, rational skeptics over what is perceived as an imposition of religion where it does not belong.

No matter: since NIHR's Faith and Medicine program in the 1990s, enough momentum has been gained that these curricular innovations are well institutionalized. By 2004, according to a review in *JAMA*, the number of medical schools incorporating religious and spiritual content into medical education had reached eighty-four;[120] by 2010, as noted earlier, the proportion of schools exceeded 90 percent.[121] Learning experiences include lectures, small group discussions, and practice at conducting patient interviews,[122] the latter an important way to elicit information on religion in the clinical setting but fraught with challenges that inhibit some physicians.[123] Classroom teaching is multifaceted: reading and discussion of published studies, presentation of cases, acquisition of interview and communication skills, and learning about healthcare chaplains and the health-impacting beliefs, practices, and cultural traditions of the world's religions.[124]

This sea change in medical education is an instructive case study in how educators can recognize an oversight in how physicians train, then successfully and in a short amount of time do something about it. In this instance, medical educators saw that a focus on the etiology of disease and prescription of effective therapies, which of course is essential in medical training, does not need to happen "at the expense of fostering caring and humane concern for patients."[125] In less than a generation, the traditional organization of undergraduate medical training has been reconstructed in other ways too, aimed at producing more well-rounded practitioners skilled in delivering more compassionate whole-person care to patients. Acknowledging that humans are spiritual beings facing more than just physical and mental challenges has nudged medicine in a direction that has resulted in rethinking how doctors learn to practice their trade.

Residency programs, too, especially in psychiatry, have developed objectives for teaching about spirituality, with an emphasis on developing requisite knowledge, skills, and attitudes to competently care for patients.[126] This emphasis entails performing spiritual assessments, incorporating spirituality into treatment plans, encouraging residents' self-reflection about how their own beliefs influence their clinical decision-making, learning to implement certain spiritually based therapeutic models, and understanding when to make pastoral referrals.[127]

Over the past decade, reports in the medical literature and popular media describe how such coursework and learning experiences make a difference in how physicians in training see their calling and respond to challenging situations in the clinic. Some examples:

- *Medical school.* At Albert Einstein College of Medicine, the first-year Introduction to Clinical Medicine class and third-year Patient, Doctors, and Communities class contain units on how patients' religious beliefs influence treatment decisions, how to communicate with patients from diverse religious backgrounds, and how to make chaplaincy referrals.[128]
- *Residency training.* At Morehouse School of Medicine, physicians in the public health/preventive medicine residency program participate in a longitudinal community practicum in partnership with a faith-based organization, learning to conduct a community health needs assessment and design an intervention tailored to needs of underserved populations.[129]
- *Graduate school.* The list of training competency clusters for the graduate program in clinical psychology at Loma Linda University School of Medicine includes "proficiency in the appropriate use of religion/spirituality in clinical practice," encompassing requisite knowledge, attitudes, and practice skills that account for the religious and cultural diversity of patients.[130]

Many more examples can be found in North America and overseas, notably in the United Kingdom[131] and Brazil.[132] Among fellowship training programs, there has been less progress. A review of such programs in palliative medicine, for example, found that while they unanimously incorporate spirituality within their curricula, in some fashion, they have not incorporated robust or systematic methods of delivering educational content or evaluating effectiveness.[133]

Nursing schools have also developed innovative ways to incorporate teaching on religion within undergraduate and graduate programs,[134] in the United States[135] and other countries.[136] Spirituality content has been introduced into coursework on nursing practice, health assessment, public health nursing, and working with geriatric, psychiatric, and obstetric patients.[137] To achieve the best results—training knowledgeable and compassionate nurses—material on religion and spirituality should be "threaded" longitudinally throughout nursing curricula.[138] This can only be achieved with strong support from nursing school and university administrators,[139] something maybe more likely to occur in faith-based institutions, such as Baylor or Liberty University.

Content on religion, faith, and spirituality are integrated into educational curricula in many settings, not just medical or nursing school classes. Other places where one finds teaching on religion and health or religion and medicine is within the academic health sciences, including graduate and undergraduate programs in the medical humanities, graduate schools of public health, and complementary and integrative medicine centers within medical schools.

Medical humanities is a relatively new interdisciplinary field at the intersection of the biomedical sciences, medical education, clinical practice, and the core humanities disciplines, namely philosophy, history, literature, religion, and the arts. Also included are non-biomedical professional fields that affect medicine and healthcare, such as law, ethics, and public policy. Medical humanities emerged in the 1970s and 1980s in response to the observed overmedicalization of the physician-patient relationship and the looming crisis of technology dominating healthcare treatment at the expense of human caring. The promise was to infuse humanistic values into medical education and the healing arts, producing medical professionals attuned to whole-person care—to a view of humans as a nexus of body, mind, and soul.

From the beginning, consideration of human spirituality has been featured in efforts to define the scope of the medical humanities,[140] one of the few spaces within academic medicine where such discussions have been ongoing and valued. By now, medical humanities programs, centers, and institutes have been established at many academic medical centers, often also providing instruction in bioethics, history of medicine, spirituality, and other subjects. These programs sponsor medical education courses and electives, postgraduate education, and the training of academic scholars. At some institutions, religion and health centers and medical humanities centers—and centers for medical ethics—are one and the same, or have merged together from separate programs over time. Among the oldest (since 1982) and most prominent is BCM's center, discussed earlier. Medical humanities and religious studies are both highlighted within its listings of faculty expertise.[141]

Prominent medical humanities centers with medical education offerings on religious subjects include the McGovern Center for Humanities and Ethics at the University of Texas Health Science Center at Houston; the Institute for the Medical Humanities at the University of Texas Medical Branch; the Trent Center for Bioethics, Humanities, and History of Medicine at Duke; the Center for Medical Humanities, Compassionate Care, and Bioethics at SUNY Stony Brook; and the Program in Health and Humanities at Emory. Content is delivered through required courses, blue-book electives, independent study classes, field research, clinical shadowing, lecture series and symposia, and dedicated internship and externship programs.

The medical humanities field has a professional association, the American Society for Bioethics and Humanities, that counts religion as one of its core disciplines. Accordingly, it sponsors a Religion, Spirituality, and Bioethics affinity group, and includes sessions on religion and spirituality in its annual scientific conference and continuing education events.[142]

As the medical humanities field has continued to gain traction, it is becoming recognized that a significant and unmet need for more expansive content exists earlier in the educational trajectory of medical and healthcare students, specifically in the premedical years. This recognition is fueled by widespread changes in contemporary medical school curricula aimed at introducing more humanistic, whole-patient-oriented, and problem-based learning experiences, and by greater sensitivity to cultivating cross-cultural competence in students. To adapt to this changing environment, undergraduate degree programs have begun appearing in the United States.

The earliest of these at a major university (since 2004) is the Medical Humanities Program at Baylor University. At Baylor, as well as the estimated seventy-plus other undergraduate programs, religious content is present, as required courses or electives, including professional shadowing experiences in healthcare settings.[143] Many programs are offered at faith-based colleges and universities.[144] Baylor has a required course on Christian spirituality and healthcare, and I have given an upper-level undergraduate seminar course on the history of religious healing, a subject taught in other courses throughout the country in departments or programs outside of medical humanities, such as anthropology or religious studies.[145]

Religious coursework and content are also located within schools of public health, besides those at Emory and Harvard. An outstanding resource here is psychologist Doug Oman's book *Why Religion and Spirituality Matters for Public Health*,[146] which details public health education on religion within leading graduate schools of public health. These include the public health programs at Berkeley,[147] Boston,[148] Michigan,[149] Drexel,[150] and the University of Illinois at Chicago.[151] This is an interesting development as public health is a field historically more progressive and secular and populated by programs at public universities, in comparison with the medical humanities degree programs found at so many private Protestant and Catholic colleges and universities. Teaching about religion in schools of public health points to a growing realization of the consonance of certain faith-based values, such as communitarianism and social justice, with the core distinctives of public health.[152]

Another place in which religion is incorporated in medical education is within academic centers for complementary and integrative medicine. Formerly known as alternative medicine and, before that, as holistic medicine, the complementary and integrative medicine community in the United States has been a welcoming home for medical education on the subject. By convention, the term *spirituality* is used here, rather than *religion*, perhaps because the former is considered more inclusive and less tied to institutional faith traditions. The etymology and history of these concepts as used in medicine has been parsed, debated, and critiqued,[153] but notwithstanding the preferred terminology, undergraduate and postgraduate training and continuing education on religion, health, and healing have been a cornerstone of this field since the early 1990s.

In 1992 the NIH held its first major conference on alternative medicine and commissioned proceedings that became known as the Chantilly Report.[154] Coedited by Dave Larson, the NIH identified seven fields of practice, one of which—mind-body interventions—was based in part on the literature on spirituality, religion, and health, drawing heavily on Larson's own reviews as well as mine.[155] Major integrative medicine centers at Duke, Arizona, Stanford, Michigan, Columbia, and elsewhere have treated spirituality as an essential component of therapeutic practice and as a subject that must be engaged to ensure cultural competency in practitioners.[156] Research and education on spirituality and health have been integral to efforts by freestanding private institutions as well, such as IONS in Petaluma, California,[157] and the recently closed Samueli Institute in Alexandria, Virginia.[158]

Besides classroom instruction and practicum experiences, learning occurs in settings outside of formal degree-granting institutions. Faith-based professional organizations sponsor conferences for students and continuing education for practitioners. Examples include the Christian Medical and Dental Associations,[159] the locally organized Maimonides Society,[160] the Islamic Medical Association of North America,[161] and the United Kingdom's Christian Medical Fellowship.[162] The Nurses Christian Fellowship,[163] which publishes the *Journal of Christian Nursing*, and the American Holistic Nurses Association,[164] which publishes the *Journal of Holistic Nursing*, offer conferences, academic scholarships, and educational content on spirituality.

Additionally, religious safe spaces exist at most academic medical centers for patients and families, as well as for faculty, staff, and students. These include places for prayer, reflection, and meditation, and are associated with local ministries, institutional healthcare chaplaincy, or chapels located within hospitals. Learning events may be held at these sites. At TMC, for example, a large Catholic Student Ministry sponsors worship, fellowship, and service activities and educational programs across many institutions throughout the medical center.[165] There is also a Chabad House at TMC, offering a similar menu of services to the Jewish community, as well as direct support to patients and families.[166]

Also, throughout TMC, nearly a dozen individual chapels, located at the various healthcare institutions, each sponsors its own schedule of activities, and numerous other prayer and meditation spaces are available.[167] These include four dedicated spaces just at Houston Methodist Hospital: the Wiess Memorial Chapel, the Muslim Prayer Room, the Outpatient Center Meditation Room, and the new outdoor Healing Garden. Whenever I am at Methodist, I try to find time for reflection at the wonderful chapel, and have visited the other sites too. Methodist may be especially attentive to the diverse spiritual needs of its constituencies compared to other hospitals, but it is not unique in providing such spaces. Faith is a visible and accessible presence for all who pass through the doors at such institutions, whether patients, families, practitioners, or students.

The Future

The daily life of academic medical centers, especially for students and residents, is a bustle of activities, leaving little time for looking inward. Academic medical centers, including schools of medicine, nursing, public health, and other health professions, make concerted efforts to carve out spaces for faith and spirituality to coexist alongside biomedicine, science, and patient care. This practice benefits students and their education, but ultimately benefits patients and populations who will gain from well-rounded, culturally competent, and compassionate professionals to serve them.

Of all the ways that religion and medicine have come into contact and continue to partner with each other, I suspect that the depth and breadth of what is described in this chapter may be most surprising. Medical and health sciences educators have done admirably in ensuring that future practitioners and scientists have ample opportunity to develop and maintain themselves as whole persons, body and mind and soul, something so often shunted aside due to constant stress and long years of training. Even for those not inclined to spiritual pursuits, schools and training programs have ensured that curricula feature the latest research findings from clinical and scientific studies pointing to salutary effects of faith or spirituality in the lives of patients.

Considerable momentum has been gained since the 1990s, owing much to the work of Dave Larson and NIHR. The Faith and Medicine curriculum program and various research conferences and reports seeded so much of what came after, and are most responsible for growth of the various initiatives described throughout this chapter. But if Dave were still here, he would encourage forward thinking on the part of educators in order to identify ways to more effectively communicate information about religion and health to students, practitioners, scientists, and laypeople. A few suggestions that I believe would carry on the spirit of what Dave started:

- *Undergraduate medical education.* More required hours with spiritual content, especially in clerkship rotations, and more elective offerings on special topics such as religious bioethics and end-of-life care, pastoral shadowing experiences, partnerships with community faith-based groups, and research on mental health.

- *Postgraduate medical education.* More content in residency training in more specialties, including family practice, internal medicine, psychiatry, pediatrics, ob-gyn, and geriatrics, and involving spiritual assessment, chaplaincy and ethics referrals, and grand rounds with case presentations.
- *Graduate education in the health sciences.* More coursework and internship and externship opportunities, specific to educational norms of respective health sciences fields, including for health educators, nurses, clinical psychologists, and public health researchers.
- *Postdoctoral training.* More specially focused opportunities for already credentialed professionals to dig deeper and gain research expertise in religion and health, modeled after existing programs such as Duke's annual summer research workshop on religion, spirituality, and health[168] or Harvard's fellowship program in health, religion, and spirituality.[169]

At present, this may be a utopian vision. Still, at the pace this field is evolving, some changes can be expected and some are already underway. A long-term goal—besides, of course, better-trained caregivers and more effective healthcare—is translation of cutting-edge scholarship into professional competency standards and clinical standards of practice issued by specialty boards for physicians, nurses, health educators, and other healthcare professionals.[170] These standards will need to be tailored to respective professions and specialties, as each engages religion in different ways and thus requires distinct guidelines. A helpful and impressive first step is *Spirituality and Religion within the Culture of Medicine*, published in 2017.[171] The editors, Harvard professors Michael Balboni and John Peteet, solicited contributions from experts in over a dozen specialties, including pediatrics, oncology, internal medicine, and surgery, as well as from other scholarly fields such as law and ethics, each weighing in on these very issues with case reports, guidance for practice standards, and ideas for research.

All that being so, such innovations may be easier called for than accomplished. Not to throw cold water on any enthusiasm I may have generated, but I am reminded of an experience at the beginning of my teaching career. It was the early 1990s, and I was a young associate professor of family and community medicine in Virginia. I was asked to lecture first-year family practice residents during an assigned slot in the regular weekly didactic sessions, held every Wednesday. Our department chair wanted me to present the latest research on religion and health, in order to bring our residents up to speed on a subject that they likely were not exposed to in medical school.

After offering a brief and early version of the material covered in the previous chapter, a young resident approached me with a look of anguish in his eyes and plaintively lamented, "You mean there's something *else* we have ask about?" This knocked me for a loop, for just a moment, after which I was flooded with guilt. Our residents were trained to take no more than about seven to ten minutes per patient encounter, and that covered history-taking, physical examination, formulating a treatment plan, and everything else that goes into a clinical visit. Our department was strict about enforcing this time limit, yet here was a professor, who was not even an M.D., unpacking a bunch of information about a subject they had never considered might be relevant to their work.

After all these years I still remember that class session and remain earnestly sympathetic. Cultivating good listening skills, encouraging *brief* spiritual assessment where it seems appropriate, and imparting familiarity with resources for referral seem about the best that medical educators can hope for in most situations. But even these small steps are vital, as there is a price to pay for reinforcing tacit misperceptions of religion as wholly irrelevant to the prevention of illness, promotion of health, and practice of the healing arts. While forward progress has been made since my experience with our residents—this chapter provides documentation—old beliefs die hard.

Back again in the early 1990s Dave Larson told me of a small study that he hoped to write up. Alongside his series of reviews of research on religion within psychiatry and other medical fields, he had surveyed the coverage of religious topics within the many guidebooks on the market geared to self-study for the medical board exams. Only in the psychiatry guides, and only in those of a few publishers, did the words *religion, religious, spiritual*, and so on even appear in the text. Where they did, it was almost invariably as part of a list of symptoms of diagnoses of psychosis and related disorders. *Religiosity*, for example, was listed alongside drooling, twitching, bizarre ideations, delusions, and so on. Dave was aghast but never did write up his review. An informal perusal of the current state of some of these guides finds the negative connotations mostly absent, but still only perfunctory mention in most guidebooks of religion or spirituality as clinically relevant, although a few exceptions do exist.[172]

Still, I do not wish to imply pessimism. As an educator I have noted a change in the most recent cohorts of students regarding their recognition of the role of religion in health, healing, and medical care. What once seemed strange or unlikely is now part of the body of tacit knowledge related to sound medical and nursing practice, whether particular students value faith or spirituality in their own life or not. Students are able to acknowledge that such issues motivate the health-related behavior of many patients, influence their utilization of health-care services and resources, and may impact on their mental and physical health status. As the next chapter shows, religion also exerts an influence on the health-care decision-making of many patients and practitioners and on guidelines that animate medical care, informing prescriptions and proscriptions surrounding many sensitive medical and healthcare issues.

7

Prescriptions and Proscriptions

The 1970s witnessed emergence of a popular critique of the concepts and practice norms of Western medicine. Parallel to movements in politics, education, psychology, and religion, laid out in works like Alvin Toffler's *Future Shock*[1] and Marilyn Ferguson's *The Aquarian Conspiracy*,[2] calls for more humanistic, responsive, and patient-centered medical care became widespread. Among the most influential attempts to refocus the culture of the healing arts came from an unlikely source: Norman Cousins, former editor-in-chief of the *Saturday Review*, who wrote a captivating account of his experiences as a connective tissue disease patient.[3] Cousins's bestselling *Anatomy of an Illness* stimulated efforts to rethink what goes on in medical care settings—how decisions are made, for what reasons, and who gets to decide—and jumpstarted a national discussion of medical self-care, personal responsibility, holistic medicine, mind-body healing, and healthcare reform. These discussions continue today.

Cousins successfully tapped into the zeitgeist of the decade, a time when presumptions of Western medicine were being rethought, including foundations of the so-called medical model.[4] Medicine had become too reliant upon technology and too impersonal and uncaring, and popular and academic medical writers were both calling for change. Medicine was increasingly recognized as insensitive to human psychological needs, and modern physicians were characterized as "specialists without spirit."[5] How disease was defined and treated, and especially how patient values and concerns were marginalized in clinical decision-making, were being documented, mulled over, and studied.

This era of critique and self-reflection within medicine was the product of a conversation that began at least a decade earlier. Pioneering bioethicist Albert R. Jonsen described how widely hailed postwar advances in medical technology inserted "impersonal machines that intervened between doctor and patient," raising genuine questions and concerns that required summoning a set of "new intellectual resources . . . to struggle with the new questions."[6] Medical advances based on technological progress, he noted, were increasingly seen as a double-edged sword, with medicine, medical care institutions, and the medical profession on the precipice of an ideological and public relations crisis:

> As the 1960s dawned, this unalloyed optimism began to falter and qualms began to tweak the conscience of those who were responsible for the advances

Religion and Medicine. Jeff Levin, Oxford University Press (2020) © Oxford University Press.
DOI: 10.1093/oso/9780190867355.001.0001

in medicine and science. Some public opinion expressed qualms about the way in which the introduction of medical technologies damages the relationship between physicians and patients by encouraging the growth of new specialties to the detriment of general practice and by making the relationship more impersonal.[7]

Throughout the decade, Jonsen added, leading clinicians and medical scientists "broke their silence . . . [and] aired their qualms of conscience at unprecedented conferences, ruminating before their colleagues and even lay audiences about the social and ethical problems involved in medical and scientific progress."[8] What began as a "slow accumulation of concerns about the ambiguity of scientific progress"[9] eventually gave birth to the field of bioethics, a term believed to have been coined in 1970 by University of Wisconsin scientist Van Rensselaer Potter.[10]

Ethical deliberations were not new to Western medicine. Writing on this subject, according to Jonsen, dates at least to English physician Thomas Percival's *Medical Ethics*, published in 1803.[11] Moreover, long-standing traditions of medical and health-related commentary are found within Roman Catholic moral theology and Protestant theological ethics, dating back centuries, as well as in the writings of moral philosophers[12] as far back as Greece and Rome.[13] A principal source of authority for clinical and biomedical decision-making was and always has been the dictates of respective faith traditions. Although not necessarily formalized within medical practice standards—and, when articulated, the idea met with resistance from apostles of a more technologically based medicine[14]—the tenets of religions, including rulings by ecclesial or clerical bodies, have always carried weight both with religious laypeople and religious physicians and nurses.

Duke's Farr Curlin elaborates on this point:

> I suspect that no reader will find it hard to believe that religion matters for medical ethics. Ethics, or *practical* reason, is that domain of reason that has to do with how we ought to act—what we ought to do in any particular case and how we ought to live in the broader sense. Religions obviously make authoritative claims about how we ought to act and how we ought to live. Where we find a medical ethics question, therefore, we will find religious answers, and religious answers will frequently differ from those that emerge from secular frames of reasoning. . . .[15]

With expansion of moral and ethical discourse on the practice of medicine throughout the 1960s and 1970s, religious voices maintained an important place at the table. This includes representatives of formal religious institutions and people of faith within the community of healthcare providers and administrators, as well as influential laypeople, including patients and policymakers. As Jonsen has made clear,

> Bioethics does not belong to the bioethicists who worry about its disciplinary status. From its beginnings, bioethics has gotten people talking. It is public discourse carried on by many people in many settings.[16]

Nor has this conversation been exclusively Christian in context. An important figure in this movement was Rabbi Immanuel Jakobovits, philosopher and former chief rabbi of the United Hebrew Congregations of the (British) Commonwealth. His Ph.D. dissertation at the University of London, published in 1959 as *Jewish Medical Ethics*,[17] established the contemporary field bearing its name and was the earliest work to reconcile ethical challenges of modern medical practice with *halachah* (Jewish law) and rabbinic teachings.[18] *Jewish Medical Ethics* was also among the foundational texts for the field of bioethics. Jakobovits made clear that he saw moral teachings of religions and practice standards of medicine as mutually impactful—each created challenges for the other. Accordingly, he sought to survey

> the attitude of Judaism, as well as of Christian and other religious teachings, to moral and religious problems in medical practice. . . . My main concern was to analyse the moral views of the major faiths on various medical procedures which may impinge on religious principles. . . .[19]

Even after his ascension to chief rabbi in 1967 Jakobovits continued to make scholarly contributions to medical ethics,[20] helping shape its engagement of religion and overall program. He is widely remembered as a significant figure in academic ethics, even among those unfamiliar with his role as revered leader of the Orthodox Jewish community of the United Kingdom and one of the most important figures in twentieth-century Judaism.

While the acknowledged father of Jewish medical ethics,[21] Jakobovits was by no means the first scholar to devote himself to medical *halachah*. The *t'shuvot* (*responsa*, or rabbinic rulings) literature in Judaism goes back centuries, and much of this writing concerns *halachic* deliberations on medical care.[22] Contemporaneous with Jakobovits, great *poskim* (rabbinic decisors) within the Orthodox world, notably Rabbi Moshe Feinstein and his son-in-law Rabbi Moshe Dovid Tendler,[23] and Israeli rabbis Shlomo Zalman Auerbach[24] and Eliezer Yehudah Waldenberg,[25] offered religious guidance regarding clinical decisions. The difference between Jakobovits's approach to medical ethics and the older tradition of medical *halachah* is that "Rabbi Jakobovits focused on moral problems raised by medicine and medical practice as opposed to those raised by Jewish law."[26] His approach, then, was in keeping with long-standing traditions of writing on medical matters with Roman Catholic moral theology and philosophy, something that distanced him in some respects from traditional rabbinic sources.[27]

Academic religious scholars such as Jakobovits and his Christian contemporaries—including Episcopalian minister Joseph Fletcher, Methodist theologian and Princeton professor Paul Ramsey, and Jesuit moral theologian Richard A. McCormick—were instrumental in the birth and growth of medical ethics as a profession and field of study.[28] Since then, another couple generations of religious and theological scholars have provided leadership to the field. These include, among many others, Kenneth Vaux,[29] from the Institute of Religion and later Garrett-Evangelical Theological Seminary; Allen D. Verhey,[30] Harmon L. Smith,[31] and Stanley Hauerwas,[32] from Duke; Gilbert Meileander, from Valparaiso University;[33] and David C. Thomasma, from Loyola University Chicago, along with his collaborator Edmund D. Pellegrino, from Georgetown, a physician and Roman Catholic lay leader.[34] Also noteworthy are John Swinton,[35] University of Aberdeen practical theologian and minister, and Stony Brook professor Stephen Post, editor-in-chief of the third edition of the *Encyclopedia of Bioethics*[36] and trained at the University of Chicago Divinity School in comparative religious ethics and moral philosophy.

In his chapter titled "A History of Religion and Bioethics" in the *Handbook of Bioethics and Religion*, Jonsen examines the tacit presumption that while religious considerations may have been seminal for bioethics, their presence as a salient force has since faded.[37] "This opinion is a commonplace among many who have opinions about bioethics,"[38] he noted, and though he draws no definitive conclusion he suggests that there has been a "revival of interest in religion"[39] within the field. I am inclined to agree. Indeed, others have argued that the rise of this field itself represented a "bioethics revival" and that this rekindling of interest in medical ethics is attributable to work by prominent Christian and Jewish theological scholars.[40]

Medical decision-making is and always has been a religiously informed space, even before there was a recognized field of bioethics.[41] Religious values influence medical decision-making in the clinical setting, across the life course, and across the world's faith traditions.[42] For controversial issues such as abortion, stem-cell research, euthanasia, test-tube babies, organ donation, and brain death, dictates of religious belief systems have influenced and continue to influence decisions made by medical care providers, patients, and families. This is so regardless of whether such deliberations are officially enshrined in policies of healthcare institutions or government or are approved by the most staunchly secular apologists of technological medical progress.

Whether the shifting sands of academic scholarship are keeping up with these trends, I cannot say. I am not a bioethicist. But I concur with sociologist John H. Evans, who observes, "Religion is inevitably a part of American public bioethics, because the public is very religious."[43] Religion, he explains, informs bioethics through informing public opinion and public policy. At the same time, religious bioethicists and the institutional faith traditions both approach decisions regarding medical conduct from a diversity of perspectives. The former have clustered around two methodological camps—casuistry and principlism[44]—and healthy debate over reconciling these positions has been ongoing for decades.[45] The latter are as fragmented in their positions on respective clinical matters as about theology and ontology.

Notwithstanding the ubiquity of religious input into biomedical and clinical policies and practices, for particular procedures or courses of action there is inconsistency across belief systems. Conclusions regarding what is proscribed or prescribed by respective religious codes differ both across and among Christian and Jewish bioethicists[46] and across other religions.[47] A notable example is the ethical status of elective pregnancy termination within the biblical faith traditions. The diversity of opinions and approaches advocated by earnest Christians and Jews underscores how substantially different conclusions may be drawn as to how God and Scripture intend for one to act in the face of respective medical challenges. I address this most contentious of bioethical issues, abortion, later in the chapter.

A Field Is Born

As noted, discussion of moral and ethical issues in the care of medical patients can be traced back centuries. A search of the National Library of Medicine's PubMed index identifies over two hundred thousand scholarly publications on the topic of ethics, including hits on *medical ethics* in English or other languages dating to the early nineteenth century. Within Western medicine, thoughtful observations on the need to train students in the ethics of medical care were published in *JAMA* almost one hundred years ago.[48] Subsequent events, such as the Nuremberg trials for perpetrators of Nazi war crimes that exposed ghastly medical experimentation,[49] also galvanized physicians, philosophers, educators, and others to more deeply reflect on good and bad, and right and wrong, within the practice of medicine.

As bioethics emerged as a formal field of study and practice, it was in a sense a joint project of professionals in various disciplines, fields, and specialties working to coalesce strands of thinking and writing and speculation within their respective intellectual communities. In Jonsen's history of bioethics, he described the key contributions of theologians focused on "rediscovering the tradition"[50] and philosophers laboring at "clarifying the concepts."[51] Each followed a particular program of work, one theological and one conceptual, and in their mutual dialogue and conversations with others (e.g., physicians, lawyers, policymakers) forged something akin to a new discipline. It is uncertain, though, whether *discipline* is an accurate term: even after half a century of work, it is difficult to identify a single master theory, set of common principles, or dominant methodology.[52] On the other hand, it is not clear that one can identify such for established disciplines such as sociology, psychology, or economics either. Suffice it to say that, functionally speaking, bioethics indeed gives the appearance of a field or discipline, even if no unanimity exists among self-identified constituents on many substantive matters.[53]

The diversity of viewpoints is no more obvious than when it comes to underlying principles—if any—said to justify particular courses of action. There is no agreement on whether such principles even exist or are useful to unpack for the field, and if the answer to both questions is yes, little consensus is present as to the content of such guidance. In *The Foundations of Bioethics*, physician-philosopher H. Tristram Engelhardt Jr. underscored this point with a marvelous reference to the "cacophonous plurality of bioethics."[54] This cogent phrase is the closest thing to a summary of the state of the field and points to special challenges facing the intrepid scholars synthesizing enormous amount of material from so many fields and sources in order to support the work of those helping people who require medical care and to inform the healthcare policymaking process.

Without disparaging the many successes and advances in bioethics that have ensued, even within the field there is considerable skepticism over whether bioethicists have succeeded in accommodating or accounting for this substantial diversity of opinion and hermeneutics. Still today, according to Engelhardt, "Bioethics remains in the plural."[55] He goes on to say, "Moral diversity is real. It is real in fact and in principle. Bioethics and health care policy have yet to take this diversity seriously."[56]

This diversity is especially, and primarily, visible when it comes to religious sources of moral guidance, notably references to God or the Divine or presumably universal principles. People of faith may be just as divided among themselves, or more so, than differences that separate the religious and secular voices weighing in on important decisions made in the clinical setting and in distribution of medical resources. Ideally, it may seem, an appeal to God "can provide the perfect answers to the perfect questions."[57] However, notes Engelhardt, "all do not listen to the Deity, or listen in the same way. As a consequence, there is general disagreement about the perfect question and their perfect answers."[58]

An honest perusal of the academic bioethics literature and of ethics statements proffered by professional and licensing organizations within medicine and healthcare and by denominational groups reveals this same cacophony of viewpoints. Bioethicists and medical care providers, especially writing from explicitly faith-based orientations, continue to expand on the same themes animating discourse in this field for decades, without reaching universal consensus or resolution. Sometimes they speak in harmony if not in unison, but more often, it seems to me, at cross-purposes. Granted, I am an outsider when it comes to this field: I consider myself well read on the subject, but am not on the front lines conducting bioethics research or offering clinical consults. Perhaps credentialed scholars and professionals in the field will disagree with these conclusions, but in my opinion they are self-evident.

Moreover, it may be pollyannaish to expect that true consensus will ever be obtainable. Principlist approaches to medical decision-making—that is, appeals to fundamental principles to inform and guide such decisions, as opposed to more situationally based guidance derived from contingencies of specific cases—may in the final analysis be impossible, if by this we mean underlying principles that imply the same thing to all possible constituencies and are interpreted the same way.[59] Again, Engelhardt weighs in:

> Different ways of articulating concerns to achieve the good or avoid evil will lead to different claims regarding what is good to do. . . . There is no single secular canonical sense of what it is to do the good, for the goods open to persons are multiple and incompatible. As a consequence, different rules for acting beneficently will conflict.[60]

Another source of conceptual confusion is competing terminology to define the field. Labels such as *bioethics, medical ethics,* and *clinical ethics* are often used interchangeably, but they do not mean the same thing. They might best be thought of as conceptually nested. That is, *bioethics* references moral and ethical issues that arise in the biomedical enterprise broadly, including research and policy-related dimensions. *Medical ethics* refers to those values and judgments that do or should govern the practice of medicine. It is more about a real or implied professional code of conduct. *Clinical ethics* is concerned with parsing discrete decisions that medical care providers must make during the clinical encounter. To some extent, these terms define distinct, if overlapping, literatures, and issues that arise in one context are not necessarily as problematic in others. Significantly, religious concerns have been brought to bear on deliberations in each context.

Religious scholarship within bioethics has evolved like other fields of study, with individuals and institutions waxing and waning in influence.[61] Since the 1970s and 1980s, important figures have included Kenneth Vaux at the Institute of Religion at Texas Medical Center and Baruch Brody at Rice University and

Baylor College of Medicine. Also significant was the Park Ridge Center for Health, Faith and Ethics,[62] established by Martin Marty and described in Chapter 6. The Kennedy Institute of Ethics at Georgetown University,[63] founded in 1971 and currently directed by Daniel Sulmasy, and the Hastings Center,[64] founded in 1969 by philosopher Daniel Callahan,[65] both were instrumental in establishing bioethics as a field and have sponsored conversations on the salience of religious and secular themes and perspectives in bioethics.[66]

Since the 1960s, parallel to the advent of bioethics as a field, hospitals have convened ethics committees or boards charged with vetting controversial clinical decisions. The idea was slow in taking hold.[67] By 1983, according to national survey data, only 1 percent of U.S. hospitals had formed such committees;[68] by the turn of the century, over 90 percent had done so;[69] and by 2007, about 100 percent of large hospitals were on board.[70] Today, these committees are mandated by accreditation bodies—including, since 1992, the Joint Commission on Accreditation of Healthcare Organizations[71]—so compliance is close to universal, although the effectiveness of such committees has remained a point of contention,[72] perhaps due to an absence of consistent and specific standards.[73] They routinely, if inconsistently and hesitatingly, must slog through complicated moral issues requiring the parsing of religiously informed and defined considerations, such as in the disposition of human beings at the beginning and end of life. Healthcare chaplains are often represented on these boards in order to give voice to religious concerns in general and to sectarian perspectives, where applicable. Hospital ethics committees exist throughout the world, including in Europe, Asia, and the Middle East.[74]

Of similar vintage are institutional review boards (IRBs) at academic medical institutions, convened to vet the use of human subjects in clinical and other health-related research protocols.[75] Since passage of the National Research Act of 1974,[76] an IRB's presence is mandated for recipient institutions by federal funding agencies, including the NIH.[77] I was privileged to be appointed as graduate student representative on the IRB at the University of North Carolina School of Public Health from 1982 to 1983, and served as secondary reviewer on several projects. It was not uncommon for religiously contested concerns to arise, but at the time no clear roadmap was available on how to proceed systematically.[78]

Today, bioethics is a substantial professional and academic enterprise. Since 1998 a membership society exists, the American Society for Bioethics and Humanities (ASBH), which evolved out of three former organizations for bioethicists.[79] The ASBH has eighteen hundred members and sponsors an annual conference. The field supports many prominent academic journals, such as the *AMA Journal of Ethics*; the *American Journal of Bioethics*; the *Hastings Center Report*; the *Journal of Law, Medicine, and Ethics*; the *Journal of Medical Ethics*;

the *Journal of Medicine and Philosophy*; the *Kennedy Institute of Ethics Journal*; and *Theoretical Medicine and Bioethics*. At present, there are nearly one hundred academic centers in the field,[80] and more than seventy certificate, degree, or fellowship programs.[81]

It is not a simple matter to track how many of these centers and programs feature events, research projects, or scholars focused on religious themes. But an informal audit of colleagues at some of these institutions suggests that religion, broadly defined, is ubiquitous throughout the institutional field of bioethics, although not consistently central to the work of respective institutions or people. Another indicator of the continued importance of religion is the presence of religious content across the four editions of the *Encyclopedia of Bioethics*. From the first edition, published in 1978,[82] to the fourth edition, published in 2014,[83] the number of entries whose titles or headings include explicitly religious or theological categories or words has remained at about forty. To me, this fact indicates consistent interest in and recognition of the importance of religion as a foundation of contemporary bioethics, and suggests that the presupposition of a waxing and waning (and waxing again) of religious bioethics may not be completely accurate. It has been there all along.

Notwithstanding evidence of the growth of bioethics as a field and a continued presence of religious scholarship, scholars, and content, an unsettling awareness of Jonsen's "cacophonous plurality" is never far away. In a news story about the founding of the Park Ridge Center in 1986, Martin Marty laments, "Medical ethics is a sophisticated and promising field, but it has often developed independently of religious concerns. You don't have Mormon blood-transfusions or Baptist brain-surgery, yet every story on medical ethics has a religious dimension."[84] This is a fact of life in the clinical encounter. Yet despite how much bioethics has evolved and grown over the past three decades, religious and theological concerns still confront medical ethics scholars and professionals no less than physicians and other medical providers responsible for care, as well as the laypeople and patients who receive this care.[85]

Fortunately, efforts have been made to provide focused guidance. Besides the academic works cited earlier, such as Guinn's *Handbook of Bioethics and Religion*,[86] another great resource is the Religious Beliefs and Health Care Decisions handbook series published by the Park Ridge Center in the 1990s, a set of religion- and denomination-specific guides.[87] The Jewish volume, for example, written by Rabbi Elliot N. Dorff, is two dozen pages and contains a detailed unpacking of historical and *halachic* perspectives on a wide range of healthcare issues requiring clinical decisions and policymaking.[88] Within Judaism, helpful denomination-sponsored material also is available, such as a series of bioethics monographs published by the Reform movement under the editorship of Rabbi Richard F. Address.[89]

Rights and Wrongs, Dos and Don'ts

Within bioethics, notwithstanding the plurality of viewpoints and perspectives, theoretical models have been proposed to organize and inform ethical decision-making in the clinical encounter and with respect to healthcare policy. Most prominent has been the model that philosopher Tom L. Beauchamp and theologian James F. Childress have proposed.[90] They identified four moral principles, described as "moral norms," which "derive from the common morality, though they certainly do not exhaust the common morality."[91] They go on to explain, "Most classical ethical theories accept these norms in some form, and traditional medical codes presuppose at least some of them."[92]

These principles are respect for autonomy, nonmaleficence, beneficence, and justice.[93] According to Beauchamp, *autonomy* is defined as "the obligation to respect the decision-making capacities of autonomous persons," *nonmaleficence* as "the obligation to avoid causing harm," *beneficence* as "obligations to provide benefits and to balance benefits against risks," and *justice* as "obligations of fairness in the distribution of benefits and risks."[94]

The four-principles model has become "canonical" for the field,[95] although the model is not without its critics. Like any principlistic approach, it may be less helpful at the bedside, in the context of clinical ethics, where a more casuistic (case-based) approach has been proposed.[96] Some observers see casuistry as better accommodating the pluralism of beliefs and values unavoidable in medical ethics.[97] The four-principles approach, however, has defenders[98] who endorse it as a valuable means for "doing good medical ethics"[99] and honoring the "goals of medicine,"[100] notwithstanding that it is not universal. The casuistry-versus-principlism debate has animated scholarly discussion within bioethics for the past quarter century and, while intellectually stimulating, is a bit beyond the concerns of this chapter.

Of greater relevance here is the significance of religion as a consideration for each principle. It should not be surprising to discover that respect for autonomy of patients, provision of healthcare as a justice-contexted issue, and the imperative to do good and not do harm are widely found in the ethical teachings of religions, something noted, for example, as a common feature of Catholicism, Islam, and Judaism,[101] in addition to other faiths.[102] But the different ways that these principles are understood within respective religions, and differences in their relevance and salience for courses of health-related action, complicate their clinical application. Some scholars considering those factors that are relevant to Muslims[103] and Jews,[104] for example, question whether the principles are as culturally neutral and cross-culturally applicable as purported, concluding otherwise. Other scholars disagree, identifying the Beauchamp and Childress principles in the belief systems and moral codes of major faith traditions,[105] including in medieval Islamic teaching[106] and, to some extent, rabbinic writings.[107]

Aasim Padela provides a reasonable summary of this issue:

> The approach of each faith to medical ethics is strikingly similar. They all relate ethics to sacred law utilizing the religious texts to provide the general principles and moral code that is to be observed. Each faith then uses the machinations of the sacred law to further extrapolate the principles to the modern context, creating rules and codes governing the etiquette of the clinical encounter and the permissible and impermissible therapeutics. While the details of the medical ethics within each faith are different, there are large areas of overlap within the rulings and even within [the] process of law-making.[108]

Religious values, stated or unstated, explicitly or implicitly, have influenced the "healing transaction" and medical decision-making for as long as there have been medical care providers.[109] For the past half century, at least, theological scholars have systematically weighed in on procedures or courses of action proscribed or prescribed according to exegeses of sacred writings or interpretations or rulings made by religious or ecclesial authorities, such as Roman Catholic moral theologians and Jewish *poskim*.[110]

Among leading medical ethicists in the West are well-known contemporary Protestant,[111] Catholic,[112] and Jewish[113] theological scholars. Among *poskim*, for example, *t'shuvot* have been issued regarding abortion, stem-cell research, euthanasia, test-tube babies, autopsy, transplantation, cloning, and other clinical matters.[114] While this is not a scientific survey, I have on my bookshelves nearly fifty volumes on the subject of Jewish medical ethics from across the Jewish denominational spectrum, in Hebrew and translation, from esteemed *poskim* and contemporary scholars. This selection includes important works by rabbinic and secular scholars, in Israel and the diaspora, commenting on clinical challenges that arise in making patient care decisions, including at the beginning and end of life, and on larger issues of healthcare policy, such as distribution of finite resources. Further, a PubMed search on "Jewish medical ethics" or "Jewish bioethics" turns up over seventy-five academic medical references on this subject since 1970. One would likely obtain similar results, or identify an even larger literature, for other religions.

At present, bioethical literatures in English are rapidly emerging from contemporary Hindu,[115] Buddhist,[116] Muslim,[117] Sikh,[118] and Taoist[119] scholars. The scope of this literature maps onto long-standing Christian and Jewish writing in bioethics, including material on the calculus of decision-making involved in treating challenging clinical cases and discussion of principles derived from sacred writings that provide guidance for physicians. Engelhardt has even described a framework for a secular-humanist bioethics, outlining features and limitations of such a perspective for informing the spectrum of medical decision-making from the clinical setting to the healthcare policy arena.[120] A religious critique of the proposal to secularize bioethics also has emerged.[121]

The new field of psychiatric ethics also has a substantial religious basis, as seen by attention devoted to the subject in *The Oxford Handbook of Psychiatric Ethics*.[122] An entire section is titled "Religious Contexts of Psychiatric Ethics," including chapters on ethical challenges for psychiatric practice from Muslim, Jewish, Catholic, Protestant, Buddhist, Confucian, and Hindu perspectives. This helpful reference opened up a significant frontier for bioethical scholarship and commentary. Significantly, these chapters underscore the diversity of approaches and justification for action, differentiating how these faith traditions proceed in their encounter with mentally ill patients.

Besides the *Handbook of Bioethics and Religion*,[123] *Religious Methods and Resources in Bioethics*,[124] *Religious Perspectives in Bioethics*,[125] and other books and articles already referenced here, material on religion is found in regular bioethics encyclopedias, handbooks, and dictionaries, including in each edition of the *Encyclopedia of Bioethics*. Whether or not religion is indeed experiencing a revival in bioethics, it remains a salient influence on deliberations made at the bedside, in the lab, and in legislative and judicial contexts. This may be something to celebrate or lament, depending upon one's perspective, but religious concerns are nonetheless ever-present when considering courses of action involving people's health and lives. Religious concerns come into play for patients and families, as well as for those who care for them. Religion may be an illuminating factor and source of guidance, or a complicating factor and nuisance, but these issues are real and impactful and cannot be wished away.[126]

A frontier for religious bioethics is the complicated issue of healthcare as a basic human right.[127] Secular and religious support for this concept exists, on grounds of justice.[128] Commentators, including physician and humanitarian Paul Farmer, have weighed in on the moral scandal of societies providing insufficient care for the poor—while providing an overabundance of specialized care only for the affluent who can afford it.[129] Laurie Zoloth, former dean of the University of Chicago Divinity School, has provided a religious Jewish perspective on this issue.[130] This conversation is important not just for substantive insights into healthcare justice but for expansion of bioethical scholarship beyond the narrower focus on clinical decision-making regarding medical procedures for individual patients to issues involved in community and preventive medicine and environmental and public health. This latter context, incidentally, seems more in keeping with Potter's original motivation for proposing a field of bioethics—to establish an interdisciplinary field of ethics concerned with ensuring ecological survival.[131]

A sequela of this discussion is the extension of bioethical writing to themes bearing on public health and the well-being of populations. An insightful analysis by Jesuit priest Michael D. Rozier,[132] at the time a doctoral student in public health at the University of Michigan and currently on faculty at Saint Louis University, advocates for moral theology to weigh in on ethical deliberations in public health. He exemplifies this by applying virtue ethics to issues such as vaccination policy and promotion of a balanced diet. Another example is an article of mine from 2012 that outlines ten biblical or rabbinic concepts that I hoped would inform the debate on healthcare reform.[133] These concepts are *b'rit* (covenant), *k'dushah* (holiness), *tzedek* (justice), *chesed* (mercy), *mip'nei darkhei shalom* (for the sake of peace), *pikuach nefesh* (to save a life), *k'lal* (peoplehood), *tikkun olam* (repair of the world), *t'shuvah* (repentance), and *yovel* (jubilee).[134]

Sadly, there is a lacuna of bioethical guidance for matters related to public health policy and intervention,[135] as opposed to volumes of published writing on the ethics of discrete clinical interventions. Others also have noted this discrepancy, along with the challenging change of perspective required "when populations become the patient."[136] At the same time, evidence suggests that this situation is improving, by necessity, since the recent healthcare reform debate in the United States. The bioethics field has been encouraged—forced by circumstance, really—to broaden its vision beyond the individual patient encounter to consider healthcare's organization and delivery.[137] Religious guidance regarding more communal issues related to healthcare reform and population health appears in detail in the next chapter.

Another important issue for bioethics in the new century concerns empathy in response to suffering.[138] Informed by earlier discussions of suffering in medicine,[139] especially in a theological context,[140] this issue is central to ethical deliberations over end-of-life issues such as removal of care.[141] An essential scholarly take on suffering came from Anglican theologian John Bowker in his *Problems of Suffering in Religions of the World.*[142] Bowker detailed the encounter with suffering—its origins and manifestations, and responses to it—within contemporary belief systems, including Judaism, Christianity, Islam, Hinduism, Buddhism, Zoroastrianism, Jainism, and even Marxism. Suffering, including and especially through experience of illness, is a ubiquitous part of human life, and because of this ubiquity, "religions give to suffering a place of central importance or consideration—indeed, it is often said that suffering is an important *cause* of religion, since the promises held out by religion represent a way in which men can feel reassured in the face of catastrophe or death."[143] The faith traditions are unanimous in imploring caregivers—and all of us—to respond to suffering others with selflessness and compassion, just as we would have others respond to us. Ideally, the tenets of religion inspire such a response, both from individuals and communally.

This discussion underscores budding recognition of the importance of compassion as a value for medical decision-making, which has implications not just for the subject matter of bioethical scholarship—for example, the clinical encounter—but also for how bioethical scholarship is conducted and how people are taught and trained as bioethical scholars. Note, for example, that the academic bioethics center directed by Stephen Post at Stony Brook University contains "compassionate care" in its name,[144] a first for the field. Its mission statement also explicitly places value on other-regarding virtues, namely "empathy, compassion, respect, humility, justice, loyalty, benevolence, diligence."[145] Post is making an overt statement here that these things matter for medicine no less than the various –ologies, such as pathophysiology, immunology, etiology, nosology, and all the rest. He is not alone: others, notably patients, have identified compassion as largely absent in today's medical care.[146]

Hard Choices at the Beginning and End of Life

The hottest of hot-button issues in bioethics involves termination decisions at the beginning and end of life, complicated by competing viewpoints among religions.[147] How to negotiate such life-and-death decisions constitutes the "dilemma of modern medicine."[148] What is the calculus involved, and where do faith traditions come down on these matters? The lack of uniformity here among and even within religions, substantively and hermeneutically, leads to great confusion and distress for medical practitioners, healthcare institutions, and families. This state of affairs, along with the presence of high-profile cases, has led to the insertion of politicians and mass media, exacerbating tensions and confusion.

Consider, for example, elective abortion, the voluntary termination of pregnancy. This has been the most contentious, publicly debated issue in bioethics for nearly half a century in the United States, since the Supreme Court's decision in *Roe v. Wade* in 1973 decriminalized the practice.[149] The politics of human embryos and their disposition—including through cloning and stem-cell research—has been described as "the third rail of bioethics."[150] Decades on, it continues to be challenged and defended with a ferocity unmatched by almost any other issue in public life in the U.S.

Even without the controversy surrounding the Supreme Court's ruling, reproduction is especially sensitive. Adjudicating medical decisions regarding the course of pregnancy inherently butts up against closely held beliefs and attitudes about personal autonomy, women's rights, the sanctity of human life, the limits of medicine, the sovereignty of the nuclear family, authority of the government and courts, the common good, and more. Religious considerations, as well as people's heartfelt understandings (and misunderstandings) of what sacred writings have to say or suggest about abortion, inform and direct action in support of these competing beliefs and attitudes, sometimes leading to violent confrontation.

Contemporary bioethical debate about such emotion-laden decisions during pregnancy has been ongoing for decades.[151] Discussions in the medical literature even predate *Roe v. Wade*. An editorial in the *British Medical Journal* titled "Ethics of Abortion, Sterilization, and Birth Control" was published in 1932.[152] Ethical choices present themselves not just prenatally but perinatally, such as in the newborn nursery.[153] At the time of this writing, leading U.S. politicians are debating normalization of a form of abortion that some people consider infanticide; legislation has been passed and signed into law in New York State.[154] This, in turn, has led to speculation that the governor of New York may be, or should be, excommunicated from the Roman Catholic Church, although church leadership has indicated that such an action would not be forthcoming.[155] Such legislation would have been unanticipated even by abortion rights supporters a few years ago, underscoring how the national conversation about pregnancy, abortion, and when life begins is a continually shifting playing field, with new issues arising, new reasons for respective constituencies to become offended, and emotions as raw as ever. As such, abortion remains an intellectually stimulating subject for bioethics scholars, but also one that may carry some professional and personal risk.

For laypeople of faith, a pertinent question regarding abortion is whether scriptures and other sacred writings provide any guidance as to how to proceed. For religious Jews and Christians, for example, does the Bible speak to what is and is not permissible and under what circumstances? The answer is yes, in a way, but how to interpret this guidance is not uniformly agreed upon and is, as a result, a source of great public and political debate.

In Deuteronomy 30:19, we are implored to "choose life." Earlier, in Exodus 20:13 (20:12 in some Bibles), the Ten Commandments includes the famous prohibition "Thou shalt not murder." For many Christians, notably Roman Catholics, evangelicals, and other conservative Protestants, these passages (in conjunction with others) are taken to forbid termination of any pregnancy between the time of conception and birth for almost any reason. For most liberal mainline Protestant denominations, abortion is generally discouraged, but is acceptable under certain circumstances—for example, if a pregnancy is due to rape or incest, the mother's health or well-being is threatened, or the fetus is deemed unviable, and only if the pregnancy has not reached the third trimester. For Catholics and many evangelicals, these latter exceptions are believed arbitrary and without basis in scripture.[156]

For still other religious believers, notably observant Jews, interpretations of Bible passages and guidance from other canonical writings (e.g., the Talmud) call into question whether human life necessarily begins at conception, rather than at birth, and also treats the life of the mother as taking precedence over that of a fetus. According to Rabbi Avraham Steinberg, in his authoritative *Encyclopedia of Jewish Medical Ethics,*

> A negative attitude toward abortion is expressed unanimously among the rabbinic decisors and commentators. Nearly all agree that some type of prohibition is involved in the performance of an abortion. However, there are differing views as to the nature of the prohibition, its seriousness, and the reason for the prohibition.[157]

For non-Jews, this absence of consensus among rabbis may seem odd, but for Jews it is hardly unanticipated. Just as in Christianity, there is within Judaism a spectrum of denominational affiliations and thus a wide range of opinions generated on many important moral issues. But even among those rabbinic decisors committed to ruling according to *halachah*, such as within the Orthodox and Conservative rabbinates, there is considerable hermeneutic plurality and flexibility, and always has been.[158] *Halachah* may be immutable in one sense, but not in another. That is, according to academic religious scholar and attorney Dena S. Davis, "All decisors work with the same body of literature and the same basic principles, but the way in which they apply the sources is inescapably interpretive."[159]

For Orthodox and many Conservative Jews, induced abortion is forbidden in all instances except in those rare cases when needed to save the life of a mother who would otherwise die if made to take a baby to full term.[160] This is so up until birth,[161] supported almost without exception by traditional *halachic* sources[162] and contemporary *halachic* rulings,[163] although there is some debate as to whether this is a biblical or rabbinic prohibition.[164] In instances of mortal hazard to a pregnant mother, abortion is not just permissible but required, regardless of trimester.[165] But this only applies if a mother's death is imminent—threats to her health or mental health or well-being or quality of life are generally not held as sufficient to mandate or permit termination of pregnancy. Moreover, for many Orthodox rabbinic authorities, exceptions for rape or incest are impermissible,[166] although the Reform and Conservative rabbinates have ruled otherwise,[167] as have a minority of Orthodox rabbis.[168] In Israel, abortion under these circumstances is permitted by law.[169]

A critical consideration in permitting or mandating abortion in certain circumstances is that according to Jewish law the fetus in the womb is not yet a living person. It does not yet possess a *nefesh* (soul) in the sense that other faiths describe "ensoulment." Before birth, it is thus not yet a living person and does not yet have the same legal status as a living person.[170] "Feticide, then," according to Rabbi David M. Feldman, "does not constitute homicide, and the basis for denying it capital-crime status in Jewish law—even for those rabbis who may have wanted to rule otherwise—is scriptural."[171] At the same time, as a soon-to-be person, the fetus's "right to life" is inviolate unless it threatens the life of its mother, in which case it is considered a *rodef* (pursuer), a threat to the life of a living person, the mother. In nearly all other circumstances, killing the fetus is a "moral offense and cannot be justified."[172]

Accordingly, abortion is forbidden by Judaism, across most of the denominational spectrum, for most other reasons, including the possibility of delivering a baby with a life-threatening disability, although some rabbinic authorities would permit abortion in that instance in strictly delimited circumstances.[173] Even among many liberal rabbinic authorities, justifying abortion for still other reasons, such as population control, post hoc contraception, expediency or convenience, or "on demand"—rationales that are prevalent among secular Americans, including secular Jews—would be widely rejected[174] or even considered "repugnant."[175]

The calculation and parsing involved in deducing an appropriate course of action from sacred texts, canonical commentaries, and a multiplicity of rabbinic rulings must clearly entail an enormous amount of complexity. For religious Jews, according to Jakobovits, while the judgment to be made "may be based on medical evidence, [it] is clearly of a moral nature."[176] He goes on to explain,

> The decision on whether, and under what circumstances, it is right to destroy a germinating human life depends upon the assessment and weighing of values, on determining the title to life in any given case.
>
> Such value judgments are entirely outside the province of medical science. No amount of training or experience in medicine can help in ascertaining the criteria necessary for reaching such capital verdicts, for making such life-and-death decisions. Such judgments pose essentially a moral, not a medical problem. Hence they call for the judgment of moral, not medical, specialists.[177]

To summarize, traditionally religious Jews are thus, in certain respects, more liberal than the most liberal mainline Christians—notably when it comes to requiring an abortion up until delivery, if needed to save a mother's life. Yet at the same time Torah-observant Jews are as ardently pro-life as the most devout Catholics, such as when it comes to forbidding abortion in almost all other circumstances. Many liberal Jews, by comparison, tend to express positions that fall more in line with liberal Protestants or secular Americans, although they may take a harder line in favor of what Roman Catholics and evangelicals refer to as "sanctity of life" issues than do liberal Protestants, but just define this concept differently.[178]

Perspectives of clergy and members of other faith traditions fall somewhere between the poles of *halachic* and liberal Judaism. Buddhism, like Roman Catholicism, affirms that human life begins at conception and thus forbids abortion, although in practice some Buddhist nations recognize situations requiring leniency, such as to save a mother's life or when pregnancy results from rape.[179] Hinduism condemns abortion and most Hindus likewise disapprove, but not as absolutely as in other traditions, and in practice it is legal and increasingly accepted in India.[180] Islam endorses the sanctity of all life, including that of the fetus, but recognizes extenuating circumstances in which abortion is permissible, such as a threat to the life of a mother; as in Judaism and Christianity, opinions and practices vary widely.[181] Sikhism considers abortion as taboo but does not contain teachings that explicitly forbid it, besides promoting respect for life; thus abortions are permitted and occur, not just to save a mother's life.[182] Among Christians, the simplest way to summarize opinions and practices regarding abortion is to note that it is "an issue on which Christians are widely and strongly divided,"[183] as reflected in the contentiousness of public debate in the U.S.

At the other end of the life course are serious bioethical issues no less challenging and nuanced as abortion. None are subject to more heated disagreement than euthanasia, the intentional termination of life through physician assistance, whether passive ("pulling the plug," or withdrawing care) or active (including assisted suicide).[184] As with abortion, the major religious traditions are all over the map, although none countenances any kind of on-demand or state-sponsored ending of life, as approved in some European nations, including the Netherlands.[185]

Euthanasia as a possible course of action generally arises in two contexts: first, among the elderly undergoing the dying process or others in the midst of decline from a terminal disease; second, among younger folks with catastrophic medical challenges or those with severe depression or difficult life circumstances that make living too much to bear. Recently, other rationale for euthanasia have been advanced, much more extreme and with almost no traction in public opinion, such as for means of population control or even to voluntarily self-exterminate the human species.[186]

Unlike with abortion, politicians have been loath to involve themselves here. It is a no-win situation for them, and even potential gains of political capital may not be worth the trouble. For everyone pleased with the position one takes on a particular case, there are others upset, no matter which side one takes. Also, this issue is not as easily deconstructed into black and white, good and evil, and right and wrong as religious and political partisans have done with abortion. Euthanasia and end-of-life decision-making generally are more shaded and do not correlate as precisely with right-left polarities within politics and theology as does abortion. Yet this has not stopped political interference. Consider the fa-mous and tragic Schiavo case; religious factors were involved here, no less prom-inently than the messy clinical and legal issues.[187]

In 1990 Terri Schiavo, a twenty-six-year-old woman from Florida, suffered cardiac arrest, brought about by an eating disorder, and became comatose. After developing hypoxic-ischemic encephalopathy, she exhibited no higher-level cortical function, imaging showed cerebral atrophy, and other testing found no brain activity. In the vernacular, she had flatlined, although she had some reflexes left and did not appear to be suffering.[188] A percutaneous endoscopic gastros-tomy (PEG, or feeding) tube was inserted, and Schiavo's condition deteriorated into a persistent vegetative state, where she remained, living in a skilled nursing facility and then a hospice for the rest of her life. Neurologists universally deter-mined that she had irreversible neurological damage.[189] These pieces of the story are not contested; almost everything else is.

With no living will or durable power of attorney, Schiavo's husband was ap-pointed as her legal guardian with no objection from her parents. In 2000, sev-eral years after the husband and family had a falling out, a protracted legal battle ensued, pitting husband and family against each other. The former, in light of the irreversibility of her condition, wished to remove her feeding tube; the latter protested and sued for guardianship. The parties then entered into a contracted legal dispute over whether to withdraw care. One point of contention was whether Schiavo's own wishes were indeed indeterminate; another was whether she was truly in a terminal state. Medical expert witnesses retained by the family tried to cast doubt on the permanency of Schiavo's condition, although none had ever "personally examined the patient, reviewed the medical records in any detail, considered the medical opinions of the consulting neurologists, nor reviewed the CT scans or EEGs."[190]

Numerous partisan religious and political organizations weighed in, and the case became an ongoing media circus, just like previous such spectacles including the O. J. Simpson trial. Politicians soon became involved, including Governor Jeb Bush and his brother, President George W. Bush, and the tragedy of this young woman's situation became fodder for angry rhetoric, no less so than the public discourse on abortion.[191] Eventually, after multiple hearings, trials, and appeals, the Florida Supreme Court ruled that Schiavo's artificial nutrition and hydration were to be removed, and after two weeks she died.[192] Her family celebrated a Roman Catholic funeral Mass, her husband later had her cremated and buried in a separate service, and the story was soon gone from the news cycle.

There was perhaps little to distinguish this case from hundreds of others, ex-cept that it garnered national attention and played out in public, almost on a daily basis. Moreover, it devolved into what has been termed "a political farce when elected representatives with little medical knowledge attempted to play both doctor and judge."[193] Unfortunately, with all the parties weighing in, including inflammatory television commentators and leaders of partisan religious organizations, none connected to the case, we never heard from Schiavo herself. Even the voices of her husband and family members were "largely drowned out by a very loud, self-interested public debate"[194] dominated by individuals and organizations without direct access to the medical facts of the case and who saw its unfolding as a means to advance their respective causes, whether "right to life" or "right to die."[195]

The Schiavo case became a flashpoint for national debate about end-of-life care, euthanasia, assisted suicide, spousal and parental rights, healthcare proxies or surrogates, and myriad other issues central or peripheral to the facts of the clinical case. The way these issues were described and discussed in the popular media was much distorted, which troubled bioethicists—but then so did the sad facts of the case itself, which exposed a lacuna of theoretical frameworks to apply in such a complex situation.[196] Interestingly, public opinion survey data revealed that religious opposition to removing the feeding tube was correlated with, and conflated with, opposition to elective abortion.[197]

This observation itself is provocative and inconsistent with how the major faith traditions view the ethics of end-of-life decision-making when confronted with terminal illness, brain death, or artificial hydration and nutrition. While sharing a general disdain for euthanasia, at the same time Hinduism, Buddhism, Islam, Christianity, and Judaism countenance withdrawal of life support for a patient whose life is being prolonged entirely by artificial means and has no hope of recovery. Each religion weighs in differently and with different rationale and criteria, but none absolutely forbids such action under all circumstances, as long as the patient's intentions can be gauged.[198] Within Christianity[199] and Judaism,[200] there is a range of opinions, varying by denomination, but notwithstanding, considerable overlap still exists. Even within Roman Catholicism and Orthodox Judaism there are circumstances that would justify withdrawing certain forms of care if it is believed that death is imminent, however defined.[201]

For example, Orthodox Jewish bioethicist Baruch Brody states bluntly that careful reading of authoritative rabbinic texts on withdrawal of life support suggests that the view of *halachah* "is obviously not a sanctity-of-life position. Instead it is a nuanced balancing of many values."[202] Brody draws upon several sources, including Rabbi Feinstein's views on futile cases. Feinstein concluded, "If physicians have no means of healing a terminal patient or of improving his quality of life by reducing his pain, but do have the ability to keep him alive for a limited time, then they should not do so."[203] Rabbi Steinberg concurs and reviews the range of rabbinic opinion, but also notes the universality of rabbinic opposition to withdrawing food or fluids to hasten death.[204] A critical concern here is the issue of what constitutes "futility,"[205] a difficult concept that bioethicists struggle with in other contexts.

With the continued proliferation of new high-tech forms of medical treatment, these sorts of religiously contexted or -mediated life-and-death issues will not fade away. The challenges confronting us now and down the road are not unlike those faced by the pioneers of bioethics decades ago who lived through the postwar technological revolution in Western medicine. There likely will be new controversies we cannot foresee. Some may be related to manipulation of the human genome. Will they be resolved by individuals in consultation with medical caregivers and clergy, or will the heavy hand of the state dictate the final say?

In 1990 James P. Wind, former editor of the Park Ridge Center's journal *Second Opinion*, asked, "What can religion offer bioethics?"[206] That the question had to be asked, Wind suggested, signified an "enigma present within bioethics and within American society as a whole."[207] Specifically, most of us "make room for individuals with religious perspectives at the same time that we conduct our daily affairs as if those perspectives made little difference."[208] Three decades later, the same question could rightly be posed for bioethics.

Medicine cannot afford to move forward without thoughtful deliberation over appropriate courses of conduct, in terms of the contingencies of individual cases and progress of medical science in overcoming disease and restoring well-being. Nor can such deliberation wisely ensue without the most compassionate human values brought to bear through the sage input of theologians, philosophers, suffering patients, and others with a stake in this issue who labor to discern what is right and good. This is no disparagement of the good intentions of most physicians, biomedical scientists, and healthcare administrators, but a soulless, technocratic future uninformed by thoughtful moral reasoning and with little regard for the human spirit is not a utopian future for medicine.

8

Policies and Programs

The impetus behind the growth of bioethics and clinical medical ethics as professional fields and areas of scholarship, as noted, has been to establish parameters for ethical research and clinical practice. The religious bases of this work likewise have emphasized practicalities of decision-making for physicians and patients confronted with challenging situations demanding morally imbued deliberations about life and death. Such deliberations about larger issues related to public health policy and population health have been comparatively sparse, regardless of faith tradition,[1] although Roman Catholic and Jewish bioethicists have given passing attention to the issue.

Jewish and Catholic writing on communal obligations for healthcare evinces significant shared values. Aaron L. Mackler, professor of theology at Duquesne University, Conservative rabbi, and expert on Jewish-Catholic dialogue on bioethics, has succinctly described these commonalities:

> A foundational text in each tradition is the teaching in the book of Genesis that God created humans in God's image. This concept powerfully expresses the intrinsic value and dignity of each human being. . . . Although Jews and Catholics acknowledge God's ultimate sovereignty, they are called to exercise stewardship in acting to help other persons and to improve the world. These values support provision of health care to people in need.[2]

Rabbi Elliot Dorff explains that Judaism endorses "the clear duty to try to heal, and this duty devolves upon both the physician and society. . . . [H]owever, Jewish sources on distributing and paying for health care are understandably sparse."[3] This is not unique to Jewish scholarship. For clinical ethics in general, according to Catholic bioethicist Edmund Pellegrino, social responsibility for "deficiencies in distribution, quality, and accessibility of even ordinary medical care for the poor, the uneducated and the disenfranchised" has long been a significant lacuna in the medical literature.[4] Thankfully, this situation is resolving in Judaism, Catholicism, and other traditions.[5] Recent discussions elaborate on the religious foundations of communal obligations regarding public health and healthcare, motivated by contemporary legislative debates on healthcare reform.

The ramped-up political conversation surrounding healthcare reform in the United States beginning in the early 1990s supplied a ready-made focus

Religion and Medicine. Jeff Levin, Oxford University Press (2020) © Oxford University Press.
DOI: 10.1093/oso/9780190867355.001.0001

for religiously motivated concerns at the intersection of theodicy, biomedical ethics, public policy, and population health. These concerns, in turn, gave birth to, defined, and shaped the national discussion on healthcare rights. This was first widely visible in the debate over what came to be known as Hillarycare— what might be termed Healthcare Reform v. 1.0. Associated legislation, officially known as the Health Security Act,[6] was drafted in 1993 and introduced in the House (and identically in the Senate) in 1994, but ultimately failed, meeting with substantial resistance from both the political right, on account of industry reaction to its perceived overreach and the stridency and closed-door nature of deliberations,[7] and the political left, on account of retaining market-based features and failing to endorse a single-payer system.[8] The bill was soon withdrawn by the Democrats' leadership when they determined that the legislation was doomed.[9] Fallout for the Clinton administration was severe, and the resulting anger on both sides of the political aisle is believed by some analysts to have contributed directly to the Republican takeover of the House in 1994.[10]

Significantly, the debate over Hillarycare, especially regarding its ethical foundations, was informed in part by religious lobbying: formally, through membership by faith community leaders on a panel of thirty-two ethicists advising the Task Force for National Health Care Reform that helped assemble the legislation, and informally, by white papers and policy statements issued by denominational and other religious organizations. Among the former were Rabbi Dorff, Monsignor Charles L. Fahey, and at least a couple of Protestant ministers;[11] remaining members "had secular backgrounds."[12] A notable example of denominational statements was a position paper titled "Judaism and Health Care Reform," issued by the Commission on Social Action and Public Policy of the United Synagogue of Conservative Judaism.[13] This document included a resolution on universal healthcare ratified at the Conservative movement's Biennial Convention in 1991, a declaration advocating for healthcare reform on the basis of *halachah*, a selection of rabbinic texts with commentary from Rabbi Dorff, a call to advocacy for Jewish congregations and laypeople, and bibliographic resources.

Concurrently, in 1993 the United States Conference of Catholic Bishops issued a Pastoral Resolution titled "A Framework for Comprehensive Health Care Reform."[14] This document advocated for legislation prioritizing three moral principles: protecting human life, promoting human dignity, and pursuing the common good.[15] It built on an earlier pastoral letter issued by the bishops in 1981,[16] and on the papal encyclical *Pacem in Terris*, issued by Pope John XXIII in 1963, affirming "the right to be looked after in the event of ill health."[17] Although these efforts failed to produce ratified legislation during the Clinton years, they were significant cornerstones for the Bishops' advocacy efforts a decade and a half later when a renewed push for healthcare reform surfaced under President Barack Obama.[18]

The subsequent Obamacare debate, beginning in 2009—call it Healthcare Reform v. 2.0—was an opportunity for advocates of reform to reboot their efforts and learn from past missteps. A significant difference in the lead-up to introduction of legislation between the Hillarycare and Obamacare efforts was a substantially larger mobilization of organized religious advocacy for and against features of the second round of proposals before Congress. Religions and denominations across the spectrum—Christian, Jewish, Muslim, and others—including competing branches of respective religions, weighed in through well-organized efforts and well-crafted policy statements. The number of such statements was legion—far more than can be summarized here—yet despite competing theological foundations there was considerable overlap and agreement on identifying moral imperatives for healthcare reform enabling better access to care among all Americans and greater allocation of resources to ensure primary prevention of disease and promotion of health and well-being.

Religion and Healthcare Reform

Faith-based expressions of advocacy for health policy reform in the United States did not originate with the Hillarycare debacle. Nor did religious denominations and faith-based organizations (FBOs) lobbying for legislation and issuing substantial policy statements come to its first widespread public attention during the subsequent Obamacare debate. Moreover, nor was the first example of federal support for faith-based programming and initiatives in healthcare preceded by establishment of a White House faith-based office and satellite office in the Department of Health and Human Services (DHHS). The narrative on health-directed partnerships between the faith community and government is a much older story than perhaps most observers are aware. Moreover, large-scale national reform efforts in the healthcare sector did not just start in the 1990s, and the religious community has been a major player in policy-related healthcare advocacy since the beginning.[19]

Organized efforts to reform healthcare and government social services go back over a century, and religious people and institutions were instrumental in advocating for change and formulating appropriate responses, including philanthropic and legislative. Churches and faith-based charities were a significant presence in provision of social welfare services during and after the mid-1800s, playing a proportionally larger role than even today.[20] The Roman Catholic Church was especially active in promoting social reform.[21] Long before the advent of the welfare state, people of faith mobilized personal and institutional resources to establish social services programs in the United States. The government welcomed such volunteer-sector participation, including from religious organizations, as, prior to the New Deal, public programs for caring for the poor and needy were "fragmentary, locally diverse, and continually changing."[22]

Jane Addams, for example, raised as an evangelical and churchgoing Presbyterian, cofounded Hull House in Chicago in 1889, the nation's first settlement house, and was a leading activist for numerous progressive social reforms, including efforts to improve the health and living conditions of those in poverty.[23] Her relationship to institutional religion became complex and ambiguous, gravitating to Unitarianism and humanism, but her early faith and education at Rockford Seminary instilled a Christian conviction foundational for her subsequent efforts, and "she found in the history of the early Christians a new model for cross-class living."[24] This was similar to the spirit that infused an active social consciousness in Protestants early in the twentieth century, giving rise to the social gospel movement.

Formal lobbying by faith groups played a significant role in the formulation of New Deal and Great Society programs,[25] including healthcare and civil rights legislation. Political activism was framed as a moral imperative supported by religious views, and religious advocates encouraged or even demanded collective action in the public sphere for the greater good. Initiatives were viewed as a way to externalize the prophetic and pastoral mission of respective religious belief systems, acting in obedience to sacred teachings in order to serve as "champions of the poor."[26] This activist ethos is similar to the motivating forces that led to establishment of hospitals and hospices, medical missions and healthcare ministries, pastoral care and healthcare chaplaincy, and congregational disease-prevention programming and community-wide health initiatives, as documented in previous chapters. Ironically, according to an economic analysis, religious advocacy beginning during the New Deal era effectively led to a "crowd-out" of faith-based charity during the Depression,[27] which may be instructive for future projections on how government faith-based initiatives may affect benevolent church giving.

A push to revisit the healthcare reform debate began soon after the failure of Hillarycare. Advocacy for reform was more bipartisan than histories of that era have recorded. According to a report issued by the conservative Heritage Foundation, "The need for health care reform has never been questioned by health care policy analysts on either side of the political spectrum."[28] Proof of this was introduction of several pieces of legislation by Republicans in the House and Senate offering alternatives to the bill proposed by Democrats that became known as Obamacare. Examples just from the 111th Congress included Rep. Mark Kirk's Medical Rights Reform Act of 2009 (H.R. 3970), Rep. Paul Ryan's Patients' Choice Act (H.R. 2520), Rep. John Shadegg's Improving Health Care for All Americans Act (H.R. 3218), Rep. Tom Price's Empowering Patients First Act (H.R. 3400), and Sen. Tom Coburn's Patients' Choice Act (S. 1099).[29] These bills never made it out of committee, their existence denied in partisan political grandstanding and media accounts excusing the overreach of the Obamacare legislation on grounds that it was the only option available since Republicans had refused to propose any alternatives.[30] Ironically, other legislation proposed by Democrats likewise received minimal traction or publicity, such as Rep. John Dingell's Affordable Health Care for America Act (H.R. 3962).

The official name of the law that emerged from the Congress's revisiting of healthcare reform was the Patient Protection and Affordable Care Act (PPACA) (H.R. 3590), often abbreviated as the Affordable Care Act. After reconciliation in the Senate the revised bill was titled the Health Care and Education Reconciliation Act of 2010 (H.R. 4872). The respective bills were passed and then enacted into law in March 2010.[31] The legislation has been a source of controversy ever since, among Republicans opposed to it from the beginning and among progressive Democrats who believe that it did not go far enough. In recent years, efforts have been made to chip away at certain of its provisions, most (but not all) unsuccessfully. Despite assertions to the contrary, the healthcare reform debate in the U.S. is still ongoing. Indeed, toward the end of his term in office in 2016, President Obama penned an op-ed piece in *JAMA* that boldly laid out follow-up plans to expand on Obamacare legislation with additional reforms.[32] With the Trump administration, those plans are on indefinite hold.

Religious participation in the national discussion leading up to passage of the PPACA preceded the legislative push beginning in 2009, and in fact dates back to efforts undertaken during the Clinton and George W. Bush administrations. Involvement of the faith community in advocating for and participating as a major player in reform of healthcare delivery was advanced as consistent with the prophetic role of churches and religious bodies to advocate for justice and compassion and maintain an active role in the public square. In 2008, for example, the White House hosted one of its monthly Compassion in Action Roundtable meetings on the theme of Community-Based Solutions for Health Needs.[33] Speakers and participants included representatives from Muslim and Christian communities, as well as representatives from DHHS and the Centers for Disease Control and Prevention (CDC), the event keynoted by the acting Surgeon General of the United States.

The meeting was held because the Bush administration recognized that "[a]mong the most pressing needs faced by many low-income communities is access to quality primary healthcare."[34] The White House sought "to advance a broad-based reform agenda that regards frontline nonprofit organizations as central players in addressing poverty, disease and other great needs."[35] Presentations highlighted existing efforts taking place across the country in which "faith-based and other community organizations are among the central actors in driving creative solutions to these complex issues."[36] These efforts included private-sector initiatives involving medical care systems, clinics, and academic medical centers, and federally directed programs involving myriad agencies, including the U.S. Agency for International Development, DHHS, and the Department of Veterans Affairs (VA).

But this gathering, at the tail end of the Bush administration, was not the first effort to give voice to this issue. In 2001, at the start of the administration, a report was issued by the U.S. Bureau of Primary Healthcare summarizing a national conference on the theme of Communities in Action: Reforming the Health Care System from the Inside Out. Authored by Jay F. Hein, public policy analyst from Indiana, the report argued for community-based solutions addressing lacunae in healthcare access and quality through systemic, integrated, patient-centered, and evidence-based approaches. Existing programs from throughout the country were described, the report concluding that "communities aren't waiting for the federal government to solve their health care crises, and (better news) . . . they don't need to."[37] Hein was later appointed domestic policy adviser in the Bush White House and director of its faith-based office, and at the time of writing is president of the Sagamore Institute, a social policy think tank.

Going back further, in 1997 the Clinton administration held a forum cosponsored by the CDC and the federal Agency for Toxic Substances and Disease Registry. Its published report, *Engaging Faith Communities as Partners in Improving Community Health*, included a keynote address by the Surgeon General of the United States, panels on issues related to church-state separation and scientific evidence for faith-health links and efficacy of faith-based programs, and presentation of case studies on existing faith-based partnerships in HIV prevention, breast and cervical cancer education, cardiovascular risk factors in adolescents and women, smoking cessation and health screening, and international outreach in Jamaica and Kenya.[38] The takeaway point, which could be a byword for the present chapter, was simple: "Partnerships between faith organization [sic] and the health system, be it medical care or public health, are not new."[39]

These efforts to shine a light on the issue during the Clinton and Bush years mobilized a diversity of religious denominations and FBOs. The election of President Obama in 2008 galvanized liberal mainline denominational groups to take seriously the opportunity to inform political debate and the ensuing policy-making process for healthcare reform. But, to be clear, official statements and white papers in support of particular legislative agendas began appearing several years prior to the new president's inauguration in 2009, and they originated from across the religious spectrum. Indeed, if the religious community had been this responsive and involved years earlier, and had the Clinton administration's task force been more open to outside input, the failed attempt of Hillarycare might have had a different outcome.

In the lead-up to drafting the PPACA and its subsequent vote and passage, statements came from numerous North American religious denominations. Most have lobbying arms, many with offices within the Washington beltway, and the respective documents served as implicit action plans to influence the content of legislation and outcome of what was expected to be a contentious legislative battle. On the whole, these statements were influential at all stages of the policy-making process during the healthcare reform debate. The eventual legislation bears the mark of most of them, although not every group got everything they demanded. While these documents mostly agreed about the broad strokes of healthcare reform legislation, the various reports indicated substantial differences on contentious issues such as public funding of contraception, abortion, and euthanasia.

The Roman Catholic position on healthcare reform was discussed earlier. Protestant denominations also ensured that their voices were heard.

In 2008 the United Methodist Church adopted into its Book of Resolutions a statement titled "Health Care for All in the United States," emphasizing issues related to access, quality, and cost, and endorsing a single-payer system guaranteeing healthcare for all Americans.[40] Since its earliest days going back to John Wesley, the document noted, "Methodists have believed that providing health care to others is an important duty of Christians." They strongly endorsed the Obamacare legislation and lobbied for its passage. This resolution was amended and readopted in 2016.

The Evangelical Lutheran Church in America began considering a proposed social statement on healthcare reform at its Churchwide Assembly in 1999, for presentation at its next Assembly in 2003.[41] The discussion touched on familiar themes of limited access among the poor, equity and justice issues, insurance reform, and the necessity of building a health and healing ministry in keeping with Jesus's example. After considerable negotiation, Social Policy Resolution CA09.04.18, titled "Health Care Reform," was adopted at the 2009 Assembly. It stated simply:

> RESOLVED, that the Evangelical Lutheran Church in America, in Assembly, commit this church in all of its expressions to the premise that "each person should have ready access to basic health care services that include preventive, acute, and chronic physical and mental health care at an affordable cost" and be it therefore further RESOLVED, that this assembly request that the ELCA Washington Office, in partnership with synods, congregations and members of the ELCA, convey the urgency and sense of this resolution to Congress and the White House.[42]

The Presbyterian Church (U.S.A.) has long spoken out about healthcare issues and in favor of a national health plan. Major documents include *Life Abundant: Values, Choices, and Health Care—The Responsibility and Role of the Presbyterian Church (U.S.A.)*,[43] a policy statement adopted by the 200th General Assembly in 1988; and *Resolution on Christian Responsibility and a National Health Plan*,[44] adopted at the 203rd Assembly in 1991. The first statement acknowledged that healthcare in the U.S. was in crisis, the church has a corporate responsibility to work for health and healing as a part of its witness, and professing Christ requires working for "a national health policy that does justice for all."[45] The second statement laid out a national health plan that was quite radical—more akin to Hillarycare than to the PPACA. It called for a mandatory, government-controlled system funded through progressive taxation and with strict top-down controls rationing care on the basis of bureaucratic decision-making.[46] Subsequently, in 2008, the church pushed the envelope even further and endorsed a publicly financed, single-payer, universal national health insurance system.[47]

The Southern Baptist Convention, by contrast, opposed the Hillarycare and Obamacare legislation, but at the same time strongly advocated for healthcare reform and was very much involved in the policymaking process since the earliest days of the first healthcare reform debate. In 1994 it passed a "Resolution on Health Care Reform" that stated clearly the moral obligation of Christians to speak out about healthcare injustices, including underinsurance of segments of the population.[48] The Southern Baptists championed reforms of the healthcare delivery system so as to "provide affordable care for all those in need," in keeping with the historic presence of Christians at the forefront of "compassionate health care ministry."[49]

The resolution was light on specifics but did make note of several "morally objectionable provisions" in the Clinton legislation, including public funding of abortion, distribution of contraceptives to minors, rationing of medical care for economic reasons, government interference in the physician-patient relationship, and "inadequate conscience clauses which fail to protect religious persons, institutions, organizations, and medical facilities from participating in a health care system which would condone and support morally objectionable practices."[50] A subsequent resolution, adopted in 2012, condemned the absence of protections for religious freedom in the PPACA, especially regarding mandatory coverage of abortion and contraception.[51]

Other Christian denominations issued statements or otherwise lobbied on behalf of healthcare reform, either offering proposals or weighing in on provisions of the legislation that became the PPACA. The list of religious bodies is longer than can be detailed here, and includes the Episcopal Church,[52] United Church of Christ,[53] Mennonite Church USA,[54] Church of God in Christ,[55] Church of the Brethren,[56] and Christian Church (Disciples of Christ).[57] These were not the only institutional religious groups to participate in this process. Non-Christian religions also lent their voice. Prominent among these was the Islamic Society of North America, which issued a position paper on healthcare reform in 2009.[58] This document endorsed the legislative initiatives of President Obama, including universal coverage, uniform insurance premiums, a national health insurance exchange or marketplace, and a public option for health insurance coverage. Each of these features of prospective legislation was deemed "essential" to true healthcare reform.

Especially influential were a spate of position papers, policy reports, and resolutions advocating for or against features of healthcare reform originating from across Jewish denominations and organizations,[59] and from Jewish academic bioethicists such as Laurie Zoloth.[60] In her *Health Care and the Ethics of Encounters*, published in 1999, Zoloth drew on Jewish religious texts, historical tradition, and a hermeneutics of *halachic* analysis in a lively critique of the debate about healthcare justice, which she acknowledged had "faltered . . . in the face of intellectual and political paralysis."[61] Her specific recommendations were mostly liberal, politically speaking, emphasizing distributive justice and critique of the morality of market-based approaches, but her method was grounded in traditions of debate in and about Jewish law and its authority, and she herself is Orthodox. Jewish denominations drew on a similar pool of texts and interpretive traditions, yet came to conclusions that differed from each other in significant ways.

The Union for Reform Judaism adopted a resolution in 2007 supporting health insurance for all Americans.[62] It was less concerned with advocating for a single-payer system, as opposed to a better-regulated market solution, than stressing that, regardless of the specifics of a legislative solution, *halachah* obligates a community to provide health services for all citizens. The resolution labeled the current system "a disaster," and besides supporting policy advocacy called on congregations to survey the health needs of their members and offer a range of wellness programs. A resolution adopted in 1993 was more aggressive in its approach, affirming support for the Hillarycare legislation and advocating explicitly for a single-payer system of nationalized medical care.[63]

The United Synagogue of Conservative Judaism adopted a resolution at its biennial convention in 1991 endorsing "a comprehensive national health care plan that ensures adequate coverage for all Americans."[64] It was published as a formal position paper in 1993, as described earlier in this chapter. In contrast to the Reform movement's resolution, the Conservatives' document contained a detailed unpacking of rabbinic and other theological principles supporting a communal obligation to provide for healing as well as distribution of scarce resources for this purpose. These principles included *hatzalat nefashot* (the saving of human life), *shemirat ha-briyut* (preventive care), *tzedakah* (communal obligations to meeting basic human needs), and *bikkur holim* (visiting the sick).

The Rabbinical Council of America, the professional organization of Modern Orthodox rabbis, issued a policy in 1999 on healthcare reform.[65] As did the Reform and Conservative movements, it supported "access to universal coverage with realistic fiscal controls." But it departed from the other movements in a strong statement on the sanctity of life that could have come from the Catholic bishops or the Southern Baptist Convention:

> Judaism teaches us to the infinite value of each human life and of our obligation to preserve life. However, we must be concerned that in the quest to restrain costs, new health care initiatives may not give due consideration to the sanctity of human life and to ethical and religious imperatives that seek to protect such sanctity.[66]

The statement also urged that "physicians must be permitted sufficient flexibility in selecting the form of a patient's treatment in order to provide them with the optimum capability for preserving life," as well as "sensitivity to ethical and religious imperatives in the formulation of any guidelines related to allocation and selection of medical treatments, procedures and resources."

A more religiously traditional Orthodox group, Agudath Israel of America, issued a public letter to President Obama in 2009, articulating its own position on healthcare reform.[67] Authored by Rabbi Abba Cohen, vice president for Federal Affairs and Counsel, the letter endorsed universal coverage, in common with other Jewish movements. But it departed from the more liberal groups, even more stridently than the Rabbinical Council of America, on the matter of religious liberty.

Rabbi Cohen made clear a "conviction that the preservation of life and the promotion of good health and well-being are *religious imperatives* that emanate from the inherent sanctity of human life."[68] Moreover, for any legislation to be acceptable it must accommodate the religious rights of patients, providers, and employers; their religious and moral beliefs; and the decision-making authority of physicians, which must not be usurped or preempted by government or federal panels. The letter was especially concerned about medical decisions made via calculations of cost-effectiveness or quality of life, rather than its inherent sanctity, and enforced by agents of the government with hostility toward needs of individuals. A more recent document, issued in 2015, reiterated Agudath's opposition to "any health care reform proposal that would force a religious entity or individual to violate their religious beliefs," especially with respect to the PPACA's contraception mandate and concerns about end-of-life decisions.[69]

During the lengthy congressional debate regarding what became the Obamacare legislation, many Jewish communal and membership organizations weighed in with their own advocacy statements. Each represented constituencies with a stake in the final product, and some organizations had been involved in discussions of healthcare and welfare reform going back many years. These included the Jewish Federations of North America,[70] the Jewish Council for Public Affairs,[71] B'nai B'rith International,[72] and the National Council of Jewish Women.[73] These organizations almost unanimously supported features that became enshrined in the PPACA bill, except where they believed that the legislation did not go far enough. On the whole, these groups continue to take politically liberal positions on the organization, delivery, and public financing of healthcare.[74]

To summarize, these documents reveal distinctive but unsurprising differences of opinion. For example, the Southern Baptist Convention and the United States Conference of Catholic Bishops were mostly in agreement on human life issues, such as opposition to public funding for abortion and euthanasia, and at odds with liberal Jewish organizations and most liberal Protestant denominations. But, to reiterate, there was also broad agreement across all religious groups: the healthcare system is a mess, and authentic discipleship calls on believers, regardless of creed, to intervene. These statements, on the whole, called for specific healthcare policies on the basis of moral imperatives grounded in respective scriptural and faith traditions. This form of public advocacy was viewed as consistent with the prophetic role of these institutions—their divinely mandated obligation to call the world out of complacency and sin and to right injustices and act with compassion[75]—whether grounded in *halachah*, Catholic social teaching, or some other sacred value system that mandates and directs moral action. Call it social justice, *tikkun olam*, obedience to God, speaking with a prophetic voice—no matter, the call was the same.

Government Faith-Based Initiatives

Just as FBOs have played a role in government initiatives in healthcare and public health, so too has government extended its hand in partnership with the faith-based sector in its own health-related initiatives. Such involvement over the past four federal administrations in Washington has been a source of political controversy. The origins of these efforts, however, differs substantially from the received story, which goes something like this: when President Bush took office in 2001, his evangelical fervor led him to establish a White House faith-based office to give government funding to the religious right in order to subvert the Constitution and replace our democracy with a Christian theocratic state.

Variations on this narrative were typical of the reporting at the time.[76] None of it was remotely true.

The history of the federal faith-based initiative began with a provision on "charitable choice" drawn up by Sen. John Ashcroft for federal welfare reform legislation introduced in 1996. The Personal Responsibility and Work Opportunity Reconciliation Act of 1996 (P.L. 104-193) (PRWORA), included in Section 104 a clause authorizing "services provided by charitable, religious, or private organizations."[77] This provision was described as follows:

> The purpose of this section is to allow States to contract with religious organizations, or to allow religious organizations to accept certificates, vouchers, or other forms of disbursement . . . on the same basis as any other nongovernmental provider without impairing the religious character of such organizations, and without diminishing the religious freedom of beneficiaries of assistance funded under such program.[78]

In other words, *charitable choice* refers to federal enablement of FBOs to compete on equal footing alongside secular agencies for grants and contracts to provide human services. An analysis of PRWORA noted, "This provision significantly changes the historic relationship between the religious community and the public sector by opening the door for mixing religion and publicly supported social services."[79] The original bill (H.R. 3734, 104th Congress) passed with bipartisan support in the House, 256-170, and in the Senate, 74-24; President Clinton signed it into law in 1996.[80] Note that this occurred five years before a White House Office of Faith-Based and Community Initiatives (hereafter, "the office") was formally established through Executive Order at the start of President George W. Bush's first term in 2001.[81] In 2009 the initiative was retained by President Obama and rebranded as the Office of Faith-based and Neighborhood Partnerships.[82]

The first full-time director under President Bush was John J. DiIulio Jr., a University of Pennsylvania political scientist, Roman Catholic, and lifelong Democrat; the President's Advisory Council on Faith-Based and Community Initiatives, an oversight body for the office, was chaired by Indianapolis mayor Stephen Goldsmith, who is Jewish.[83] The office functioned under authority of the White House Domestic Policy Council, reporting to the White House chief of staff.[84] Faith-based offices also were established within nearly a dozen federal cabinet departments, including DHHS. where it was known during the Obama administration as the Center for Faith-Based and Neighborhood Partnerships, or Partnership Center, for short. I am proud to note the important leadership role played by individuals with ties to Baylor University, including Jay Hein, Distinguished Senior Fellow at the Baylor Institute for Studies of Religion, who directed the office under President Bush, and Melissa Rogers, Baylor graduate, who directed the office under President Obama.

Readers may recall attendant controversies early on in the history of the office, such as contentious public debates over church-state separation. Concerns were raised about the purpose and function of the office,[85] such as whether public funds would be used to underwrite religious proselytizing. These were legitimate concerns and would have been troubling if true. But, to repeat, they were groundless. The Bush administration's motivation was quite straightforward: to marshal personal and institutional faith-based resources and religiously motivated generosity, as part of a compassion agenda, in order to develop a multifaceted grassroots response to widespread social problems not being ameliorated by government action alone.[86]

Notwithstanding the received narrative, the office was established to serve primarily as a clearinghouse promoting charitable choice as a means to better provide for social services, including "health support services."[87] The most commonly voiced criticism of the office—that it entailed distributing tax money to churches and religious groups, which could, in turn, use these funds to support sectarian activities such as proselytizing—was, at best, simply false, a product of having failed to read the official documents that established the office. At worst, this was a distortion intentionally ramped up to sink the office and embarrass the Bush administration. Since the Clinton years, contentiousness about charitable choice has been manufactured in part to score political points with respective constituencies, left and right. Attacks on the office made for strange bedfellows:

> One may recall the unusual tag team of [Christian conservative] Dr. Pat Robertson and [secular liberal] Norman Lear working together to scuttle the initiative right out of the gate. The religious right was especially opposed to the form the initiative took in the first term of President Bush, due in part to its refusal both to limit access for Eastern or non-Christian faiths and to create a most-favored status for ultra-conservative Christians. The secular left was opposed to the initiative, on principle, as an attempt by the religious right to gain access to public funding. As noted, the reality was quite the opposite; the religious right attempted to derail the initiative.[88]

Since its origins, charitable choice has had broad bipartisan support. This includes not only from President Clinton, who signed the original bill into law, but also from Vice President Al Gore; his own vice presidential running mate, Sen. Joe Lieberman; Democratic governors, such as former governor Jim Hunt of North Carolina; and Democratic cabinet officials, such as Henry Cisneros, former secretary of Housing and Urban Development.[89] The office has continued throughout the past three administrations, while criticisms from left and right, respectively, tend to wax and wane depending upon which party is in power.

To be clear, the office did not allocate a single federal dollar to any faith-based group—it had no budget to fund any programs—and forbade federal monies received through an agency or department grant or contract from being earmarked to support religious activities. An Executive Order issued in 2002 made these points explicit, while clarifying the purpose of the office:

> Consistent with the Free Exercise Clause and the Free Speech Clause of the Constitution, faith-based organizations should be eligible to compete for Federal financial assistance used to support social service programs and to participate fully in the social service programs supported with Federal financial assistance without impairing their independence, autonomy, expression, or religious character. Accordingly, a faith-based organization that applies for or participates in a social service program supported with Federal financial assistance may retain its independence and may continue to carry out its mission, including the definition, development, practice, and expression of its religious beliefs, *provided that it does not use direct Federal financial assistance to support any inherently religious activities, such as worship, religious instruction, or proselytizing.*[90]

To ensure that these points were not missed with respect to health-related programs, Secretary Tommy G. Thompson of DHHS issued a Final Rule in 2004 that further clarified the specifics of the regulatory provisions derived from Bush administration Executive Orders.[91] It reiterated participation of FBOs in competition for department grant funds; forbade use of department funds for "inherently religious activities, such as worship, religious instruction, or proselytization";[92] underscored the independence of FBOs to carry out their religious mission, provided it is not done with federal funds; made clear that such recipients do not forfeit exemption from federal law prohibiting employment discrimination on the basis of religion; prohibited recipients from discriminating against prospective program beneficiaries on the basis of their religion or religious beliefs; and required recipients to carry out all program activities in strict compliance with department guidelines forbidding financial support of religious activities. The document also included several additional pages of detailed comments on and explanations of each of these concerns, especially regarding what is and is not permissible regarding religious organizations receiving federal funds from DHHS.[93]

In 2010 an Executive Order issued by President Obama amended President Bush's prior order from 2002 and reaffirmed the same points, using very similar language:

> Faith-based organizations should be eligible to compete for Federal financial assistance used to support social service programs and to participate fully in the social service programs supported with Federal financial assistance without impairing their independence, autonomy, expression outside the programs in question, or religious character. Accordingly, a faith-based organization that applies for, or participates in, a social service program supported with Federal financial assistance may retain its independence and may continue to carry out its mission, including the definition, development, practice, and expression of its religious beliefs, *provided that it does not use direct Federal financial assistance that it receives (including through a prime award or sub-award) to support or engage in any explicitly religious activities (including activities that involve overt religious content such as worship, religious instruction, or proselytization), or in any other manner prohibited by law.*[94]

Not to belabor this further, but note that establishment of a White House faith-based office was not the product of a devious Republican plot to undermine the U.S. Constitution and create a theocracy. The office passed muster with President Obama, progressive Democrat and former constitutional law instructor at the University of Chicago, who retained and built on President Bush's model. Moreover, charitable choice, which formed the basis for the office, was signed into law by President Clinton, also a Democrat and former law professor at the University of Arkansas. Charitable choice also received further constitutional vetting in law review articles[95] and in a report from the nonpartisan Congressional Research Service.[96] Additionally, a report from the liberal Brookings Institution, coauthored by Melissa Rogers, University of Pennsylvania–trained attorney, affirmed the legal and Constitutional parameters that should be met in operating federal faith-based initiatives and partnerships.[97] By now, the question of the constitutionality of charitable choice and the White House office is a nonissue, as much as anything can be in Washington—which means, at best, for the time being. The office, by all accounts, is "here to stay,"[98] unless and until some future president chooses to scuttle it.

For the first year and a half of the Trump administration, no announcement was made regarding the office, and many people in government speculated that the president had scrapped the concept. Its unsettled status led some to wonder— sadly or hopefully, depending upon their perspective—whether the office had been abolished for good. Bipartisan optimism about the office, especially since its renewal under President Obama, seemed to have vanished.

Finally, in May 2018, through Executive Order, the office was reestablished, modestly rebranded as the White House Faith and Opportunity Initiative (WHFOI).[99] It is similar to prior incarnations, with a few twists: (a) it is no longer a formal office run by a director, but an initiative led by an adviser reporting up through the assistant to the president for domestic policy; (b) it includes in its portfolio an explicit emphasis on religious freedom; and (c) it serves in a broader advisory function, providing recommendations regarding aspects of the administration's policy agenda and helping integrate aspects of this agenda "that affect faith-based and community programs and initiatives."[100] Beyond that, most everything else is unchanged, including a significant focus on healthcare. In November 2019, prosperity gospel preacher Paula White was appointed as the adviser for the WHFOI. Additionally, a formal Request for Information was earlier issued by DHHS, requesting a Solicitation of Comments, an important step in the reestablishment of the initiative's home in the department,[101] which is up and running.[102]

Despite speculation that the Trump administration was distancing itself from the faith-based concept due to its contentiousness or for other reasons, this turned out to be a serious misreading of the president. So the work continues, promoting collaboration between government and civil-society sectors. It makes sense that this would be so, as the idea of a broad-based initiative fostering opportunities "to strengthen the institutions of civil society and American families and communities"[103] across government domains reinforces themes that are held in favor by the administration, such as a commitment to strengthening infrastructure. The initiative has a lot to offer as a coordinating hub for programming already ongoing across government at all levels—federal, state, and local, as well as globally. But until the new leadership becomes acclimated and more information is made publicly available, it is not easy to anticipate how it will function or be received. As with much about the Trump administration, predicting what will transpire and how particular initiatives will be rolled out is difficult.

Membership and composition of the President's Advisory Council convened by each administration to support and oversee the work of the office provides insight into what each president sees as the office's religious and political parameters. During the Bush administration, the council featured mostly conservative Christians, especially evangelicals and Roman Catholics. During the Obama years, there were more liberal mainline Christians and a greater proportion of members of other religions, including representatives of Islam, Hinduism, Buddhism, Sikhism, the Bahá'í faith, Reconstructionist Judaism, and Native American spirituality.[104]

Name changes have meaning, too, in my opinion, offering a window into the perspective and values of the president. The Bush administration's "Community Initiatives" has a distinctly Chamber of Commerce feel, reflecting President

Bush's affinity for a business-oriented model. The Obama administration's "Neighborhood Partnerships," by contrast, gives off a New Urbanism vibe, consistent with President Obama's background in inner-city community organizing. The Trump administration's "Opportunity Initiative" gives the appearance of branding for a program to promote free enterprise and infrastructure development, in keeping with President Trump's career as a real estate developer.

Public reports were issued during Bush and Obama administrations outlining office accomplishments.[105] Other monthly Compassion in Action Roundtable events have highlighted office successes, such as on healthy families.[106] My Baylor University colleague Byron R. Johnson, director of the Institute for Studies of Religion, produced two valuable reports[107] summarizing and advocating for the kind of "public-private, sacred-secular partnerships"[108] supported by the office and its satellites in federal cabinet departments and agencies. Another important document, from early in the Obama administration, took stock of accomplishments of the office under President Bush and offered strategic recommendations from the President's Advisory Council on how to strengthen the work of the office and prepare for expansion and strengthening of faith-based partnerships.[109] An important focus of this report was its advocacy for religious freedom, specifically beneficiaries' "religious liberty rights."[110] This latter point is significant, as it shows that emphasis on religious liberty proclaimed in President Trump's recent Executive Order has precedent in recommendations made for the office by President Obama's advisers.

A major sector of programming for the office has been the domain of healthcare and public health. Programmatic and policy successes in community and global health during the Bush and Obama administrations were among the office's most prominent successes. Examples include the President's Health Center Initiative, which established twelve hundred community-based health centers mostly operated by FBOs; the Let's Move! Faith and Communities initiative, addressing childhood obesity through exercise and other interventions; Access to Recovery, a national program targeting substance abuse; the President's Malaria Initiative, a preventive program in fifteen countries; and myriad projects targeting hunger and nutrition assistance, at-risk youth, veterans' healthcare, HIV/AIDS, fatherhood and healthy families, violence against women, and more.[111] Not all of these efforts were under the aegis of the DHHS Partnership Center; some were overseen by faith-based offices in other cabinet departments.

The highest-profile success has been an innovative and celebrated global health program: the President's Emergency Plan for AIDS Relief (PEPFAR), originating during the Bush administration and then a centerpiece of the Obama administration's Global Health Initiative.[112] First funded by Congress in 2003 PEPFAR has been the most successful program ever established to address AIDS in the developing world. Under the leadership of Georgetown University physician Mark Dybul, beginning in 2006, PEPFAR was also the largest single initiative ever launched to address a single disease.[113] Uniquely at the time for a major global public health initiative, it was based on "a new philosophical foundation centered in country ownership, a results-based accountable approach, the engagement of all sectors, and good governance."[114]

A key to PEPFAR's success, according to Dybul, was that he was empowered to "break the rules and then rewrite them."[115] By this, Dybul meant that President Bush encouraged new ideas, "which turned the development debate on its head . . . rethinking the traditional roles of 'donor' and 'recipient.'"[116] This approach entailed establishing "a partnership between equals," fulfilling President Bush's desire to do away with the "old system laden with paternalism, postcolonial guilt, and Cold War meddling."[117] Dybul noted in 2009 that the new administration of President Obama "seems intent to build on those good ideas,"[118] which it did.[119] In 2018 PEPFAR celebrated its fifteenth anniversary of bipartisan leadership and support. Despite a mostly flat budget for the past decade, over 13 million adults and children to date have received lifesaving antiretroviral treatment.[120]

PEPFAR is significant for the present discussion because it rethought not just the conventions of development efforts and norms for faith-based interventions, but how government solves pressing social and health problems. Most efforts typically focus on funding downstream solutions, such as individual behavior-change programs, or emphasize upstream solutions, such as policy change. These are worthy approaches, of course, but distinctively top-down solutions ignore the possibility of drawing on vast private- and volunteer-sector and community resources from people and institutions that could become collaborative partners. There is thus a third way: midstream solutions involving partnerships between government and civil-society institutions, including the faith-based sector.

To this end I have been vocal in advocating for a role for the Surgeon General of the United States in leading such efforts for population health. In two published commentaries,[121] one written with Jay Hein, I made the case for the Surgeon General as a vital ally in educating Congress and the executive branch about the importance of faith-based partnerships for addressing systemic structural inequities, such as endemic poverty, at the foundation of population-health disparities.[122] There are ideological contingencies, however, especially pronounced in the current hyperpartisan Washington environment, that make this a thorny issue on which to expend political capital. It is less treacherous to advocate instead for solving such disparities via top-down, government-run programs focused on changing discrete health behaviors in individuals. This puts the burden for change on people located far downstream of structural and institutional sources of these disparities, and does so without assistance, resources, or insights from the most important, meaningful, and influential social network in many communities.

Religion and Global Health

This so-called third way—midstream partnerships with the civil-society sector including FBOs in partnership with governments, nongovernmental organizations (NGOs), and secular philanthropies—is no more evident than in global health. These represent a third domain of government and public-sector alliances and initiatives with FBOs for purposes of healthcare improvement and public health development. Christian NGOs have been especially involved in these partnerships.[123]

Such collaborative work extends beyond U.S. borders, addressing issues broader and more impactful—and more multidimensionally complex—than those involving the political calculus of domestic legislation. These include programs directed by transnational partnerships among governments, NGOs, religious bodies, and interfaith alliances. Such partnerships are not just desirable, but expedient and necessary: this is big-agenda work, often with a global or continental scope, and requires cooperation among powerful players from many sectors and nations. Especially valuable are nongovernmental bodies that can mobilize financial resources (funding), personal resources (warm bodies to do fieldwork), organizational resources (including leadership skills and acumen), and political resources (power and connections). All are required if these efforts are to succeed.

Faith-based NGOs are important players in humanitarian assistance, including healthcare, in the developing world. Among organizations that combine proselytizing with aid work, complicated ethical issues may arise.[124] For example, among communities or populations in need, such as disaster victims, proselytizing may not be a perceived need; and carried out nonconsensually, proselytizing may be exploitative of the vulnerability of victims and also a source of ill-being.[125] The counterargument is that government authorities "that decline the assistance of a faith-based NGO involved in proselytising work may deprive the needy of aid."[126] Specifically, "Agreeing to allow faith-based NGOs to operate frees much-needed resources for use in other communities, and preventing them from providing humanitarian assistance could have catastrophic consequences."[127]

The issue here is similar to what confronted the U.S. Congress and executive branch when the federal faith-based initiative was first being formulated, but the calculus is different. Whereas legislation and Executive Orders included clauses placing clear restrictions on certain religious activities, such as seeking converts, the situation confronting NGOs in international settings is more fluid and negotiable. Different nations and political bodies have different thresholds of accommodation.

Two positive examples can be identified involving the World Health Organization (WHO), which has long recognized the value of partnerships with the faith sector for addressing HIV/AIDS in Africa. A 2005 report described the Drug Resources Enhancement against AIDS and Malnutrition (DREAM) program undertaken in Mozambique by the Sant'Egidio Community,[128] a Rome-based Catholic lay movement with a heart for service to the poor, especially in Africa. The program combined Highly Active Anti-Retroviral Therapy with a comprehensive and multidimensional approach to care that is integrated into the country's National Health Service.[129] In a 2007 study focused on programs in Lesotho and Zambia, WHO reported that FBOs "play a much greater role in disease prevention, care and treatment than previously thought in sub-Saharan Africa."[130] The report offered recommendations to heighten dialogue and action between the faith and health sectors, including formal courses and joint training to develop religious and public health literacy in both sectors, increased programmatic and policy collaboration to engender respectful engagement across sectors, and collaborative research.[131]

WHO, notwithstanding, has been somewhat ambivalent in its commitment to faith-based collaboration, despite a history of successes. Perhaps this derives from politically charged perceptions of personal faith and institutional religion that differ dramatically across member nations and among professional leaders and apparatchiks in the organization. Many within WHO recognize the value of faith-based partnerships for addressing population-health goals and objectives, but powerful forces may constrain their effective advocacy. At the same time, this characterization should not be overstated. WHO has worked for decades with faith-based NGOs throughout the world in public health development and disease-eradication efforts. These include programs and initiatives addressing myriad issues: HIV/AIDS, smoking cessation, maternal and child health, diet and nutrition, the Ebola crisis, control of infectious diseases such as tuberculosis and malaria, healthcare access in underserved rural areas, undersupplies of medicines in isolated communities, and more.[132]

Through the years, WHO has worked with myriad faith-based NGOs in numerous programs, some small and focused, others broad and strategic. WHO partnered, for example, with UNICEF and the Christian Medical Commission of the World Council of Churches (WCC) to draft the 1978 Alma Ata declaration introducing the concept of "Health for All."[133] WHO's Partnership for Maternal, Newborn and Child Health has collaborated with Interchurch Medical Assistance (IMA) World Health, a U.S.-based nonprofit, in delivering healthcare services and supplies to vulnerable and marginalized people in the developing world.[134] WHO has estimated that "at least half of Africa's health care is provided by faith-based groups," including IMA World Health.[135]

In 2018 the director-general of WHO, Tedros Adhanom Ghebreyesus, delivered a remarkable address before the WCC, at an event commemorating its seventieth anniversary.[136] He reminded the gathering that WHO was founded the same year, and that both organizations had worked together on numerous projects since their beginnings. He also noted the centrality of health and healing to the ministry of Jesus and the work of churches ever since. Referencing a 1974 Memorandum of Understanding (MoU) between the organizations, he declared that "the time is right for a new MoU to mobilise faith-based organizations for universal health coverage and the SDGs [sustainable development goals]."[137]

Dr. Tedros, as he is known, prioritized joint efforts to provide universal healthcare by 2030, address widespread public health emergencies and humanitarian crises, and develop HPDP and disease-control programs in the developing world. This bold agenda will require both partners, WHO and WCC, working in tandem; it cannot be accomplished effectively in any other way. He continued, "As places of community and solidarity, churches and other faith-based institutions can play a vital role in promoting health. Faith leaders carry a voice of authority that sometimes speaks louder than that of governments and other leaders."[138] Both organizations, he concluded, shared a single vision: "'Health Promoting Churches' all over the world."[139]

This strong statement could be dismissed as a harmless keynote or stump speech before a partisan audience, but that would be mistaken. In the past, despite a long history of many ground-level alliances with churches and FBOs,[140] WHO has been reticent to make formal declarations like the one above. Their most recent report on traditional medicine strategies for the years 2014–2023, an important global initiative dating to 2002, makes no mention of churches, religion, or anything faith-based. The words do not even appear in the report.[141] I had my own experience of this institutional ambivalence in the mid-2000s when WHO contacted me from Geneva to ask for my leadership on an initiative or report (this was unclear) involving faith-based prevention of mental illness. I was very excited at the prospect, but after a couple conversations, WHO never followed up or contacted me further.

Other FBOs have developed their own multinational, cross-sector, interfaith partnership networks independently from WHO and other quasigovernmental bodies. An example is Christian Connections for International Health (CCIH), a U.S.-based organization founded in 1987. Today CCIH is a network of over three hundred Christian groups on five continents seeking "to promote global health and wellness from a Christian perspective."[142] It has several core focus areas, including community-based prevention and care, health systems strengthening, integration of faith and health, and women and child health. The latter is an initiative focusing on family planning based on voluntary prevention of pregnancy and excluding induced abortion services.[143]

Academics have become collaborative partners, both in planning, implementing, and evaluating faith-based health interventions and programs and in faith-based global health research. Graduate programs at the intersection of religion and public health have begun to appear in theological seminaries, such as joint M.Div./M.P.H. programs at Yale[144] and Emory,[145] training clergy for leadership roles in health ministries and missions at home and abroad. So much of global health is faith-infused, and so much of faith-based work in healthcare and public health is global in context. Overlap is becoming the norm, not the exception.

A prominent and important academic program in this field is located at Georgetown University. It integrates scholarship and development work in global health with the work of what it terms *faith-inspired organizations* (FIOs). The World Faiths Development Dialogue (WFDD) describes itself as "a secular, academic, non-profit research organization"[146] with two main institutional objectives:

> [T]o reinforce, underscore, and publicize the synergies and common purpose
> of religions and development institutions addressing poverty; and to explore
> issues on which there is little consensus and where common ground is unclear
> among different faith traditions, within faiths, and between faiths and develop-
> ment institutions.[147]

The WFDD was founded in 1998 by the president of the World Bank, James D. Wolfensohn, and the archbishop of Canterbury, Lord George Carey. Its academic home is at Georgetown's Berkley Center for Religion, Peace, and World Affairs under the direction of Katherine Marshall, professor at Georgetown's Walsh School of Foreign Service and former World Bank official. Marshall has written and lectured extensively for many years on topics at the interface of religion and global development,[148] including on population health and institutional faith-health partnerships.[149]

According to its most recent annual report, WFDD and its collaborative partner at the Berkley Center, the Religion and Global Development program, "occupy a significant position in the complex fields where religion, development, peacebuilding, and humanitarian relief intersect."[150] The WFDD has participated in and coordinated numerous initiatives throughout the world, on five continents, including projects related to population health. Through the years, it has been prolific in producing reports, policy briefs, and working papers detailing its project-specific work and its strategic efforts.

In a 2012 report, funded by the Tony Blair Faith Foundation, the WFDD summarized the ongoing work of the faith community targeting global health issues in Africa.[151] This was, in essence, a gigantic literature and program review. The report provided an overview of existing efforts by FIOs to provide healthcare throughout the African continent. It defined a faith-inspired organization as "a network, organization, program, project, facility, congregation, community, small group of individuals, faith leader, or other individual with links to or inspired by religion or spirituality, and a faith or denomination and the structures or individuals within it, providing or supporting social services."[152] The report was an insightful and devastating critique, but ultimately hopeful.

To begin, the report noted that "information on faith-inspired organizations is not systematic or comprehensive, and there are many substantial gaps in knowledge about FIOs."[153] In this respect, the situation is no different than for congregational HPDP programs and health-related faith-based initiatives in the United States. These gaps in knowledge matter, substantively, and not just to academics, because "without solid information and understanding of important health care providers, national and international organizations cannot make optimal choices on health policy, practices, and investments."[154] Accordingly, the report made an obligatory call to "develop evaluation methodologies that better assess the faith aspects and distinctive features" of the work of FIOs in global health development.[155]

The report also offered a glance at the amazing scope of the collective global effort, noting "there are *tens of thousands* of faith-inspired organizations working on health, representing different faiths and denominations, with great variation in size, structure, and other characteristics."[156] Another estimate enlarged this: over one hundred thousand FIOs are involved in health work just in Africa, and are the predominant nonprofit-sector providers of healthcare in many African countries.[157] Existing programs, moreover, cover a wide range of foci and outcomes, besides providing primary care, including health advocacy, behavior change communication, HIV/AIDS, malaria, major childhood diseases, maternal and child health, medical and nursing training, mental health, pharmaceutical and medical supplies, and tuberculosis.[158] The report concluded that while articles and reports typically "lament how little is known about faith-inspired work" on healthcare throughout the world, in reality, "substantial research, data, and knowledge exists."[159] What remains problematic is how few practitioners are aware of this work and available data.

An important outgrowth of WFDD is the Ahimsa Forum, a biennial roundtable event sponsored by the Ahimsa Fund, an organization seeking "to instigate change and implement innovative global health projects that are accessible to the poor and to create an international network of communities."[160]

The 2017 conference was cosponsored by WFDD on the theme of "Global Health, Social Entrepreneurship, and Faith-Inspired Communities," and Katherine Marshall was a featured speaker. The first Ahimsa event, in 2013, also cosponsored by WFDD, addressed a similar theme: "Global Health and Faith-Based Communities." Its panels focused on strategies by which FIOs can address a host of issues: poverty; healthcare growth inequity; faith-health partnerships for development; social resource scarcity, including infrastructure deficits; intersector communication challenges; tension between charity and sustainability; and empowerment of local faith-based communities, among other topics.[161] The second event, in 2015, followed up on the same topic,[162] and again the WFDD played a major role. Through these events, the Ahimsa Fund serves as "an incubator, an accelerator and a matchmaker" for collaborative projects, the most recent of which seeks to defeat noncommunicable diseases.[163]

Numerous other academic and philanthropic efforts, including cross-sector initiatives and government health diplomacy, are ongoing throughout the world. The best resource that summarizes existing work and unpacks the complexity of issues arising at the interface of religion and global health is *Beholden: Religion, Global Health, and Human Rights*, by Harvard's Susan R. Holman.[164] This book is highly recommended for anyone who wishes a thorough history and overview of this subject, written by an academician uniquely credentialed in both religious studies and public health and with years of experience in the field. *Beholden* underscores how governments, religions, and service organizations must negotiate their way through uniquely constructed sets of political, ideological, and cultural barriers. The idea of beholden-ness, according to Holman, ought to "shape a vision for what is possible at the intersection of religion and global health,"[165] grounded in a conviction that

> human rights history and ideas should matter for people of religious faith and that anyone engaged in faith-based aid organizations has a fundamental responsibility to understand something about this issue and be familiar with resources that are available to help foster such accountability.[166]

The Future of Faith-Health Partnerships

Despite complexities and controversies defining the intersection of religion and religious institutions with medicine and healthcare in the policy sphere, faith-based institutions have much to offer as we strive to build a healthier planet. Moreover, we probably cannot achieve all that we need without participation from such institutions. An analysis published in 2016 reported that the most conservative estimate of the annual economic value of FBOs to the U.S. economy is $378 billion. Correcting for the fair-market value of goods and services provided puts the annual value at about $1.2 trillion.[167] "The faith sector," the authors conclude, "is undoubtedly a significant component of the overall American economy, impacting and involving the lives of the majority of the U.S. population."[168] This includes substantial contributions to healthcare and health.

The contentiousness of these efforts may just come with the territory and must be accommodated or otherwise dealt with as difficult ideological and turf-related issues arise. Perhaps there is no way around it. But as the recent history of health-care reform and domestic and global health–related advocacy establishes, this path is worth traveling, as much social good can come from such partnerships and initiatives, at least when partners are working harmoniously toward the same identified end.

The takeaway from this chapter, however, should not be overstated. The intersections among religion, medicine, and government programs and policies are not all rosy and civic-minded. History reveals a nefarious dimension too.

Consider, for example, Operation Whitecoat, a classified project that involved conducting biodefense research on test subjects drawn from among Seventh-day Adventist conscientious objectors.[169] Readers unfamiliar with this project may find the details hard to believe.

Beginning in 1954, a top-secret experimental program was initiated at Fort Detrick, Maryland, directed by the U.S. Army Medical Research Institute of Infectious Disease, in which over two thousand human volunteers were infected with dangerous pathogenic agents believed to be candidates for Soviet biological weapons. Exposures included developmental vaccines or actual virulent agents for tularemia, yellow fever, plague, Q fever, Rift Valley fever, anthrax, chikungunya, sand fly fever, staphylococcal enterotoxin B, multiple versions of equine encephalitis, and a few other diseases.[170] Volunteers were largely drawn from among conscientious objectors and members of the Seventh-day Adventist Church. The program operated for nearly twenty years and had the enthusiastic support of the church, which viewed Whitecoat as an extension of its long-standing humanitarian mission and a meaningful way for its noncombatant membership to contribute to their country's defense.[171]

Decades later, a controlled, retrospective cohort study examined surviving volunteers and found no significant and lasting health deficits, at least within the substantial limitations of the follow-up study, which examined only a fraction of participants.[172] This result is gratifying, especially for the brave men who took part and their families. But it does beg the question as to the sophistication of the original experiments: these men, after all, were being used as guinea pigs for testing presumably dangerous biological weapons. Did these weapons even work? Were they tested correctly? Were they ever a significant threat to the population? After all of this, is the United States any safer than before?

In this strange and obscure episode in the history of the United States (and the history of medicine and the history of religion), the federal government in conjunction with the defense establishment implemented a policy that exploited religious ties of its citizens in a way that threatened to do great harm to their health, promoting it as service to the common good—and enabling the military to develop covert weapons that could potentially harm the health of citizens of other nations.[173] Knowing what we do now about other morally dubious projects involving the government and the health of Americans—the U.S. Public Health Service's racist and genocidal Tuskegee Syphilis Experiment[174] and the CIA's notorious MKULTRA mind-control program[175] come to mind—perhaps something like Whitecoat is not difficult to imagine. What sets it apart, however, is the willing accedence of a religious denomination that encouraged participation among its members and that to this day praises the episode as patriotic and heroic.

Thankfully, such episodes have been rare, presumably. It pays to recognize, though, that government involvement can co-opt, preempt, or otherwise compromise medicine. It can do the same to religion. Yet government involvement also can serve to align religion-medicine partnerships with strategic goals and objectives, enabling them to have the greatest reach and do the most good. The programs described in this chapter underscore this point. But such involvement also can mean government control, which threatens to derail and subtly shift the motives animating the original intent. Perhaps the best and most promising religion-medicine alliances evolve organically and function outside the purview of government agencies.

FBOs and people of faith have critical roles to play in healthcare policy and delivery, but may be more effective the more independent they can remain from government sanction and oversight. Alliances with local, state, and federal agencies can be fruitful without ceding command and control authority to the state. Agents of government do not need to serve as final decisors in such partnerships for there to be successful outcomes, but this requires civil-society institutions to withstand the temptation to submit to government control as a condition of funding. This is an underrepresented dilemma in current discussions of the challenges and dangers of faith-based involvement in charitable choice.

At the same time, as much as governments stand to gain from healthcare alliances with faith-based institutions, religious people and organizations have more to gain from participation in the political life of the nation and world. Service to humankind, writ large, requires people and institutions of faith to take on an advocacy role, fulfilling the prophetic function of calling out governments for their endemic torpor and injustice in meeting the needs of citizens. The deck may be stacked against the faith community in such transactions—other players, government included, may have more decision-making authority and more power to dictate outcomes—but compassion and justice require that their voice be heard. Indeed, cultivating and encouraging moral and ethical action in the public sphere is an essential and ubiquitous function of religions.[176]

Religious voices are among the most passionate and articulate champions for domestic and global health justice. Mixed successes of organizations such as the National Religious Partnership for the Environment (NRPE), an interfaith alliance of religious groups advocating for political action addressing climate change and environmental justice,[177] demonstrate that it is possible for Catholics, evangelicals, mainline Protestants, and Jews to make common cause for health-directed advocacy. The NRPE, through its ethical stance identifying a biblical grounding for integrating ecological concern with social justice activism, has been moderately effective, according to the title of an insightful sociological analysis, in promoting the "greening of mainline American religion."[178] Recent commentaries have identified shared themes in moral theology across faiths supporting health-related efforts of both small and large scale. These include supporting policies that seek compassion and health justice for victims of the 2014 Ebola outbreak[179] and grand alliances seeking international cooperation in creating health infrastructure in the developing world.[180]

As long as religion has existed, it has ensured that its voice be heard in the public square. Sometimes its presence in public discourse is articulate and a force for good. Other times, its words are incoherent and disruptive. Religion can be a unifying influence, bringing out the best of what humans have to offer, or its representatives can be apostles of divisiveness. Regardless, people and institutions of faith are and always have been at the forefront of U.S. social change, whether promoting positive transformation in social policy, as in the civil rights movement, or ramping up collective hatred, as in the current backlash against Muslim-American citizens.[181]

In their edited collection, *Religion Returns to the Public Square: Faith and Policy in America*, political scientist Hugh Heclo and historian Wilfred M. McClay describe religion's ever-present place in American public life.[182] Religion and faith have been factors in the political calculus since the time of the founders, although generalizations about their constructive and destructive influences are hard to come by.[183] Heclo tells the story of "the profound, troubled, and inescapable interaction between religious faith and government action in the United States."[184] This interaction occurs across three domains, or rather from three interrelated perspectives: institutional, involving federal and state governments; behavioral, involving religious identities and beliefs that motivate personal actions; and philosophical, involving ways that religion, generally, and specific religions inform "broad policy outlooks on the social order."[185]

We can observe the interaction of religion and public policy in each of these three ways within numerous public policy domains, including and especially related to healthcare and public health. For example, as we have seen, religious denominations lobbied strongly for healthcare reform legislation, Catholic bishops and evangelical pastors have spoken out against taking the life of the unborn, and interfaith organizations have offered a unified front articulating why respecting the natural environment is a universal spiritual value and sacred obligation. We can also observe how the complicated, multidimensional dance between faith groups and policymakers plays out uniquely within government, political, and civil-society sectors, which overlap and interact with each other in myriad ways, overtly and covertly. Heclo notes that connections between religion and public policy are "profound and unavoidable," specifically because "both claim to give authoritative answers to important questions about how people should live."[186] He describes this as an "inescapable coupling"[187] but reminds us that religion and policy are distinctive, with different functions and worldviews, and thus "mark a continuous flash point in public life."[188] This is obvious in any retrospective look at contemporary and unending debates over healthcare reform and the federal faith-based office.

At the risk of resorting to a cliché, and despite many challenges and barriers manifest throughout global faith-health partnerships,[189] I believe that the future is bright. For one, existing work has achieved measurable successes, even if program evaluations are often unsophisticated and large-scale evaluative research lacking. But I also believe in the potential for such collaborative work because the situation demands it. These efforts are especially vital in light of the accelerated global connectedness of the world's population and ongoing resource scarcity that shows no sign of abating. This work will succeed because it *has* to—we have few other options, and governments alone cannot meet the need. Only continued and expanded intersector cooperation, however configured, can marshal the requisite personal, financial, and tangible resources. To use a financial metaphor, I would buy futures in faith-based global population-health work. This is the next chapter in the historic alliance between religion and medicine.

9

Challenges and Choices

Efforts to establish and maintain alliances between religion and medicine, as we have seen, are multidimensional and have existed for centuries, or longer. But continued functioning of such partnerships, especially those operating under professional oversight of institutional medicine, face persistent challenges. Foremost is ongoing competition between the medical and faith-based sectors to define the terms of engagement and exert final decision-making authority on playing fields where they compete. At present, this encounter is one-sided:

> Medicine, in the final analysis, calls the shots and jealously guards its turf, uneasy about sharing decision-making authority with faith even in matters where said domain possesses expertise that better equips it than medicine to make informed judgments. Where faith maintains a say (e.g., in bioethics, healthcare chaplaincy, medical missions) it is only because medicine lets it. More could be said, but suffice it to add one note: the dynamics of the faith-medicine relationship, as manifested in all sorts of research and scholarly endeavors and in all manner of professional activities, is complex and a function of dynamic forces both historical and political.[1]

Many of these forces are outlined in this book. Negotiating their dynamics is a continual undertaking, just as since the first encounters between religion and medicine thousands of years ago. Will these institutions ever be best friends, contented partners characterized by happy and copacetic relations? This seems unlikely—too much is currently at stake. Both institutions control a wide domain, exerting respective decision-making authority over matters of spirit and flesh,[2] although in parts of the developed world religion's dominance is not as state-sanctioned now as in the past.[3] Increasingly, medicine—and science, generally—is an arbiter of the most important issues facing civilization. Scientists and physicians are deferred to in matters of gravest import involving our collective future, supplanting religious leaders as moral decisors and lead agents of social control.[4] This medicalization of morals has been seen as a marker of the secularization of society.[5]

Actually, waxing and waning of medicine's and religion's spheres of influence have been everpresent, like a constantly undulating *yin-yang* symbol, throughout

Religion and Medicine. Jeff Levin, Oxford University Press (2020) © Oxford University Press.
DOI: 10.1093/oso/9780190867355.001.0001

history. At no point has ascendancy of one source of authority extinguished the influence of the other. If circumstances are right, they can find a way to do business.

An interesting historical account of the Society for the Suppression of Vice in early nineteenth-century England[6] describes its effort to redefine and regulate "moral insanity" from a quasiscientific perspective.[7] According to the authors, "The doctrine of moral insanity arose from an attempt to reconcile theological concerns to sustain the notion of the corrupt and immaterial soul with a burgeoning medical science. . . . As a body of discourses, medicine legitimated and encoded morality through its status as science."[8] This movement was instrumental in the origins of psychiatry and psychology later in the century, but ultimately unsuccessful in smothering the authority of religion. The new nosological understanding of mental disease offered a "science of morality, which transcended but did not displace religious doctrine."[9] Any emerging conflict between competing religious and medical authority was "partially reconciled . . . through the endorsement of theological morality by the medical profession."[10]

The complementarity of medicine and religion is exemplified in the story of the Vice Society: each player had something valuable for the other. Medicine provided religion with a rational and ostensibly science-based validation of its moral position. Religion enabled medicine to expand its reach into the realm of human behavior. Each party benefited. Summarizing the history of the encounter between religion and medicine by asserting a correlation of medicalization and secularization is to oversimply a more complicated, nuanced, and dynamic narrative. Sociologist Peter Conrad, leading expert on medicalization, emphasized this point over twenty-five years ago: "While it is true that medicine is in important ways nudging aside religion as our moral touchstone, the interface of medicine and religion is more complex than a simple secularization thesis would suggest."[11] Another recent consideration: preeminent sociologists of religion have begun questioning whether evidence for secularization even exists.[12]

Not to overstate, but religion and medicine continue to function as rivals. Whether friendly rivals or locked in a death struggle, or something in between, this depends upon the context and circumstances of a particular encounter. The terrain upon which these institutions compete to exert their respective authority determines how medicine wields its upper hand, and how heavy-handed it does so.

At present, the conversation between religion and medicine—what academics call a "discourse"—is more like two separate conversations.[13] In one, religion is a problematic, or focus of concern, for medicine, the best example being the research studies described in Chapter 5. The methodologies of medical research are employed to document the impact of religion on the health of people or populations or on healing. In the other conversation, medicine is the problematic, or focus, for religion, characterized by bioethics, healthcare delivery, medical missions, and pastoral care. Perspectives drawn from pastoral, moral, or practical theology, for example, are applied to issues that arise in the practice of medicine or in public health. For good reason, the corpus of scholarly writing at the intersection of religion and medicine has been described as "a tale of two literatures."[14] As I hope this book has made apparent, *religion and medicine* may be a useful label for naming an area of scholarship or tracing the history of relations between two meta-institutions, but does not define a single undifferentiated phenomenon. It is not one thing, but many.

Perhaps it is unrealistic to expect that relations between religion and medicine will ever be substantially better than they are now. Anyway, the world is too complex and fractured for a single model of their underlying relationships— for example, the complementarity spoken of throughout this book—to hold sway across faith traditions, systems of medical care, and global cultures. This fracturing suggests there may be multiple futures to consider. In some places and settings religion and medicine may remain at odds, antagonists working at cross purposes. Elsewhere they may function in tandem, or maintain separate domains but with minimal contention, each recognizing and accepting the other's boundaries. Elsewhere still, they may come together into some new creation acknowledging their separation as illusion and envisioning an ideal future where they are one: healing as sacred calling, and spirituality as healing journey.

Then, too, there is the familiar observation that Western medicine has bifurcated into two paths that define respective and distinctive futures.[15] There is the technological approach of academic Western medicine that defines biomedical research and institutional medical care: high-tech diagnostic equipment; genomics and genetic manipulation in the lab; personalized "designer" pharmaceuticals; increased use of artificial intelligence in the clinical encounter, from history-taking to diagnosis to devising treatment plans; and so on. Undergraduate medical education is reducing contact with real people with real diseases, substituting standardized patients; doctor-patient contact, when real, is becoming virtual, as with telemedicine.

By contrast, there is the call for a more humanistic approach to medicine,[16] with evidence that it is finally gaining traction. Signs point to a quickening: changes in medical curricula, with patient contact beginning in year one; changes to the MCAT, which now tests for knowledge from psychology and social science; growth in university programs and majors in the medical humanities; team-based clinical practices placing a premium on whole-person care; and mainstreaming of previously "alternative" therapies, including spiritually based approaches, into models of integrative medical practice.

Medicine thus seems headed in two different directions simultaneously. Each idealized future is like a vector shooting toward the horizon, accelerating forward, the two paths speeding further apart with time. Each future expresses a distinctive worldview: one valuing science and technology as the ultimate arbiter of medical decision-making and parameters of our collective future, the other prioritizing cultivation of healthy relationships and moral consensus in mapping how we can heal and become whole, as individuals and a society. The former has no place for religion, spirituality, or faith in the calculus defining health, healing, or medical care; for the latter, it is a cornerstone. Some hope has been expressed that these two futures can be reconciled,[17] but I am withholding judgment. I am hopeful, but not optimistic.

Relations between religion and medicine are just as polarized and unsettled elsewhere in their wider encounter. Divergent futures can be envisioned for religion not just within clinical practice and medical education. Especially as the organization, delivery, and financing of medicine and healthcare become matters of national policy and global outreach, how the institutions of religion and medicine are able to cooperate is becoming a matter of public debate. Further separation and alienation are possible, as is an enthusiastic embrace of new alliances. None of us has a crystal ball, so none of us can state definitively what the future will resemble. But we can identify significant challenges whose negotiated resolution will go a long way toward determining whether the future of the religion and medicine story is one of continued conflict or renewed cooperation and partnership.

To restate, religion and medicine have a history of encounter extending back a long time. This is not in doubt. But that is not to say that every important issue has been settled. Serious questions remain, and choices must be made regarding the near and mid-term future of alliances between religion and medicine. By this I mean strategic relations between the faith-based and medical sectors, broadly defined, as well as functional relations between people, professions, organizations, and initiatives representing these two worlds.

Unpacking such issues in their entirety is beyond the scope of this chapter. But prominent challenges and concerns are discussed here in the form of questions meriting thoughtful consideration by medical practitioners, religious professionals, academic scholars, and policymakers. These questions do not all originate with me; others have broached them also. For some, answers have already been proposed. But for the most part these matters still need resolving. The issues are raised here to help frame the evolving conversation between religion and medicine.

Legal and Constitutional Challenges

Multisector partnerships between the private and civil-society sectors and government agencies, as described in Chapter 8, play an expanding role in public health interventions and community-wide healthcare programs. Federal funding of faith-based initiatives involving local congregations and religious denominations remains subject to political debate,[18] despite judicial vetting during the Clinton, Bush, and Obama administrations.[19] Careful efforts were made to delineate parameters of what is and is not permissible in such partnerships, fueled by public voicing of concerns when the White House faith-based office was established. The charitable choice doctrine, formulated under President Clinton, and federal funding of faith-based programs, which predates by decades establishment of a White House faith-based office under President Bush, create administrative, legal, and ethical challenges that persist despite repeated efforts to clarify what is acceptable.[20] While the contentiousness of these disputes has died down, key questions remain.[21]

What are or should be parameters surrounding federal funding of faith-based initiatives and partnerships in health?

This is the most widely voiced question that continues to be raised, even two decades after charitable choice became public policy. Debate continues on both sides of the political aisle, with proponents and opponents among both Republicans and Democrats.[22] Despite the continued successes of such partnerships, their lower-profile and relative lack of media attention compared to a decade ago have rendered them out of sight and out of mind as far as the general public and academic community are concerned. Continual parsing of this question is no longer a high priority for public debate (although it continues in Washington and state houses), so widespread controversy over this initiative has diminished. Nonetheless, the federal government maintains a formidable stake in a faith-based role in healthcare and public health, even if its presence is less publicized.

The ambiguity of the current status of the initiative is best exemplified by one unusual fact: faith-based offices still exist in about a dozen cabinet-level departments and federal agencies and still actively pursue their mission, including the DHHS Partnership Center,[23] yet a White House office was not established until almost halfway through the present administration. At the time of this writing, the office does not even appear in public documentation of the White House's executive administrative structure.[24]

Before the question posed above can be answered, it would be helpful to clarify the status of the White House faith-based initiative and the administration's intent to maintain support of federal faith-based initiatives in health. The DHHS center continues to operate, and in keeping with current priorities now focuses on the opioid crisis, childhood obesity, and severe mental illness; is explicit in its intention to "champion religious liberty"; and is directed by an attorney with a background working for conservative think tanks.[25] This is a break with the Obama and Bush administrations, when the DHHS center was led by individuals with professional expertise in administering health- or human-services-related programs. This suggests, possibly, that the current administration envisions a more politically driven role for the DHHS center, although under the Obama administration it was also engaged in politically partisan efforts, including promotion of the PPACA legislation.

Who defines acceptable behavior—of a religiously partisan nature—on the part of funding recipients?

This issue was debated at length at the outset of the Bush administration. As detailed in the previous chapter, presidential Executive Orders,[26] law review articles,[27] and other policy-related documents[28] adjudicated parameters of permissible behavior, and as noted, public outcry seems to have died down. Moreover, vetting these parameters is oftentimes depicted by proponents of a federal role in promoting faith-based partnerships as indicating that the matter is settled. But this may be an overstatement, for two reasons.

First, few things are ever settled in national politics; parsing and renegotiation are never-ending, or at least appear as such in order to play to various constituencies. More importantly, concerns continue to be expressed about the boundaries of current efforts—that is, what constitutes going too far, in a faith-based sense—due to reports of questionable behavior on the part of funding recipients. A case in point involves a federal court ruling that an evangelical prison ministry program in Iowa misused federal funds by violating the Constitution's Establishment Clause forbidding state funding of sectarian religious activities.[29]

Second, religious liberty has become such a political hot potato of late that renewed questioning of official federal neutrality regarding religion—whether such neutrality exists or should exist—adds a dimension of controversy to consideration of any federal interface with the faith-based sector. This issue pits features of the PPACA, which establishes legislatively approved entitlements, against features of the Religious Freedom Restoration Act of 1993 (RFRA). The highest-profile court case to date has involved Hobby Lobby, a company owned by an evangelical Christian family who argued that the PPACA's contraception mandate required it to pay for employee coverage of certain contraceptive methods that violated the religious beliefs of the company's owners. After district and appeals court rulings, *Burwell v. Hobby Lobby* was taken up by the U.S.

Supreme Court, which found in favor of Hobby Lobby.[30] Yet another dimension of this debate entails conflict between the healthcare rights of patients and religious freedom of medical care providers who dissent from performing certain procedures on grounds that they are protected by a conscience clause.[31]

An interesting historical reminder that may seem paradoxical in the currently polarized political climate: the major pieces of legislation establishing contemporary federal accommodation of the faith-based sector were *all* signed into law by President Clinton, not by a Republican. These include RFRA,[32] the bill creating the Office of International Religious Freedom,[33] and the charitable choice provision that was the basis for the White House faith-based office.[34] The parameters of what is and is not acceptable when it comes to religion's encounter with the federal government, whether as a funding recipient or in political advocacy, were first laid out in detail and vetted during the Clinton administration in the 1990s. Subsequent administrations have provided mostly restatement and clarification but not a dramatic rereading of these boundaries. This reality is obscured in the convoluted political narratives on the proper role of religion in the public sphere subsequently and still advanced in Washington.

How does society balance the religious liberty of faith-based organizations (FBOs) with entitlements regarding public funding and access to healthcare?

This is the most prominent point of contention in the current debate over government faith-based initiatives. It is the poster child for what can go wrong when religion intrudes upon otherwise secular domains, such as the medical sector. In contemporary discussions of a potential rapprochement between religion and medicine, the skeptical narrative has mostly focused on moral, ethical, or legal issues related to easily sensationalized phenomena, such as parents denying medical treatment for children on religious grounds, acts of violence against abortion clinics, phony television faith healers, and doctors praying with patients. Since passage of the PPACA and the political battle to repeal or replace it, the most heated and visible point of contention has become a perceived conflict between provisions of this legislation and the religious freedom of persons and organizations opposed to certain provisions on grounds of conscience. This issue was not on the radar when charitable choice was signed into law; indeed, it passed without much public notice.[35]

The Hobby Lobby case underscores the contentiousness of this issue, and also the difficulty in parsing respective political support for and opposition to underlying issues in historically predictable ways. For example, a recent law journal article offered a "liberal case for *Hobby Lobby*,"[36] arguing that the reflexive liberal reaction to the Supreme Court ruling was "misguided" as "the decision is rooted in principles liberals should find deeply attractive."[37] Liberal Harvard law professor Alan Dershowitz concurred, noting that the decision is "monumentally insignificant" because "it was not a constitutional decision, it was a construction of a statute," and "not a single woman will be denied contraceptive care . . . and won't be burdened in any way."[38] Interestingly, he supported the ruling while strongly disagreeing with Hobby Lobby's stance on contraception and also supported passage of the PPACA.[39]

Political and Policy Challenges

Centuries-long traditions of medical care and health-directed work, as described in Chapters 2, 3, and 4, originated with religious organizations and people. Religious institutions and leaders built the first hospitals, established the first medical missions, and set up the first congregational health clinics and community-based health programs. Alliances with public health agencies are more recent in origin, but have become more visible in the new century. Strategic population-health objectives for the United States continue to be met through working relationships between the religious and public-health sectors.[40] While this is not unappreciated within public health circles,[41] the how of such partnerships remains a work in progress, especially for faith-based efforts with global partners.[42] To nurture these relationships, this conversation requires thinking through important questions.

How can the public-health sector best work with FBOs to reduce population-health disparities?

According to a consensus of public health practitioners, scientists, and historians, there is no stronger determinant of the health of populations than social class or socioeconomic status.[43] This finding is a hallmark of social epidemiology.[44] A recent review implicated poverty, social-class disparities, and poor social conditions as "the world's most pervasive public health problems. They are salient and consistent determinants of population-health status, according to various measures, and are thus responsible for an enormous toll in health-related suffering."[45] The effects of poverty on health are consistent, ubiquitous, and of substantial magnitude:

> Poverty is associated with a greater risk of chronic degenerative and acute and chronic infectious diseases; it mitigates access to preventive health services and medical care; and it causes and interacts with other social dysfunctions that themselves heighten population-health risk and are associated with deficits in subjective well-being. People in poverty live shorter lives, suffer a greater

disease burden, experience more symptomatology and pain, endure greater disability, have higher rates of depression, lose more work days, and receive less and worse medical care than those with sufficient material resources.[46]

These findings hold true for the United States and globally. They are even observed ecologically, across nations: wealthier and more educated countries have lower mortality and greater physical and psychological well-being; poorer and less educated countries do worse.[47] This has been acknowledged by WHO,[48] which also notes, regrettably, "The failure of publicly financed health care to reach the poor in almost all developing countries, an issue that deserves serious attention from governments and aid agencies."[49]

Accordingly, there is no more critical priority for public health policy, including in the United States, than implementation of a systematic antipoverty agenda featuring outside-the-box thinking to marshal "cross-sector partnerships."[50] Institutional resources are available from within the civil-society sector, including private, nonprofit volunteer organizations.[51] These can be utilized to strengthen community infrastructure, fill in gaps left by inadequate government social programs, and establish new alliances to create enduring structures for meeting local needs. Such agendas have been proposed as a matter of social policy for decades, but not been explicitly positioned as central to strengthening national infrastructure in public health. Only recently has this issue been raised in earnest.

In a commentary published in 2017 in *Public Health Reports*, the official journal of the U.S. Public Health Service, I advocated for "a renewed emphasis on antipoverty efforts . . . as a focal point of a national public health agenda."[52] A defining feature of my proposal was for a national policy emphasizing solutions featuring interventions drawing on midstream (that is, civil-society sector) resources alongside upstream solutions (for example, government policies) and downstream solutions (for example, behavior change programs), the norm for most government public health efforts. I noted that

too often public health occurs either exclusively far downstream, via programs focused solely on modifying discrete lifestyle behaviors, or exclusively far upstream, via florid national policy recommendations mandating top-down regulatory bodies. The midstream domain is typically overlooked, and outreach to potential institutional allies in redressing community- and population-wide health inequalities is neglected. Moreover, midstream intervention serves as a functional bridge linking social and health policy with the behavior and lives of people.[53]

Former U.S. Surgeon General David Satcher also advocated for a national public health strategy comprising all three levels of intervention.[54] An especially underutilized midstream resource is the faith-based sector: the totality of religious congregations, denominations, agencies, and volunteer organizations providing human services, meeting needs, and reaching underserved people and communities that government fails to adequately accommodate. There is precedent for partnerships between FBOs and public health agencies,[55] as described in Chapter 4, and current or previously existing programs have focused on disease prevention, health promotion, primary care, health policy advocacy, and other areas of public health and preventive medicine.[56] An expansion of such efforts should be part of a renewed national strategy of public health reform.[57]

What opportunities are there for DHHS agencies and offices to work in conjunction with the faith-based sector to meet national health objectives?

The answer depends on the willingness of the leadership of DHHS and respective DHHS agencies and offices to work in collaboration with FBOs. That willingness has been present during the past four presidential administrations. The Partnership Center has been a valuable resource for connecting specific religious entities with specific resource partners and respective government bodies in order to address national objectives. Over the past decade, such partnerships have targeted many issues of public health importance, including pregnancy and maternal and child health, fatherhood and healthy families, obesity and exercise, access to healthcare, HIV/AIDS, and opioid addiction and mental illness.

More systematic efforts are possible, involving partner agencies and offices throughout DHHS. This may be a worthwhile way to expand present efforts and take better advantage of vast personal and tangible resources that populate the faith community in the United States. In establishing the White House's faith-based office, President Bush spoke famously of "armies of compassion."[58] But in the domain of healthcare and public health, these armies have functioned less effectively than they could have, had their efforts been better coordinated and focused. For example, in the 2014–2018 DHHS strategic plan, implemented during the Obama administration, there was only a single, nonspecific reference to leveraging collaborations with faith-based groups in fostering public-private partnerships.[59]

There is reason, however, for optimism. In the most recent DHHS strategic plan, for 2018–2022, issued by the Trump administration, FBOs are mentioned in numerous places: as partners in cross-agency collaborations, in efforts to increase access and use of healthcare benefits, and in identifying best practices to meet consumer needs and public health priorities, enhancing cultural competence of departmental communications and population health literacy, engaging with at-risk populations to improve medical decision-making and healthy lifestyle choices, addressing mental health problems and substance abuse, strengthening emergency preparedness and response, responding to economic and social needs of refugees, promoting independence among people with disabilities, supporting caregivers, and implementing programs and research on accident prevention, dating violence, youth mentoring, healthy marriage and relationship counseling, child development, and many other community health issues.[60]

Elsewhere in DHHS there has been some strategic outreach to the faith community. The Office of Global Affairs (OGA) was established to "foster critical global relationships, coordinate international engagement across HHS and the U.S. government, and provide leadership and expertise in global health diplomacy and policy."[61] Through OGA and its predecessors, DHHS implements various strategic agendas. One of these is its Global Health Strategy,[62] a four-year plan that lays out partnerships among U.S. government agencies, national governments, multilateral organizations, and civil-society and nongovernmental groups, including faith-based groups that provide humanitarian service.[63] The OGA is also a principal U.S. governmental player in the Global Health Security Agenda,[64] a worldwide partnership among sixty-seven nations and numerous NGOs, including FBOs that contribute to particular projects, such as HIV/AIDS prevention and maternal and child health.

One place within DHHS where a more substantial engagement of religion and FBOs might pay substantial dividends is the Office of Disease Prevention and Health Promotion (ODPHP), which oversees national health goals. The most recent strategic plan, known as Healthy People 2020, identifies over forty topic areas, including major causes of death (e.g., cancer, heart disease and stroke, HIV, diabetes, accidents) and upstream issues such as social determinants of health, preparedness, public health infrastructure, global health, environmental health, and access to health services.[65] Each topic has associated objectives, interventions and resources, and national statistics. A new version of Healthy People is issued every ten years, the closest thing to an official public health plan for government, consumers, policymakers, and researchers.

A helpful recommendation, in my opinion, would be to use Healthy People as "a template to help delineate and organize a full range of public health activities that involve faith-based resources, both people and institutions, in various types of partnerships across the determinants of population health (i.e., social, environmental, behavioral), across the levels of public health action (i.e., upstream, midstream, downstream), and across particular public health issues."[66] DHHS could produce a summary document and associated online resource that includes a comprehensive review of evidence summarizing the impact of religious and faith-based variables, interventions, and organizations in each respective topic area. Evidence would come from various sources: epidemiology, health services research, community health education, health policy, and elsewhere. Such a companion document to Healthy People could serve an important function:

> It would provide for the first time, by documenting faith-based efforts and resources and any evaluative evidence, a complete catalog of historical and ongoing public health programs and initiatives with significant faith-based content. It would also provide a useful baseline for the development of detailed goals, objectives, and implementation plans for federal faith-based efforts related to each Topic Area over the course of the Healthy People 2020 implementation period and beyond.[67]

I have offered this suggestion on a few occasions,[68] including in a commentary in *Public Health Reports*.[69] I also communicated the idea a few years ago to a senior administrator at DHHS, and the recommendation was well received. But, given the existing political realities of the previous administration, I was told that the idea would have to come from outside the department. With the current administration, it will be interesting to observe whether a presumably more faith-friendly environment will welcome such an effort. A small but positive sign: in the planning document for the forthcoming Healthy People 2030 project,[70] among the list of "stakeholders" recommended for developing objectives, setting priorities, and identifying data needs are "Faith-based communities."[71]

Another location within DHHS that would benefit from an alliance with the faith community is the Office of the Surgeon General (OSG), administered by the Surgeon General of the United States. That person is not, as commonly believed, the "nation's doctor" or chief medical adviser to the president, nor is it just a ceremonial position. By statute, the Surgeon General is the operational commander of the Commissioned Corps of the U.S. Public Health Service and provides public health policy analysis and advice to the executive branch and to the American people.[72] Among the most important public roles of the Surgeon General is the bully pulpit provided by OSG to communicate health-promoting messages. Each Surgeon General has utilized the office to prioritize one or more respective health topics of special concern, including smoking, childhood immunization, AIDS, health disparities, and obesity.[73]

In an article with Jay Hein, we offered "a faith-based prescription for the Surgeon General,"[74] outlining an agenda by which OSG can leverage faith-based resources by advocating for collaborative efforts to solve "both acute public health crises and more chronic deficiencies in preparedness and response to longer-standing population health risks."[75] Our main action items entailed partnerships with religious organizations and institutions consistent with the historic mission of the U.S. Public Health Service:

- Informing the public, raising risk awareness, and changing behavior.
- Identifying public health needs and eliminating health disparities in under-served populations.
- Delivering preventive healthcare.
- Strengthening the national resolve to bolster the public health infrastructure.
- Meeting the nation's global health responsibilities.[76]

These ideas were fleshed out in a follow-up article underscoring "the consonance of the public health ethic and the communal and social-justice ethos of the major faith traditions."[77] To date, aside from public statements supporting partnerships between the public health and faith communities,[78] or public events at which the Surgeon General and director of the White House faith-based office shared a panel,[79] the OSG has not taken much advantage of the potential of such alliances. This remains an untapped resource.

Professional and Jurisdictional Challenges

As described in Chapter 3, medical practitioners and religious clergy have respective domains of responsibility in patient care settings, where they often interact. In the clinical environment, these relations are governed by an implicit decision-making hierarchy that places hospital administrators and physicians at the top, with others, including healthcare chaplains, further down the ladder. Sometimes relationships between these domains and functionaries are stable and collegial; sometimes they are transient and troubled. Their dynamics are reinforced by stated and unstated institutional guidelines governing professional jurisdiction and other turf-related issues.[80] In negotiating these sensitive interactions, certain questions arise.

For medical care and pastoral care providers, are misperceptions of the professional mission and boundaries of the other profession resolvable?

Answering this question depends in part on how one responds to other questions. For example, does the decision-making authority of the medical profession exceed that of all other professions in the clinical setting? As part of the "healthcare team," are pastoral professionals ever considered equal partners? Is their role fully understood and accepted by medical care staff and administrators? A recent review recognizes that healthcare chaplains are "key personnel" who play a pivotal role in delivering faith-based and faith-sensitive pastoral and spiritual care.[81] At the same time, the authors acknowledge that "their contribution is not always clearly understood by medical and healthcare staff,"[82] and also, "the extent of the provision and staffing of chaplaincy service internationally is unclear."[83]

This is borne out by a pair of commentaries from the United Kingdom in 2013. One stated that churches, rather than the National Health Service (NHS), ought to be funding hospital chaplains.[84] This was not on account of disapproval of healthcare chaplaincy, but quite the opposite: that chaplains instead be "accountable to God and their church, and not to a formal employer such as the NHS."[85] A rejoinder, from the president of the College of Health Care Chaplains, sensitive to ongoing concerns over professional status and funding, affirmed that NHS chaplains are "professional members of the multidisciplinary healthcare team" and essential to provision of quality care to patients.[86]

What can be done? One approach, from within the healthcare chaplaincy profession, has been to develop new practice standards prioritizing evidence-based spiritual care and encouraging research and evaluation.[87] A special emphasis is on conducting outcomes research, testing effectiveness of interventions, and evaluating spiritual assessment and screening tools.[88] Such research, ideally, serves multiple purposes: providing empirical validation for professional efforts, keeping chaplains well informed of best practices, and creating an environment supportive of continuous quality improvement.[89]

Since the start of the new century, this evidence-based approach has become institutionalized within the profession. A review of survey data from diverse chaplain samples—Veterans Affairs, Department of Defense, and civilians— suggests considerable support for this new approach, but not universally.[90] Still, for the chaplaincy this has been something of a "paradigm shift,"[91] and a reasonable response to a need for documentation to maintain and solidify its position in an increasingly rationalized, controlled, competitive, and expensive medical care environment. The expressed hope is that renewed emphasis on research and evaluation will add stability to the chaplaincy within the hospital and healthcare environment. While that is the intention, other dynamics may be in play.

In the early 1990s, when I was teaching medical school, I was invited to lecture each incoming class at the National VA Chaplains Training Center, in Hampton, Virginia. Every six weeks I would speak about the emerging research literature on religion and health. The administrators were enthusiastic, and asked for input in constructing a research agenda fundable by outside sources. They felt increasingly burdened to justify their continued presence in terms of endpoints that their institution valued, such as through medical outcomes and health services research. My sense was that they felt their position in the system was tenuous,

maybe more so since medical care had begun vectoring toward a high-tech future more focused on the bottom line, in both contexts—medical outcomes and
costs. I cannot speak to the present situation within the VA, but profession-wide
and compared to thirty years ago, healthcare chaplaincy is on stronger footing,
thanks to substantial efforts to establish a programmatic research field.[92]

How are vision or values conflicts negotiated?

Medical and pastoral professionals operate under two distinct professional worldviews, each with its own characteristic set of values and associated
functions, idealized endpoints, specialized training, and distinctive skill set.
Both are focused on obtaining the best outcome for people under their care, but
how this is defined and what is done to achieve this may substantially differ between them. This, in turn, affects how they view their unique role, how hospitals
and healthcare institutions may differentially value them, and how patients
understand what it is that each provides. Mutual mistrust may go both ways.[93]
"Each profession," it has been noted, "carries with it a unique symbolic quality."[94]
Is this necessarily a source of conflict, or can a complementarity of functions be
normalized?

As spiritual assessment, for example, becomes widely diffused across certain
medical specialties,[95] including psychiatry, family medicine, and palliative care,
some have wondered if this creates complexities that threaten care of patients,
no matter the positive intentions behind its recommendation. This issue was
unpacked succinctly by two pastoral care professionals:

> So should physicians expand their already crowded medical training schedule
> to include several condensed semesters of ethically sound, theologically based
> training to understand the inner workings of their patient's souls? Should nurses
> require parish training regardless of their personal spiritual inclinations? These
> solutions also seem on the surface to be far beyond the capacity or ethics of any
> medical curriculum today. The problem seems insurmountable and all sides
> have lofted a few barrages at one another over the years in defense of their re-
> spective roles.[96]

The authors proposed that physicians become versed in spiritual assessment,
but spiritual screening requires more sophisticated and specialized training
and will remain the province of chaplains, who are best situated to serve as resources for follow-up spiritual care and intervention.[97] Pastoral and medical
care professionals have different competencies that address distinctive clinical concerns, and chaplains are encouraged "to prioritize their time where it is
needed most"[98] and does not overlap with existing medical functions.

A very good analysis, published in the *Hastings Center Report*, suggested that healthcare chaplains labor at a work of "'translation' between the worlds of the patient and of hospital medicine."[99] The authors compared and contrasted the work of chaplains and physicians:

> While medical professionals focus on patients' medical conditions, chaplains seek to read the whole person, asking questions about what people's lives are like outside of the hospital, what they care about most, and where they find joy and support in the world. Chaplains offer a supportive presence that serves to remind patients and caregivers that people are more than just their medical conditions or their current collection of concerns. Some chaplains are skilled at translating patients' experiences and sources of meaning in real time, allowing medical teams to better understand the person they are treating.[100]

This work of translation is fraught with challenges as healthcare chaplains continue to "map out their territory."[101] These include an absence of clear professional jurisdiction in the medical sector; disagreements among chaplains as to their proper role; perceptions of turf infringement on the part of social workers and local clergy; no consensus as to best practices; and a skillset that emphasizes "soft" skills, such as caring, in contrast to "hard" skills, such as curing, which are more valued by power players within the healthcare system.[102]

For healthcare chaplains, turf issues arise through boundary conflicts not just with medical care providers but with members of local faith communities.[103] Chaplains may be marginalized by pulpit clergy who nonetheless lack the requisite professional training and background to provide services that chaplains do. On top of the dismissal of the relevance of religion and of their role that they may experience from medical colleagues and administrators,[104] such potential conflicts add to the perception among some chaplains that they are taking fire from both sides. A high level of personal resilience is thus a valued and requisite trait for healthcare chaplains, for reasons beyond garden-variety concerns with job stress.

How can medical practitioners best be made aware of faith-based resources that may positively impact on healthcare or health status?

This is a different sort of question, unrelated to medical-pastoral relations in the clinical setting, but a similar issue in one respect: how to connect patients to spiritual resources that might aid in recovery, prevent subsequent illness, or meet functional needs that arise. Community resources—personal and organizational—exist to help patients, especially those with ongoing health challenges, to regain their well-being.[105] Many are faith-based in origin, as described in Chapter 4, and focus on the needs of older adults and the underserved. Faith community nurses are an especially valuable support for community-dwelling elderly folks requiring aftercare and without other tangible resources,[106] and also a substantial source of cost savings.[107] Medical care providers ought to be aware of such resources and prepared to connect patients with people and groups that offer assistance, whether secular or faith-based. Most large hospitals have staff available to facilitate postdischarge referrals, including social workers and patient liaisons, but not all medical practices are attuned to such needs. This begs a broader question: Should physicians concern themselves with such things, much less patient spirituality and beliefs, if evidence suggests a positive impact on mental or physical health?

The answer, in my opinion, surely is yes. That is not to say that physicians must be trained to handle the nuts and bolts of these matters; others are better equipped, including chaplains.[108] But clinicians ought to be aware that maintaining continuity in one's spiritual life may be important for recovery once many patients return home. Facilitating their reintegration into religious networks, or at least connecting them with faith-based home care, can serve a vital salutogenic function. Religious hospitals may understand this implicitly, and are ahead of the curve in establishing transition programs that recognize that readmissions may in part be a function of "social issues and lack of support,"[109] whether secular or faith-based. But somewhere higher up in the administrative structure, including within medical staff leadership, there ought to be recognition of the value of personal faith and congregational networks for the well-being of patients. Such things may not matter to the practitioner nor be relevant in his or her life, but may be vital and life-giving resources for one's patients.

The best place to inculcate this awareness is in medical school and residency training. Accordingly, the past two decades have witnessed a significant change in medical and premedical education in North America, with lectures, coursework, rotations, and electives on social dimensions of the patient experience, including the role of spirituality, faith, and religion across the life course and natural history of disease now commonplace in medical schools.[110] These curriculum changes were instituted with an understanding that without recognition of the significance of personal faith and faith-based resources in the lives of patients and their recovery of health, the training of medical care professionals is lacking. Trainees are now at least exposed to things like spiritual assessment, community referrals, and healthcare chaplains, and many students work in community-based settings as part of multidisciplinary healthcare teams alongside pastoral professionals. Outcome evaluation of such teaching and practice innovations awaits longitudinal follow-up, but current evidence is a mixed bag: despite these advances, the best predictor of physicians engaging such issues seems to be their own level of spirituality.[111] Physicians who value faith are more likely to consider it a significant factor and resource for their patients.

Ethical Challenges

In addressing ethical challenges that arise in the clinical encounter, as described in Chapter 7, religious prescriptions and proscriptions are often influential in decision-making for individual physicians and patients. This has always been so throughout history, a normal and expected, if sometimes inconvenient, variable impacting on the practice of medicine. Ethics consults are available at most large healthcare institutions,[112] and pastoral care staff are available to help navigate bioethical concerns.[113] But aside from this, ethical challenges also arise in the clinical encounter *between* religion and medicine. This phenomenon is more recent, historically speaking, since the advent of biomedicine diminished the authority of ecclesial bodies over care of the sick.[114]

Today, such conflicts are liable to appear for reasons related to situations that may arise during patient care, such as while conducting or recommending a spiritual assessment, making a referral to a pastoral care provider, discussing an end-of-life decision, praying with a patient, or delivering spiritual care.[115] The spiritual beliefs of the physician and other members of the healthcare team add another layer of complexity to a difficult clinical decision that may be perceived as morally compromising.[116] The potential clash of religious worldviews between medical staff and administrators, on the one hand, and patients and families, on the other, is yet another obstacle to overcome.

Conflicts sometimes exist between a patient and his or her family or among family members, such as regarding responsibility for a comatose loved one who did not leave clear instructions through medical directive and power-of-attorney documents. This adds yet another impediment to care. As difficult as it may be for a physician to determine the correct course of action, it may become even more difficult when there is uncertainty as to which party—patient or family member—one must confer with in making a final decision. These cases often end up in litigation and neither party gets to make the final decision, which is deferred instead to a court of law. The tragic Schiavo case comes to mind here.[117]

Notwithstanding difficult and contentious issues that regularly arise, often unexpectedly, physicians have no choice but to negotiate such matters in order to truly practice "compassionate medicine,"[118] defined as doing "what is best for the patient."[119] This mirrors the passage in the Hippocratic Oath whereby new physicians swear to "do no harm."[120] Efforts to sort through the complexity of religion's encounter with medicine and medicine's encounter with religion are never-ending, and all physicians confront these issues at some point during their career. This may be a challenge, but is not a bad thing in and of itself. Working through such predicaments is a necessary and welcome part of the mission of being a doctor, and is referred to by Keith Meador in explicitly religious terms as "redeeming medicine."[121] He defines this as "a practice of caring," informed by religious principles, that seeks "to challenge the 'powers and principalities' of medicine."[122] Religion confronts medicine with many such challenges, among which the following questions—one clinical, one policy-related—are representative.

Is it ever appropriate for medical caregivers to pray with patients? Under what circumstances?

The possibility of physicians praying for patients animates popular discourse on religion and medicine as much as any other subject. Pro or con, it is a heated topic of discussion among laypeople and physicians.[123] Among skeptical critics of research on religion and health, of the type discussed in Chapter 5, everything always comes back to this one issue: that these studies are dangerous because they will encourage people to substitute prayer for proven medical care, or will encourage religious doctors to impose their beliefs on patients.[124] For the record, the studies objected to do not even remotely address such issues. It is hard to imagine how an epidemiologic study showing, say, lower five-year proportional mortality rates for heart disease among monthly female church attenders in a statewide population sample would cause doctors or sick patients to turn away from medical care. But such concerns underscore what a touchy issue this is for gatekeepers of the medical profession and scientific medicine.

When I happen to mention to a colleague or layperson that my work involves scholarship on religion and medicine, or religion and health, more often than not the first thing that I am asked to discuss is my research on faith healers. When I respond that I never have conducted any such research, the next comment is usually something along the lines of, "Oh, so you must study doctors who pray for patients." My answer is the same. These two subjects, incidentally, have been the source of most media inquiries that have come my way over the past thirty-plus years. Underlying these mistaken assumptions is a very real concern about what, for some patients and practitioners, is a very consternating phenomenon. The idea of physicians praying for healing, alongside their more conventional clinical tasks, evokes a kind of cognitive dissonance that has fed expressions of public concern (or support), stimulated debate within the medical profession, and been grist for the mill of dozens of papers on physician spirituality published in the medical literature.[125]

To begin, we should dispense with a couple of basic points: First, there always have been doctors who pray for their patients, regardless of their religion, since the beginning of time. Second, few would deny the right of medical care personnel to pray for those under their charge, if done so on their own time and silently within their own mind or spirit. So this is not a new phenomenon; nor is anyone suggesting legal or professional sanction against those exercising a right to pray privately. The matter that provokes such widespread debate and controversy involves whether physician prayer during patient encounters should be allowed or forbidden, and how to set parameters around such an activity done publicly and openly within the clinical setting. Who decides? Who initiates it?

Internist Dale Matthews thoughtfully unpacks this issue in *The Faith Factor*.[126] Matthews is a committed Christian and supportive of physicians praying for patients, if both parties are amenable. But even he recognizes a need to tread lightly and carefully so as to avoid creating conflicts, upsetting patients, and violating professional and institutional guidelines. This, he acknowledges, is a complicated issue. Matthews explains:

> The prospect of discussing religion—particularly subjective spiritual experiences—makes many doctors feel uncomfortable. If doctors are asked to pray with patients—in the examining room, before surgery, or at the hospital bedside—most feel completely out of their "professional" realm. Yet many people urgently want to talk about their faith when they are sick. When illness brings patients into our offices, they seek relief of their physical symptoms, but many seek more. They want to know: "*Why* am I sick? Am I being punished? What does God have to do with this? Is it okay to ask God to heal me? Will it make any difference if I do?"
>
> No doctor can answer these questions definitively, but I believe we can learn to listen openly and compassionately to our patients' spiritual concerns. If we are willing and the situation is appropriate, we can do more, perhaps pointing out a scripture verse, perhaps sharing a prayer or insights from our own faith journeys, or encouraging counsel with a member of the clergy.[127]

If the situation is appropriate. What precisely does this mean? Family doctor Dana King, in *Faith, Spirituality, and Medicine*, cites research indicating that half of Americans actually want their physician to pray with them, and many physicians are amenable.[128] However, a recent review of over fifty studies from around the world suggests a mismatch between what patients and physicians have in mind here.[129] The former may be looking for additional prayers of healing from a religious person of likeminded faith; the latter may be looking for a thoughtful way to be spiritually supportive and honoring. King offers helpful guidelines for negotiating such interactions, and contends that thoughtfully and compassionately engaging spirituality in this way is part of what makes for a "healing practitioner."[130]

A few specialty boards have weighed in with official guidelines addressing spirituality in some fashion, such as regarding spiritual assessment,[131] but guidance about prayer is lacking. Neurosurgeon Teo Forcht Dagi proposed that prayer be permitted in the operating room only "with the express permission of all present, including the patient, but without requiring the participation of anyone present."[132] Guidelines for general practitioners in the United Kingdom state simply that praying for patients is appropriate so long as it is "tactful."[133] Perhaps the most accurate statement on the nuanced propriety of patient-practitioner prayer was captured in the title of an article by Balboni and colleagues: " 'It Depends.' "[134] However this issue may be parsed and resolved, it remains a focal concern for patients and their physicians.

What responsibilities does the federal government have to the American public to enforce healthcare regulations in the face of resistant private faith-based entities?

This question could be rephrased: What responsibility does the government have to its shareholders (read: taxpayers) when one right (involving a class, legally speaking) seems to conflict with another right, that of an individual or multiple parties? The specifics of *Burwell v. Hobby Lobby* were touched on earlier. But now let us zoom the lens out and examine the larger issue of religious freedom in the context of healthcare.[135] What happens to religious freedom when its exercise seems to conflict with enforcement of laws that may have established a positive right to certain forms of healthcare or even, as some would assert, a right to health?[136] This is not just a point of contention in the United States, but has become a global debate.

In 2018 Reading University philosophy professor David S. Oderberg drafted a document titled "Declaration in Support of Conscientious Objection in Health Care."[137] At the time of this writing, it has over five hundred signatories, among them prominent physicians and academics from throughout the world, as well as religious leaders and organizations. The declaration is a statement on freedom of conscience and "the right to *withdraw from* or *withhold participation* in" certain medical activities or practices on moral or religious grounds.[138] The author makes clear that freedom of conscience has limits, that the declaration does not seek to impede society from funding medical and public health procedures that it sees fit to support, nor does it wish to prevent medical practitioners from delivering care nor patients from receiving care. It simply asserts a right to dissent from participation, which it affirms as consistent with Article 18 of the UN's Universal Declaration of Human Rights. The Reading declaration is thus, according to its author, consistent with "fundamental rights in any liberal, democratic society professing pluralism and tolerance."[139] It has been characterized as a primary document for a new " 'medical conscience' civil rights movement."[140]

A significant concern for many Americans across the political spectrum is that transnational global governmental bodies such as the United Nations or WHO may be granted authority, by treaty, over decisions regarding public funding of entitlements created by fiat within sovereign nations, negating the legislative will of existing representative bodies.[141] For example, global enforcement—whatever that might look like—of a positive right to healthcare or even health may compromise the presumably inalienable First Amendment right of Americans to freely exercise their religion. Such treaties may also be read as a legal mechanism enabling foreign governmental bodies to force American taxpayers to fund healthcare for citizens of other nations, including medical procedures that individual Americans may not approve of, such as related to reproductive issues or end-of-life termination. Preciously held religious values may conflict with social or health policies supported by such treaties, making it impossible for some people of faith to live according to these principles without coercion.

As advocated by a multinational group of legal and ethical scholars, one example of such global governance is a proposed framework convention for universal health coverage to be convened by WHO.[142] The authors' rationale is straightforward:

> At present, the understanding of the right to health is shrouded in vagueness. This hinders accountability to international human rights obligations. A framework convention on global health would bring clarity and precision to norms and standards surrounding the right to health, including states' duties. . . . The treaty would ensure adequate financing and an enabling legal and policy environment.[143]

Under such a scenario, member states would be bound to tax their citizens to underwrite a global infrastructure for medical care delivery and public health development. This may be good and just, according to many among us, but we should understand why many well-meaning people would be wary, for reasons that have nothing to do with nationalism or xenophobia or lack of compassion. To restate, such a mechanism would tax American citizens to fund programs outside the United States and outside of congressional oversight, and these programs may promote medical procedures that some Americans find objectionable, even abhorrent, and would never support voluntarily. Is this really a wise and prudent path to follow?

Even within the United States, as *Burwell v. Hobby Lobby* demonstrated, conflict between healthcare rights and religious freedom creates seemingly intractable situations in which one group of people is pitted against another, compelled to underwrite procedures that violate earnestly held religious beliefs. Further, such a precedent may be applied by the state to enforce procedures performed on

minors against the wishes of parents or legal guardians, such as pregnancy termination, immunization, or life-saving surgery or emergency medical care, including intubation or blood transfusion. For good reason, this conflict has aptly
been described as a "clash of rights."[144]

To be clear, there may be compelling reasons, morally speaking, for a legislatively affirmed healthcare entitlement for the many to outweigh the personal
religious convictions of the few. Anyway, such legislation as the PPACA was
approved through the democratic process. But we should recognize that use of
political power to subordinate a constitutional right in favor of a legislatively
created entitlement risks stirring up a divisive row that may only be resolvable
through factious and costly litigation. For some parties, this may be a necessary and acceptable price to pay for progress, but one should not presume that
opposition to the political entitlement is necessarily grounded in opposition to
the social good represented by healthcare for all. It may reflect an affirmation,
by some, that religious freedom and freedom of conscience are more precious
rights.

Research and Evaluation Challenges

Several categories of research, described in Chapters 5 and 6, have been used to
investigate the broad intersection of religion and health. These include clinical,
population-based, biomedical, social, behavioral, and health services studies. Of
these, the relatively small number of clinical studies, especially the controversial
experimental trials of prayer, have received the most attention, especially among
the media. The much larger number of observational studies using population
samples, totaling in the thousands, have received relatively less attention. Even
many physicians are unaware of the scope and depth of this research.

But another category of studies has received the least attention of all.
Program evaluations and evaluative research of faith-based interventions in
congregations and communities, described in Chapter 4, are the most needed
yet most overlooked type of research on religion and health. Compared to the
thousands of basic research studies, there has been "relatively little" work done
to evaluate faith-health partnerships.[145] Yet applied research studies assessing
evidence from myriad projects and interventions conducted in numerous communities through partnerships between health agencies and religious organizations are precisely what is required for future program planning in prevention,
if we are to make full use of institutional religious resources to improve the
health of populations. Meta-evaluations, too—the evaluative research version of
the meta-analysis or systematic review—would be most helpful in cumulating
results across such programs, but these, too, are lacking.

Issues that need evaluating here are simple, yet, to now, mostly underexplored. So much energy has been expended on vetting legal matters related to congregational and denominational programs on healthcare—including the constitutionality of federal faith-based initiatives—that more fundamental and just as important matters regarding the efficacy of programs and their wider application have been relatively ignored. Among the most urgent questions are the following:

What works and what does not work?

This question is the most direct and pressing. Yet, remarkably, we know little about the efficacy of faith-based interventions in health, generally speaking, despite the large number of programs that have proliferated throughout the country over the past forty years. Moreover, we are not just lacking in evidence that faith-based interventions measurably improve population-health outcomes over the long term, but empirical evidence on near-term impacts is a mixed bag, at best. The few reviews of published reports in this area have borne this out.

One reason why evaluative research and systematic reviews are so lacking is simply that interventions designed to enable careful evaluation of program efficacy and results are themselves lacking. In surveying the scene in the early 2000s, one reviewer noted that "evidence-based health promotion interventions in churches remain sporadically implemented."[146] Essentially the same conclusion was drawn regarding program evaluations and evaluative research on faith-based projects in general.[147] As a result, we are still awaiting systematic "empirical validation of factors associated with effective or efficacious such interventions."[148]

Even so, successes have been demonstrated. Especially frustrating when it comes to summarizing the impacts and outcomes of this body of work is that quite a bit of programming has occurred throughout the United States. Some programs have achieved great success, and such successes have been documented carefully, as described in Chapter 4. A review of mine from 2013 noted this frustration, remarking that despite an absence of systematic summaries and reviews, "more has been done and published than most public health leaders may be aware, and mounting evidence does exist for these programs' effectiveness,"[149] including in certain populations[150] and for particular disease outcomes.[151]

Despite limitations of existing sources of evidence, efforts have been made to assess what does and does not work, and why. Michelle C. Kegler and colleagues at Emory conducted an in-depth analysis of factors inhibiting the success of program partnerships between the faith-based and public health sectors.[152] They identified general barriers to collaboration (limited resources, competition/turf protection, racism, internal team conflict), barriers unique to the health sector (discomfort with FBOs, distrust of health agencies) and to faith communities (denominational diversity, fear or distrust of faith communities), and barriers related to crossing faith-health boundaries (different agendas, finding a common language, beliefs about church-state separation).[153] They also identified facilitators to collaboration, factors associated with successful faith-health partnerships (passion and commitment, importance of FBOs within respective communities, support from community and faith leaders, diversity of teams, supportive political climate, and mutual trust and respect).[154]

This careful and comprehensive review, from Emory's Interfaith Health Program, should be studied by anyone designing a faith-based community health program or intervention. It offers considerable insight into how public health agencies and healthcare institutions can effectively make use of faith-based resources, both human and organizational. Other excellent resources are available,[155] as well as informed recommendations for designing successful faith-health partnerships.[156]

What are the barriers to evidence-based evaluations being used formatively by government decision-makers?

The best of intentions and most successful of programs are not enough to change how insights from local faith-health partnerships are applied to national health priorities. Anecdotal evidence and evaluative findings, as noted, indicate that such programs hold considerable promise as a model component for national and global health policy. Marshaling resources from the civil-society sector, including congregations and FBOs, can provide a useful bridge between government policies and on-the-ground deliverables.[157] Ideally, successes and failures of existing collaborations could inform policy deliberations about public-private partnerships in healthcare delivery and public health. This conversation, in turn, could help direct distribution of scarce resources, governmental and philanthropic, to where they could do the most good. But this is easier said than done. Based on observations made as a result of meetings with members of the previous two administrations in Washington, two barriers stand in the way.

First, those appointed to political and administrative leadership positions must value personal faith and the larger faith community as defining a domain of human experience meaningful in the lives of many constituents, even if not in their own lives. Otherwise, the largest and deepest wellspring of personal and tangible resources for constructive change existing in the voluntary sector will remain overlooked and untapped. Second, leaders must be willing to exercise the political will—and perhaps expend the political capital—required to advance an agenda drawing on alliances between government and the faith sector, even in the face of official indifference or hostility.

The first request is not much to ask, and is somewhat equivalent to the expectation that physicians at least be open to accommodating patients' spiritual needs even if they themselves do not have religious beliefs or practice religion. The second request may be a lot to ask, and is contingent on an intricate political calculus that requires constant balancing of exigent circumstances, externalities, horse-trading, and constituent feedback that someone observing from a vantage point outside of government cannot fully appreciate. I am sympathetic, for sure, but obstinate enough to insist that those in power muster the courage to do the right thing to benefit the most people.

Takeaway Point, Restated

To restate the takeaway point from the beginning of this book:

> *The intersections of the faith-based and medical sectors are multifaceted and of long standing.*

The idea that religion and medicine can partner in ways to promote well-being and relieve suffering is a very old one. The Bible, for one, and other sacred Jewish and Christian texts, have far more to say about health, healing, healthcare, medicine, and even the human body and pathophysiology than most people may be aware.[158]

The intersection of religion and medicine is not newly discovered territory. Nor is it a conceptual space that implicitly connotes whatever disreputable images may be conjured by readings (or misreadings) of the activities of religious fundamentalists or New Agers, images that many within Western medicine find distasteful. Religious people, organizations, and institutions have worked hand in hand with medical and healthcare practitioners, organizations, and institutions for hundreds of years, at least—and especially since the mid-twentieth century, creating fields of academic study, professional practice, community intervention, and human caregiving that buttress the work of those laboring to advance the cause of preventive medicine and public health.

Former U.S. Surgeon General David Satcher, a widely revered public health leader, has made this very point: "Through partnership with faith organizations and the use of health promotion and disease prevention sciences, we can form a mighty alliance to build strong, healthy, and productive communities."[159] There is historical precedent for such an alliance, and informed by science and scholarship, it is in our best interest that this work continue and flourish.

Notes

Chapter 1

1. Rudolf Otto spoke of the "disposition for knowing the holy," a subjective impression of a divine ideation that cannot be understood without reference to nonrational, nonsensory antecedents and expressions that he termed *numinous* (*The Idea of the Holy: An Inquiry into the Non-Rational Factor in the Idea of the Divine and Its Relation to the Rational*, trans. John W. Harvey (London: Oxford University Press, 1923), 176). By contrast, Bertrand Russell asserted that neither morality nor beliefs and behaviors were informed by "any divine or supernatural origin," as no such thing existed, only "natural facts" ("Do We Survive Death?" (1936) in *Why I Am Not a Christian and Other Essays on Religion and Related Subjects* (New York: Touchstone, 1957), 88–93, 92).

2. This perspective is characterized by a "machinelike view of humans as nothing but a body—a sack of bones swishing about in a soup of chemicals" (Jeff Levin, *God, Faith, and Health: Exploring the Spirituality-Healing Connection* (New York: John Wiley and Sons, 2001), 207). See also Jeff Levin, "Restoring the Spiritual: Reflections on Arrogance and Myopia—Allopathic and Holistic," *Journal of Religion and Health* 48 (2009): 482–495; and Larry Dossey, *Recovering the Soul: A Scientific and Spiritual Search* (New York: Bantam Books, 1989).

3. E.g., Dossey noted, "*Modern medicine has become one of the most spiritually malnourished professions in our society.* Because medicine has so thoroughly disowned the spiritual component to healing, most healers throughout history would view the profession today as inherently perverse" ("Prayer, Medicine, and Science: The New Dialogue," in *Scientific and Pastoral Perspectives on Intercessory Prayer: An Exchange between Larry Dossey, M.D. and Health Care Chaplains*, ed. Larry VandeCreek (Binghamton, NY: Haworth Press, 1998), 7–37, 33).

4. E.g., Richard Sloan, *Blind Faith: The Unholy Alliance of Religion and Medicine* (New York: St. Martin's Griffin, 2006).

5. In 1985, Marcia Angell stated that "our belief in disease as a direct reflection of mental state is largely folklore" ("Disease as a Reflection of the Psyche," *New England Journal of Medicine* 312 (1985): 1570–1572, 1572).

6. Manly Hall, *Healing: The Divine Art* (1944; Los Angeles: Philosophical Research Society, 1972).

7. Ibid., 17–37.

8. Gary B. Ferngren, *Medicine and Religion: A Historical Introduction* (Baltimore: Johns Hopkins University Press, 2014); and Gary B. Ferngren and Katarina N. Lomperis, *Essential Readings in Medicine and Religion* (Baltimore: Johns Hopkins University Press, 2017). See also his *Medicine and Health Care in Early Christianity* (Baltimore: Johns Hopkins University Press, 2009), a subject also covered in Amanda

Porterfield, *Healing in the History of Christianity* (Oxford: Oxford University Press, 2005).

9. Ferngren and Lomperis, *Essential Readings in Medicine and Religion*, 1.

10. Morton Kelsey, *Healing and Christianity: A Classic Study*, 3rd ed. (1973; Minneapolis: Augsburg, 1995).

11. Jeff Levin, "How Faith Heals: A Theoretical Model," *EXPLORE: The Journal of Science and Healing* 5 (2009): 77–96.

12. Harold Y. Vanderpool, "Is Religion Therapeutically Significant?" *Journal of Religion and Health* 16 (1977): 255–259.

13. See discussion of traditional Asian and Western healing philosophies in Jeff Levin, "Esoteric Healing Traditions: A Conceptual Overview," *EXPLORE: The Journal of Science and Healing* 4 (2008): 101–112.

14. Jongbae J. Park, Selena Beckman-Harned, Gayoung Cho, Duckhee Kim, and Hangon Kim, "The Current Acceptance, Accessibility, and Recognition of Chinese and Ayurvedic Medicine in the United States in the Public, Governmental, and Industrial Sectors," *Chinese Journal of Integrative Medicine* 18 (2012): 405–408.

15. Asim A. Jani, Jennifer Trask, and Ather Ali, "Integrative Medicine in Preventive Medicine Education: Competency and Curriculum Development for Preventive Medicine and Other Specialty Residency Programs," *American Journal of Preventive Medicine* 49, 5, Suppl. 3 (2015): S222–S229.

16. Ariel Bar-Sela, Herbel E. Hoff, and Elias Faris, "Moses Maimonides' Two Treatises on the Regimen of Health: Fī Tadbīr al-Sihhah and Maqālah fi Bayān Baʿd al-Aʿrād wa-al-Jawāb ʿanhā," *Transactions of the American Philosophical Society* 54, 4 (1964): 3–50.

17. From the translation found in ibid., 18.

18. John Wesley, *Primitive Physic: An Easy and Natural Method of Curing Most Diseases*, 22nd ed. (1791; Eugene, OR: Wipf and Stock, 2003). For his other medical writings, see James G. Donat and Randy L. Maddox, eds., *The Works of John Wesley*, vol. 32: *Medical and Health Writings* (Nashville: Abingdon Press, 2018).

19. Jeff Levin, "The Discourse on Faith and Medicine: A Tale of Two Literatures," *Theoretical Medicine and Bioethics* 39 (2018): 265–282, 266.

20. Wesley, *Primitive Physic*, quotation x.

21. Ibid., 100.

22. Ibid., 57.

23. Fazlur Rahman, *Health and Medicine in the Islamic Tradition: Change and Identity* (New York: Crossroad, 1987).

24. Ibid., 84–90.

25. E.g., Ibrahim B. Syed, "Spiritual Medicine in the History of Islamic Medicine," *Journal of the International Society for the History of Islamic Medicine* 2 (2003): 45–49.

26. Tamara Sonn, "Health and Medicine in the Islamic Tradition: Fazlur-Raḥmān's View," *Journal of the Islamic Medical Society of North America* 28 (1996): 189–194, quotations 190.

27. Ibid.

28. Ibid.

29. Gerald Epstein, "Hebraic Medicine," *Advances* 4, 1 (1987): 56–66; Steven M. Rosman, *Jewish Healing Wisdom* (Northvale, NJ: Jason Aronson, 1997); and Matityahu Glazerson, *Torah, Light, and Healing: Mystical Insights Based on the Hebrew Language* (Northvale, NJ: Jason Aronson, 1993). The essential text is Julius Preuss, *Biblical and Talmudic Medicine*, trans. and ed. Fred Rosner (1911; Northvale, NJ: Jason Aronson, 1993).

30. Mones Abu-Asab, Hakima Amri, and Marc S. Micozzi, *Avicenna's Medicine: A New Translation of the 11th-Century Canon with Practical Applications for Integrative Health Care* (Rochester, VT: Healing Arts Press, 2013).

31. Robert T. Trotter II and Juan Antonio Chavira, *Curanderismo: Mexican American Folk Healing*, 2nd ed. (Athens: University of Georgia Press, 2011).

32. Cindy Lynn Salazar and Jeff Levin, "Religious Features of *Curanderismo* Training and Practice," *EXPLORE: The Journal of Science and Healing* 9 (2013): 150–158, 154.

33. Amariah Brigham, *Observations on the Influence of Religion upon the Health and Physical Welfare of Mankind* (Boston: Marsh, Capon and Lyon, 1835).

34. Ibid., 331.

35. Norman Porritt, *Religion and Health: Their Mutual Relationship and Influence* (London: Skeffington and Son, 1905); Horatio W. Dresser, *Health and the Inner Life: An Analytical and Historical Study of Spiritual Healing Theories, with an Account of the Life and Teachings of P. P. Quimby* (New York: G. P. Putnam's Sons, 1906); Percy Dearmer, *Body and Soul: An Enquiry into the Effect of Religion upon Health, with a Description of Christian Works on Healing from the New Testament to the Present Day* (New York: E. P. Dutton and Company, 1909); Edward E. Weaver, *Mind and Health: With an Examination of Some Systems of Divine Healing* (New York: Macmillan, 1913); James J. Walsh, *Religion and Health* (Boston: Little, Brown, and Company, 1920); Lily Dougall, *The Christian Doctrine of Health: A Handbook on the Relation of Bodily to Spiritual and Moral Health* (Cleveland: American Guild of Health, 1923); and Solomon Cohen, *Faith and Health: The True Way of Attaining Health through Faith* (Brooklyn, NY: Theistic Publishing Co., 1923).

36. G. Allison Stokes, "Ministry after Freud: The Rise of the Religion and Health Movement in American Protestantism, 1906–1945" (Ph.D. diss., Yale University, 1981).

37. Elwood Worcester, Samuel McComb, and Isadore H. Coriat, *Religion and Medicine: The Moral Control of Nervous Disorders* (New York: Moffat, Yard and Company, 1908).

38. Charles T. Holman, *The Religion of a Healthy Mind* (New York: Round Table Press, 1939).

39. Carroll A. Wise, *Religion in Illness and Health* (New York: Harper and Brothers, 1942).

40. Seward Hiltner, *Religion and Health* (New York: Macmillan, 1943).

41. Paul Tillich, "The Relation of Religion and Health: Historical Considerations and Theoretical Questions," *Review of Religion* 10 (1946): 348–384.

42. Wayne E. Oates, *Religious Factors in Mental Illness* (New York: Association Press, 1955).

43. Beginning with Academy of Religion and Mental Health, *Religion, Science, and Mental Health: Proceedings of the First Academy Symposium on Inter-Discipline Responsibility for Mental Health—A Religious and Scientific Concern—1957* (New York: New York University Press, 1959).

44. John S. Billings, "Vital Statistics of the Jews," *North American Review* 153 (1891): 70–84.

45. William Osler, "The Faith That Heals," *British Medical Journal* 1, 2581 (1910): 1470–1472. This theme was revisited in Jerome D. Frank, "The Faith That Heals," *Johns Hopkins Medical Journal* 137, 3 (1975): 127–131.

46. Alice E. Paulsen, "Religious Healing: A Preliminary Report," *JAMA* 86 (1926): 1519–1522, 1617–1623, 1692–1697.

47. Including "Mental Healing," *British Medical Journal* 1, 2581 (1910): 1483–1497, surveying miracle cures, demonology, faith healing, healing shrines, Christian science, spiritual healers, and related subjects.

48. "Religion and Health," *British Medical Journal* 1, 2315 (1905): 1047–1048, a review of Porritt's *Religion and Health*.

49. C. F. Nichols, "'Divine Healing,'" *Science* 19, 468 (1892): 43–44.

50. Daniel T. Kim, Farr A. Curlin, Kelly M. Wolenberg, and Daniel Sulmasy, "Back to the Future: The AMA and Religion, 1961–1974," *Academic Medicine* 89 (2014): 1603–1609.

51. Wendy Cadge, *Paging God: Religion in the Halls of Medicine* (Chicago: University of Chicago Press, 2012), 14.

52. See "Medieval Persecutions, Ritual Murder, and the Talmud," in Dan Cohn-Sherbok, *The Crucified Jew: Twenty Centuries of Christian Anti-Semitism* (Grand Rapids: Eerdmans, 1992), 38–50.

53. Iris Ritzmann, "Judenmord als Folge des 'Schwarzen Todes': Ein Medizinhistorischer Mythos?," *Medizin, Gesellschaft, und Geschichte* 17 (1998): 101–130, 101.

54. Paul Johnson, *A History of the Jews* (New York: HarperPerennial, 1987), 216–217.

55. Cecil Roth, *A History of the Jews: From Earliest Times through the Six Day War*, rev. ed. (New York: Schocken Books, 1970), 214.

56. Barbara Ehrenreich and Dierdre English, *Witches, Midwives and Nurses: A History of Women Healers*, 2nd ed. (New York: Feminist Press, 2010); Geoffrey Scarre and John Callow, *Witchcraft and Magic in Sixteenth- and Seventeenth-Century Europe*, 2nd ed. (Hampshire, UK: Palgrave, 2001); and Brian Levack, *The Witch-Hunt in Early Modern Europe*, 3rd ed. (London: Routledge, 2006).

57. Margot Adler, *Drawing Down the Moon: Witches, Druids, Goddess-Worshippers, and Other Pagans in America*, rev. ed. (New York: Penguin Books, 1986), 235.

58. Rodney Stark, *Bearing False Witness: Debunking Centuries of Anti-Catholic History* (West Conshohocken, PA: Templeton Press, 2016), 123–128.

59. Akile Gürsoy, "Beyond the Orthodox: Heresy in Medicine and the Social Sciences from a Cross-Cultural Perspective," *Social Science and Medicine* 43 (1996): 577–599.

60. Robert S. Mendelsohn, *Confessions of a Medical Heretic* (Lincolnwood, IL: Contemporary Books, 1979).

61. Daniel Mark Epstein, *Sister Aimee: The Life of Aimee Semple McPherson* (New York: Harcourt Brace Jovanovich, 1993).

62. David Edwin Harrell Jr., *Oral Roberts: An American Life* (Bloomington: Indiana University Press, 1985).

63. Jamie Buckingham, *Daughter of Destiny: Kathryn Kuhlman, Her Story* (Plainfield, NJ: Logos International, 1976).

64. James Randi, "Peter Popoff and His Wonderful Machine," in *The Faith Healers*, new updated ed. (Amherst, NY: Prometheus Books, 1989), 139–181.

65. Dave Ghose, "Leroy: The Miracle Man Starts Over," *Columbus Monthly*, May 2003, http://www.columbusmonthly.com/news/20170622/from-archives-leroy-jenkins-starts-over.

66. Jerry Sholes, *Give Me That Prime-Time Religion: An Insider's Report on the Oral Roberts Evangelistic Association* (New York: Hawthorn Books, 1979).

67. Alesha B. Doan, *Opposition and Intimidation: The Abortion Wars and Strategies of Political Harassment* (Ann Arbor: University of Michigan Press, 2007); and *Abortion Clinic Violence: Hearings before the Subcommittee on Crime and Criminal Justice of the Committee on the Judiciary, House of Representatives, One Hundred Third Congress, First Session, April 1 and June 10, 1993* (Washington, DC: U.S. Government Printing Office, 1994).

68. David C. Nice, "Abortion Clinic Bombings as Political Violence," *American Journal of Political Science* 32 (1988): 178–195.

69. Randall A. Terry, *Accessory to Murder: The Enemies, Allies, and Accomplices to the Death of Our Culture* (Brentwood, TN: Wolgemuth and Hyatt, 1990).

70. E.g., "National Right to Life Condemns Acts of Violence in Colorado Springs," National Right to Life (November 27, 2015), https://www.nrlc.org/site/communications/releases/2015/release112715/.

71. Ibid.

72. Nice, "Abortion Clinic Bombings as Political Violence," 187–188.

73. Mireille Jacobson and Heather Royer, "Aftershocks: The Impact of Clinic Violence on Abortion Services," *American Economic Journal: Applied Economics* 3 (2011): 189–223, 221.

74. E.g., Hans A. Baer, "The Work of Andrew Weil and Deepak Chopra—Two Holistic Health / New Age Gurus: A Critique of the Holistic Health / New Age Movements," *Medical Anthropology Quarterly* 17 (2003): 233–250; and Irwin Ziment, "Recent Advances in Alternative Medicine," *Current Opinion in Pulmonary Medicine* 6 (2000): 71–78. A "gap in values, attitudes, and beliefs" between patients and physicians likely underlies care-seeking that aims for "complementary" or "integrative" use of therapies, rather than as an "alternative" to conventional treatment (Bruce Barrett, "Alternative, Complementary, and Conventional Medicine: Is Integration upon Us?" *Journal of Alternative and Complementary Medicine* 9 (2003): 417–427, 418).

75. John A. Astin, "Why Patients Use Alternative Medicine: Results of a National Study," *JAMA* 279 (1998): 1548–1553.

76. J. Gordon Melton, Jerome Clark, and Aiden A. Kelly, *New Age Almanac* (New York: Visible Ink Press, 1991), 169.

77. T. S. Sathyanarayana Rao and Chittaranjan Andrade, "The MMR Vaccine and Autism: Sensation, Refutation, Retraction, and Fraud," *Indian Journal of Psychiatry* 53 (2011): 95–96. Because of the success of vaccines, today's parents "have limited or no experience with the devastating effects of diseases such as polio, smallpox, or measles," leading to complacency and susceptibility to misinformation (see Archana Chatterjee and Catherine O'Keefe, "Current Controversies in the USA Regarding Vaccine Safety," *Expert Review of Vaccines* 9 (2010): 497–502, 497).

78. Simon H. Murch, Andrew Anthony, David H. Casson, Mohsin Malik, Mark Berelowitz, Amar Dhillon, Michael A. Thomson, Alan Valentine, Susan E. Davies, and John A. Walker-Smith, "Retraction of an Interpretation," *The Lancet* 363 (2004): 750; Fiona Goodlee, Jane Smith, and Harvey Marcovitch, "Wakefield's Article Linking MMR Vaccine and Autism Was Fraudulent," *British Medical Journal* 342 (2011): 64–66; and Michael J. Smith, Susan S. Ellenberg, Louis M. Bell, and David M. Rubin, "Media Coverage of the Measles-Mumps-Rubella Vaccine and Autism Controversy and Its Relationship to MMR Immunization Rates in the United States," *Pediatrics* 121 (2008): e836–e843.

79. Jeff Levin, "Partnerships between the Faith-Based and Medical Sectors: Implications for Preventive Medicine and Public Health," *Preventive Medicine Reports* 4 (2016): 344–350, 345.

80. Martin E. Marty and Kenneth L. Vaux, eds., *Health/Medicine and the Faith Traditions: An Inquiry into Religion and Medicine* (Philadelphia: Fortress Press, 1982).

81. Natalia Berger, ed., *Jews and Medicine: Religion, Culture, Science* (Philadelphia: Jewish Publication Society, 1995); and Frank Heynick, *Jews and Medicine: An Epic Saga* (Hoboken, NJ: KTAV, 2002).

82. Fred Rosner and Samuel S. Kottek, eds., *Moses Maimonides: Physician, Scientist, and Philosopher* (Northvale, NJ: Jason Aronson, 1993).

83. Isadore Twersky, *A Maimonides Reader* (West Orange, NJ: Behrman House, 1972), contains entries from *Mishneh Torah, Guide for the Perplexed*, and other documents, including an epistle debunking astrology, which ends, simply, with "Amen" ("Letter on Astrology," 463–473).

84. Isaac Broydé, "Moses ben Naḥman Gerondi (RaMBaN; known also as Naḥmanides and Bonastruc da Porta)," in *The Jewish Encyclopedia: A Descriptive Record of the History, Religion, Literature, and Customs of the Jewish People from the Earliest Times to the Present Day*, vol. 9: *Morawczyk-Philippson*, ed. Isidore Singer (New York: Funk and Wagnalls Company, 1905), 87–92.

85. Naḥmanides, *Ramban: The Torah: With Ramban's Commentary*, trans., annotated, and elucidated by Yaakov Blinder in collaboration with Yoseph Kamenetsky (Brooklyn, NY: Mesorah Publications, 2010).

86. Raphael Pelcovitz, "Introduction: Ovadiah ben Yaacov Sforno," in Ovadiah ben Jacob Sforno, *Sforno: Commentary on the Torah*, trans. Raphael Pelcovitz (Brooklyn, NY: Mesorah Publications, 1997), ix–xxi.

87. Scion of a Chasidic rabbinic dynasty, Twerski's dozens of books include academic texts on mental health, addictions, and other psychiatric and religious subjects.

88. Avraham Steinberg, *Encyclopedia of Jewish Medical Ethics: A Compilation of Jewish Medical Law on All Topics of Medical Interest, from the Most Ancient Sources to the Most Current Deliberations and Decisions, with a Concise Medical and Historical Background, and a Comprehensive Comparative Analysis of Relevant General Ethical Approaches* (Jerusalem: Feldheim Publishers, 2003).

89. Moshe D. Sherman, "Levin, Yehuda Leib (1863–1926)," in *Orthodox Judaism in America: A Biographical Dictionary and Sourcebook* (Westport, CT: Greenwood Press, 1996), 133–134.

90. "Agudath ha-Rabbonim," in *Orthodox Judaism in America: A Biographical Dictionary and Sourcebook*, 225–236.

91. "Judah Levin Adding Machine," History of Computers: Hardware, Software, Internet, https://history-computer.com/CalculatingTools/Gadgets/Levin.html.

92. Herman Branover and Ilana Coven Attia, eds., *Science in the Light of Torah: A B'Or Ha'Torah Reader* (Northvale, NJ: Jason Aronson, 1994).

93. Albert Schweitzer, *Out of My Life and Thought: An Autobiography, 60th Anniversary Edition* (Baltimore: Johns Hopkins University Press, 1990); and James Brabazon, *Albert Schweitzer: Essential Writings* (Maryknoll, NY: Orbis Books, 2005).

94. Albert Schweitzer, *The Quest of the Historical Jesus: A Critical Study of Its Progress from Raimarus to Wrede*, trans. W. Montgomery (1906; London: Adam and Charles Black, 1911).

95. Bāqir Sharīf al-Qurashi, *The Life of Imām 'Ali Bin Mūsā al-Ridā*, trans. Jāsim al-Rasheed (Qum, Iran: Ansariyan Publications, n.d.).

96. In a modern edition of *al-Sahīfa al-Riḍā* (Cairo: al-Ma'ahid Press, 1921–1922), the text contains 163 *hadīths* in ten sections.

97. For Arabic readers, see M.ʿ A. al-Bārr, *al-Imām ʿAlī al-Riḍā wa-risālatuhū fī l-ṭibb al-nabawī: al-Risāla al-dhahabiyya. Awwal risāla fī l-ṭibb al-nabawī* (Beirut: Dār al-Manāhil, 1992).

98. al-Qurashi, *The Life of Imām Ali Bin Mūsā al-Ridā*, 170, from https://www.al-islam.org/printpdf/book/export/html/41669.

99. Mohamed Raza Dungersi, *A Brief Biography of Imam Ali Musa al-Ridha (A.S.)* (Dar es Salaam: Bilal Muslim Mission of Tanzania, 2012), 35.

100. Ritu Lakhtakia, "A Trio of Exemplars of Medieval Islamic Medicine: Al-Razi, Avicenna, and Ibn Al-Nafis," *Sultan Qaboos University Medical Journal* 14 (2014): e455–e459.

101. Sudhir Kakar, *Shamans, Mystics, and Doctors: A Psychological Inquiry into India and Its Healing Traditions* (Chicago: University of Chicago Press, 1982).

102. Paramahansa Yogananda, *The Autobiography of a Yogi* (1946; Los Angeles: Self-Realization Fellowship, 1974).

103. Paramahansa Yogananda, *Scientific Healing Affirmations: Theory and Practice of Concentration* (1958; Los Angeles: Self-Realization Fellowship, 1981), 18.

104. Kenneth G. Zysk, *Asceticism and Healing in Ancient India: Medicine in the Buddhist Monastery*, corrected ed. (1991; Delhi: Motilal Banarsidass, 1998), quotation first (unnumbered) page of preface.

105. John S. Mbiti, *African Religions and Philosophy* (Garden City, NY: Anchor Books, 1969), and "'If God Did Not Love Me, God Would Not Have Made Me!': Exploring

Divine Love in African Religion," in *Divine Love: Perspectives from the World's Religious Traditions*, ed. Jeff Levin and Stephen G. Post (West Conshohocken, PA: Templeton Press, 2010), 23–55. See also Kofi Appiah-Kubi, "Traditional African Healing System versus Western Medicine in Southern Ghana: An Encounter," in *Religious Plurality in Africa: Essays in Honour of John S. Mbiti*, ed. Jacob K. Olupona and Sulayman S. Nyang (Berlin: Mouton de Gruyter, 1993), 95–107.

106. John M. Janzen, "Health, Religion, and Medicine in Central and Southern African Traditions," in *Healing and Restoring: Health and Medicine in the World's Religious Traditions*, ed. Lawrence E. Sullivan (New York: Macmillan, 1989), 225–254, 232.

107. Ibid., 236–237.

108. David Cumes, "South African Indigenous Healing: How It Works," *EXPLORE: The Journal of Science and Healing* 9 (2013): 58–65.

109. Ibid., 60–61.

110. Marlise Richter, "Traditional Medicines and Traditional Healers in South Africa," Discussion paper prepared for the Treatment Action Campaign and AIDS Law Project (November 27, 2003), https://pdfs.semanticscholar.org/8359/89878408b67 007fa60bc844300a67a91317c.pdf.

111. Kenneth "Bear Hawk" Cohen, *Honoring the Medicine: The Essential Guide to Native American Healing* (New York: One World, 2003), 37.

112. Ken "Bear Hawk" Cohen, "Native American Medicine," in *Essentials of Complementary and Alternative Medicine*, ed. Wayne B. Jonas and Jeffrey S. Levin (Philadelphia: Lippincott Williams and Wilkins, 1999), 233–251, 234.

113. Ibid.

114. George Peter Murdock, *Theories of Illness: A World Survey* (Pittsburgh, PA: University of Pittsburgh Press, 1980).

115. In a study of mostly Christian college students in the United States, "supernatural" factors were identified in causal attributions for illness. These included sinful thoughts, punishment from God, the evil eye, sinful acts, lack of faith, hexes, payback for wrongdoing, and thin blood (see Hope Landrine and Elizabeth A. Klonoff, "Cultural Diversity in Causal Attributions for Illness: The Role of the Supernatural," *Journal of Behavioral Medicine* 17 (1994): 181–193).

116. Murdock, *Theories of Illness*, 26.

117. James A. Marcum, *An Introductory Philosophy of Medicine: Humanizing Modern Medicine* (New York: Springer, 2008), and "Reflections on Humanizing Biomedicine," *Perspectives in Biology and Medicine* 51 (2008): 392–405.

118. Marcum, *An Introductory Philosophy of Medicine*.

119. D. Vasant Lad, "Ayurvedic Medicine," in Jonas and Levin, *Essentials of Complementary and Alternative Medicine*, 200–215.

120. Ibid., 202.

121. Heinrich Zimmer, *Philosophies of India*, ed. Joseph Campbell (Princeton, NJ: Princeton University Press, 1951), 295–297.

122. Lad, "Ayurvedic Medicine."

123. Lixing Lao, "Traditional Chinese Medicine," in Jonas and Levin, *Essentials of Complementary and Alternative Medicine*, 216–232.

124. Ibid., 217.

125. Ibid., 218.

126. Vladimir Badmaev, "Tibetan Medicine," in Jonas and Levin, *Essentials of Complementary and Alternative Medicine*, 252–274.

127. Romio Shrestha and Ian A, Baker, *The Tibetan Art of Healing* (San Francisco: Chronicle, 1997).

128. Badmaev, "Tibetan Medicine," 256.

129. Yeshi Dönden, *Health through Balance: An Introduction to Tibetan Medicine*, ed. and trans. Jeffrey Hopkins, co-trans. Lobsang Rabgay and Alan Wallace (Ithaca, NY: Snow Lion Publications, 1986).

130. Jamil Ahmad and Akim Ashhar Qadeer, *Unani: The Science of Graeco-Arabic Medicine* (New Delhi: Lustre Press, 1998); and Alṭāf Aḥmad Āʿẓamī, *Basic Concepts of Unani Medicine: A Critical Study* (New Delhi: Department of History of Medicine, Faculty of Medicine, Jamia Hamdard, 1995).

131. Abu-Asab et al., *Avicenna's Medicine*.

132. Peter E. Pormann and Emilie Savage-Smith, *Medieval Islamic Medicine* (Washington, DC: Georgetown University Press, 2007), 1.

133. Michael Monette, "The Medicine of the Prophet," *Canadian Medical Association Journal* 184 (2012): E649–E650.

134. *Benchmarks for Training in Traditional/Complementary and Alternative Medicine: Benchmarks for Training in Unani Medicine* (Geneva: World Health Organization, 2010).

135. Wakoh Shannon Hickey, *Mind Cure: How Meditation Became Medicine* (New York: Oxford University Press, 2019).

136. Mary Baker Eddy, *Science and Health with Key to the Scriptures* (1875; Boston: First Church of Christ, Scientist, 1994).

137. Deidre Michell, "New Thinking, New Thought, New Age: The Theology and Influence of Emma Curtis Hopkins (1849–1925)," *Australian Journal of Feminist Studies in Religion* 2, 1 (2001): 6–13.

138. Alfred Whitney Griswold, "New Thought: Cult of Success," *American Journal of Sociology* 40 (1934): 309–318.

139. Hickey, *Mind Cure*.

140. Ernest Holmes, *The Science of Mind: A Philosophy, a Faith, a Way of Life* (1926; New York: Jeremy Tarcher / Putnam, 1997); and Charles Fillmore, *Jesus Christ Heals* (1939; Unity Village, MO: Unity Books, 1994).

141. Jeffrey S. Levin and Jeannine Coreil, "'New Age' Healing in the U.S.," *Social Science and Medicine* 23 (1986): 889–897; and Harold Y. Vanderpool, "The Holistic Hodgepodge: A Critical Analysis of Holistic Medicine and Health in America Today," *Journal of Family Practice* 19 (1984): 773–781.

142. Levin and Coreil, "'New Age' Healing in the U.S.," 890.

143. Thomas Sugrue, *There Is a River: The Story of Edgar Cayce* (New York: Holt, 1942); Jess Stern, *Edgar Cayce: The Sleeping Prophet* (New York: Bantam Books, 1967); and Harmon H. Bro, *A Seer out of Season: The Life of Edgar Cayce* (New York: Signet, 1989).

144. B. Ernest Frejer, comp., *The Edgar Cayce Companion: A Comprehensive Treatise of the Edgar Cayce Readings* (Virginia Beach, VA: A.R.E. Press, 1995).

145. Eric Mein, *Keys to Health: The Promise and Challenge of Holism* (New York: Harper and Row, 1989); and Daniel Redwood, *Edgar Cayce's Holistic Health Program* (New Canaan, CT: Keats Publishing, 1996).

146. William McGarey, *Healing Miracles: Using Your Body Energies* (San Francisco: Harper and Row, 1988), 13.

147. C. Norman Shealy, *Energy Medicine: Practical Applications and Scientific Proof* (Virginia Beach, VA: 4th Dimension Press, 2011), 69–98.

148. Levin, "Esoteric Healing Traditions"; and Kevin V. Ergil, Marnae C. Ergil, Peter T. Furst, Nancy Gordon, John M. Janzen, Elisa J. Sobo, and Linda Sparrowe, *Ancient Healing: Unlocking the Mysteries of Health and Healing through the Ages* (Lincolnwood, IL: Publications International, 1997).

149. Levin, "Esoteric Healing Traditions."

150. Genesis 12:1.

151. Elliot N. Dorff, *Tikkun Olam (Repairing the World)* (Woodstock, VT: Jewish Lights, 2005).

152. Lawrence Fine, "Isaac Luria: Introduction," in *Safed Spirituality: Rules of Mystical Piety, The Beginning of Wisdom*, trans. Lawrence Fine (Mahwah, NJ: Paulist Press, 1984), 61–64.

153. Byron Johnson and William H. Wubbenhorst, *Incorporating Faith and Works within a Healthcare Network: Baylor Scott & White's Office of Mission and Ministry* (Waco, TX: Baylor Institute for Studies of Religion, 2017), 11–13.

154. Jeff Levin, "Faith-Based Partnerships for Population Health: Challenges, Initiatives, and Prospects," *Public Health Reports* 129 (2014): 127–131; and "Faith-Based Initiatives in Health Promotion: History, Challenges, and Current Partnerships," *American Journal of Health Promotion* 28 (2014): 139–141.

155. Levin, "Partnerships between the Faith-Based and Medical Sectors," 345.

156. Kenneth Vaux, "Religion and Health," *Preventive Medicine* 5 (1976): 522–536.

157. See Harold G. Koenig, Michael E. McCullough, and David B. Larson, *Handbook of Religion and Health* (New York: Oxford University Press, 2001); and Harold G. Koenig, Dana E. King, and Verna Benner Carson, *Handbook of Religion and Health*, 2nd ed. (New York: Oxford University Press, 2011).

158. Levin, "The Discourse on Faith and Medicine."

159. Jeff Levin, "The Epidemiology of Religion," in *Religion and the Social Sciences: Basic and Applied Research Perspectives* (West Conshohocken, PA: Templeton Press, 2018), 259–286.

Chapter 2

1. Emile Durkheim, *The Elementary Forms of the Religious Life*, trans. Joseph Ward Swain (1915; New York: Free Press, 1965), 339.

2. Ibid., 297.

3. Ibid.

4. Peter Harrison, *The Territories of Science and Religion* (Chicago: University of Chicago Press, 2015); and Jeff Levin, "Peter Harrison. *The Territories of Science and Religion*" [book review], *Christian Century* 133, 4 (2016): 46–47, 49–50.

5. Rupert E. Davies, "Medical Science before Christ," in *Religion and Medicine: Essays by Members of the Methodist Society for Medical and Pastoral Psychology*, ed. John Crowlesmith (London: The Epworth Press, 1962), 1–17, 2–3.

6. George L. Engel, "The Need for a New Medical Model: A Challenge for Biomedicine," *Science* 196 (1977): 129–136.

7. Martin E. Marty and Dean G. Peerman, "Introduction: The Recovery of Transcendence," in Marty and Peerman, eds., *New Theology No. 7: The Recovery of Transcendence* (New York: Macmillan, 1970), 9–22.

8. Peter Berger, *A Rumor of Angels: Modern Society and the Rediscovery of the Supernatural* (Garden City, NY: Doubleday, 1969).

9. Ferngren, *Medicine and Religion*.

10. Ronald L. Numbers and Ronald C. Sawyer, "Medicine and Christianity in the Modern World," in Marty and Vaux, *Health/Medicine and the Faith Traditions*, 133–160.

11. Ari Kiev, ed., *Magic, Faith, and Healing: Studies in Primitive Psychiatry Today* (New York: Free Press, 1964).

12. H. H. Gerth and C. Wright Mills, "Intellectual Orientations," in *From Max Weber: Essays in Sociology*, trans. and ed. Gerth and Mills (New York: Oxford University Press, 1946), 45–74, 54.

13. Ibid.

14. Three entries in Mircea Eliade, editor-in-chief, *The Encyclopedia of Religion*, vol. 9 (New York: Macmillan, 1987): Vittorio Lanternari, "Medicine and Religion in Tribal Cultures," 305–312; Ilza Veith, "Medicine and Religion in Eastern Traditions," 312–319; and Darrell W. Amundsen, "Medicine and Religion in Western Traditions," 319–324.

15. Lawrence E. Sullivan, ed., *Healing and Restoring: Health and Medicine in the World's Religious Traditions* (New York: Macmillan, 1989).

16. Ronald L. Numbers and Darrel W. Amundsen, eds., *Caring and Curing: Health and Medicine in the Western Religious Traditions* (New York: Macmillan, 1986).

17. Lawrence E. Sullivan, "Introduction: The Quest for Well-Being and the Questioning of Medicine," in Sullivan, *Healing and Restoring*, 1–8, 2–3.

18. Ibid., 5.

19. Mircea Eliade, *A History of Religious Ideas*, vol. 1: *From the Stone Age to the Eleusinian Mysteries*, trans. Willard R. Trask (Chicago: University of Chicago Press, 1978), 19.

20. Ninian Smart, *Dimensions of the Sacred: An Anatomy of the World's Beliefs* (Berkeley: University of California Press, 1996), 94–95.

21. Ibid., 94.

22. Otto, *The Idea of the Holy*, 144.

23. Ibid.

24. Ibid.

25. Sir James Frazer, *The Golden Bough: A Study in Religion and Magic,* abridged ed. (1922; Mineola, NY: Dover Publications, 2002).

26. Ibid., 196.

27. Ibid., 195.

28. Ibid.

29. Ibid., 196.

30. Ibid.

31. Ibid.

32. Ibid.

33. Christian Deetjen, "Witchcraft and Medicine," *Bulletin of the Institute of the History of Medicine* 2 (1934): 164–175, 164.

34. Ibid.

35. Ibid.

36. Michael James Winkelman, "Shamans and Other 'Magico-Religious' Healers: A Cross-Cultural Study of Their Origins, Nature, and Social Transformations," *Ethos* 18 (1990): 308–352,

37. George Murdock and Douglas R. White, "Standard Cross-Cultural Sample," *Ethnology* 8 (1969): 329–369.

38. Winkelman, "Shamans and Other 'Magico-Religious' Healers," 323.

39. Kevin V. Ergil, Marnae C. Ergil, Peter T. Furst, Nancy Gordon, John M. Janzen, Elisa J. Sobo, and Linda Sparowe, *Ancient Healing: Unlocking the Mysteries of Health and Healing through the Ages* (Lincolnwood, IL: Publications International, 1997); and Hall, *Healing*.

40. Sullivan, *Healing and Restoring*.

41. Kenneth G. Zysk, *Medicine in the Veda: Religious Healing in the Veda* (1985; Delhi: Motilal Banarsidass, 1996). quotation xii.

42. Ibid.

43. Ibid., quotation xiv.

44. Ibid., quotation xvii.

45. Ibid., quotations xiv.

46. Ibid.

47. Joseph Mitsuo Kitagawa, "Buddhist Medical History," in Sullivan, *Healing and Restoring*, 9–32, 16.

48. Ibid., 16.

49. Ibid., 11.

50. Raoul Birnbaum, "Chinese Buddhist Traditions of Healing and the Life Cycle," in Sullivan, *Healing and Restoring*, 33–57, 34.

51. Ibid.

52. Ibid., 34–35.

53. C. Pierce Salguero, "Introduction," in Salguero, ed., *Buddhism and Medicine: An Anthology of Premodern Sources* (New York: Columbia University Press, 2017), xxi–xxxiii.

54. Ibid., quotation xxi.

55. Ibid., 21.

56. S. Haque Nizamie and Nishant Goyal, "History of Psychiatry in India," *Indian Journal of Psychiatry* 52, Suppl. 1 (2010): SS7–S12.

57. Albert S. Lyons and R. Joseph Petrucelli, "Ancient India," in *Medicine: An Illustrated History* (New York: Harry N. Abrahams, 1997), 104–119.

58. Kenneth G. Zysk, *Asceticism and Healing in Ancient India: Medicine in the Buddhist Monastery* (1991; Delhi: Motilal Banarsidass, 1998), 44.

59. Heinrich Zimmer, *Philosophies of India*, ed. Joseph Campbell (Princeton, NJ: Princeton University Press, 1951).

60. Mircea Eliade, *A History of Religious Ideas*, vol. 2: *From Gautama Buddha to the Triumph of Christianity*, trans. Willard R. Trask (Chicago: University of Chicago Press, 1982), 67.

61. Ibid., 68.

62. James Haughton Woods, *The Yoga-System of Patañjali or the Ancient Hindu Doctrine of Concentration of Mind Embracing the Mnemonic Rules Called Yoga-Sūtras, of Patañjali and the Comment, Called Yoga-Bhāshya, Attributed to Veda-Vyāsa and the Explanation, Called Tattva-Vāiçāradi, of Vāchaspati-Miçra* (Delhi: Motilal Banarsidass, 1914), esp. book 3: 203–296.

63. Ibid., 260.

64. Ibid., 266.

65. Ibid., quotations 278–279.

66. Paul U. Unschuld, *Medicine in China: A History of Ideas* (Berkeley: University of California Press, 1985).

67. Lixing Lao, "Traditional Chinese Medicine," in *Essentials of Complementary and Alternative Medicine*, ed. Wayne B. Jonas and Jeffrey S. Levin (Philadelphia: Lippincott, Williams and Wilkins, 1999), 219–232.

68. Guo Zhaojiang, "Chinese Confucian Culture and the Medical Ethical Tradition," *Journal of Medical Ethics* 21 (1995): 239–246.

69. A representative English translation: Maoshing Li, translator, *The Yellow Emperor's Classic of Medicine: A New Translation of the* Neijing Suwen *with Commentary* (Boston: Shambhala, 1995).

70. Lawrence I. Conrad, Michael Neve, Vivian Nutton, Roy Porter, and Andrew Wear, *The Western Medical Tradition: 800 BC to AD 1800* (Cambridge: Cambridge University Press, 1995).

71. See sections on the ancient Near East in Ferngren, *Medicine and Religion*, and Ferngren and Lomperis, *Essential Readings in Medicine and Religion*.

72. Ferngren, *Medicine and Religion*, 17.

73. Ibid.

74. Ferngren and Lomperis, *Essential Readings in Medicine and Religion*, 2.

75. Ibid., 5–9; and JoAnn Scurlock, *Sourcebook for Ancient Mesopotamian Medicine* (Atlanta: SBL Press, 2014).

76. Ferngren, *Medicine and Religion*, 20–21.

77. Ibid., 23.

78. Ibid., 24.

79. Ibid., 24–25; and Ferngren and Lomperis, *Essential Readings in Medicine and Religion*, 16–21.

80. Ferngren and Lomperis, *Essential Readings in Medicine and Religion*, 21–22.

81. Ferngren, *Medicine and Religion*, 23–24.

82. Henry E. Sigerist, *A History of Medicine*, vol. 2: *Early Greek, Hindu, and Persian Medicine* (New York: Oxford University Press, 1961), esp. 161.

83. Ferngren, *Medicine and Religion*, 29–30.

84. Ibid., 29.

85. Frank Heynick, *Jews and Medicine: An Epic Saga* (Hoboken, NJ: KTAV, 2002), 40.

86. Ibid., 26–29.

87. Ibid., 31.

88. Ibid., 29.

89. Ferngren and Lomperis, *Essential Readings in Medicine and Religion*, 30–31.

90. Levin, "How Faith Heals."

91. Preuss, *Biblical and Talmudic Medicine*.

92. Natalia Berger, ed., *Jews and Medicine: Religion, Culture, Science* (Philadelphia: Jewish Publication Society, 1995), 16.

93. Suessman Munter, "Medicine in Ancient Israel," in Fred Rosner, *Medicine in the Bible and the Talmud: Selections from Classical Jewish Sources*, augmented ed. (Hoboken, NJ: KTAV, 1995), 3–20, esp. 17.

94. Vivian Nutton, *Ancient Medicine*, 2nd ed. (London: Routledge, 2013).

95. Ferngren, *Medicine and Religion*; Guenter B. Risse, *Mending Bodies, Saving Souls: A History of Hospitals* (New York: Oxford University Press, 1999); and Conrad et al., *The Western Medical Tradition*.

96. Vivian Nutton, "Medicine in the Greek World, 800–50 BC," in Conrad et al., *The Western Medical Tradition*, 11–38, esp. 11.

97. Ibid., 11.

98. Ibid., 16.

99. Ibid.

100. Ferngren and Lomperis, *Essential Readings in Medicine and Religion*, 42.

101. Ferngren, *Medicine and Religion*, 37–40.

102. Ibid., 41–47; and L. Cilliers and F. P. Retief, "Medical Practice in Graeco-Roman Antiquity," *Curationis* 29, 2 (2006): 34–40.

103. Ferngren, *Medicine and Religion*, 50.

104. Ibid., 51.

105. For a discussion of Greek healing cults and the layout of their sanctuaries and temples, see Simon Price, "Elective Cults," in *Religions of the Ancient Greeks* (New York: Cambridge University Press, 1999), 108–125.

106. Ferngren and Lomperis, *Essential Readings in Medicine and Religion*, 37–43, 42.

107. Risse, *Mending Bodies, Saving Souls*, 31.

108. Ferngren, *Medicine and Religion*, 53.

109. Ferngren and Lomperis, *Essential Readings in Medicine and Religion*, 73.

110. Ibid., 72–73.

111. Ibid., 73.

112. Vivian Nutton, "Roman Medicine, 250 BC to AD 200," in Conrad et al., *The Western Medical Tradition*, 39–70, esp. 52–54.

113. See "Rome," chapter 3 in Ferngren, *Medicine and Religion*, 55–72; "Rome," chapter 3 in Ferngren and Lomperis, *Essential Readings in Medicine and Religion*, 70–99;

Nutton, "Roman Medicine, 250 BC to AD 200"; and Cilliers and Retief, "Medical Practice in Graeco-Roman Antiquity."

114. Nutton, "Roman Medicine, 250 BC to AD 200," 47–52.

115. Jack E. McCallum, "Roman Military Medicine," *Military Medicine: From Ancient Times to the 21st Century* (Santa Barbara, CA: ABC-CLIO, 2008), 270–273. Patricia A. Baker questions this evidence in "The Roman Military Valetudinaria: Fact or Fiction?," in *The Archaeology of Medicine: Papers Given at a Session of the Annual Conference of the Theoretical Archaeology Group Held at the University of Birmingham on 20 December 1998*, ed. Robert Arnott (Oxford: Archeopress, 2002), 69–80; and Patricia A. Baker, *The Archaeology of Medicine in the Greco-Roman World* (New York: Cambridge University Press, 2013).

116. Sarah Iles Johnston, "Illnesses and Other Crises," in Johnston, gen. ed., *Religions of the Ancient World: A Guide* (Cambridge, MA: Belknap Press of Harvard University Press, 2004), 452–469, 453, summarizes religious healing in ancient Egypt, Mesopotamia, Syria-Canaan, Israel, Anatolia, Iran, Greece and Rome, and Etruria.

117. Alfredo Morabia, *Enigmas of Health and Disease: How Epidemiology Helps Unravel Scientific Mysteries* (New York: Columbia University Press, 2014), 24.

118. Ferngren, *Medicine and Health Care in Early Christianity*, esp. chapter 2, "The Christian Reception of Greek Medicine," 13–41.

119. Ibid., 29.

120. Ibid., 35.

121. Nutton, "Medicine in Late Antiquity and the Early Middle Ages," in Conrad et al., *The Western Medical Tradition*, 71–87, esp. 73.

122. Ferngren, *Medicine and Health Care in Early Christianity*, 35–36.

123. Morton Kelsey, *Healing and Christianity: A Classic Study* (1973; Minneapolis: Augsburg, 1995), 26.

124. Amanda Porterfield, *Healing in the History of Christianity* (New York: Oxford University Press, 2005), esp. chapter 1, "Jesus: Exorcist and Healer," 21–41.

125. Kelsey, *Healing and Christianity*, 42–47.

126. Philo of Alexandria, *The Works of Philo: Complete and Unabridged*, new updated ed., trans. C. D. Yonge (Peabody, MA: Hendrickson, 1993).

127. Ibid., 698.

128. E.g., Elmar R. Gruber and Holger Kersten, *The Original Jesus: The Buddhist Sources of Christianity* (Shaftesbury, U.K.: Element, 1995).

129. Levin, "Esoteric Healing Traditions," 103.

130. E.g., E. B. Szekely, *The Essene Gospel of Peace: Book One* (London: International Biogenic Society, 1981).

131. Levin, "Esoteric Healing Traditions," 103.

132. Joan E. Taylor and Philip R. Davies, "The So-Called Therapeutae of *De Vita Contemplativa*: Identity and Character," *Harvard Theological Review* 91 (1998): 3–24.

133. Beginning with Peter's healing of the lame beggar in Acts 3:1–10.

134. Kelsey, *Healing and Christianity*, 99.

135. Porterfield, *Healing in the History of Christianity*, 27.

136. For a listing of Gospel accounts of Jesus's acts of healing, see Kelsey, *Healing and Christianity*, 42–47.

137. Ferngren, *Medicine and Health Care in Early Christianity*, 25.

138. "The Clementine Homilies," in *Ante-Nicene Fathers*, vol. 8: *The Twelve Patriarchs, Excerpts and Epistles, The Clementina, Apocrypha, Decretals, Memoirs of Edessa and Syriac Documents, Remains of the First Ages*, ed. Alexander Roberts and James Donaldson (1886; Peabody, MA: Hendrickson, 1994), 223–346, quotation from Homily IX, Chapter XII, 277.

139. "Origen Against Celsus," in *Ante-Nicene Fathers*, vol. 4: *Tertullian, Part Fourth; Minucius Felix; Commodian; Origen, Parts First and Second*, ed. Alexander Roberts and James Donaldson (1885; Peabody, MA: Hendrickson, 1994), 395–669, quotation from Book III, Chapter XII, 469.

140. Ferngren, *Medicine and Health Care in Early Christianity*, 27.

141. Ibid.

142. Christoffer H. Grundmann, "Healing—A Challenge to Church and Theology," *International Review of Mission* 90 (2001): 26–40.

143. Stanley Samuel Harakas, "The Eastern Orthodox Tradition," in Numbers and Amundsen, *Caring and Curing*, 146–172, 149.

144. Ibid.

145. Kamal Sabri Kolta, "Coptic Medicine," in *The Coptic Encyclopedia*, vol. 5: ed. Aziz S. Atiya (New York: Macmillan, 1991), 1578–1582; and P. E. Pormann, "Medicine," in *Gorgias Encyclopedic Dictionary of the Syriac Heritage*, ed. Sebastian Brock, Aaron M. Butts, George A. Kiraz, and Lucas Van Rompay (Piscataway, NJ: Gorgias Press, 2011), 282–283.

146. Stephen Muse, ed., *Raising Lazarus: Integral Healing in Orthodox Christianity* (Brookline, MA: Holy Cross Orthodox Press, 2004).

147. John G. Demakis, "Historical Precedents for Syngeria: Combining Medicine, Diakonia, and Sacrament in Byzantine Times," in ibid., 15–24.

148. Randy Stice, *Understanding the Sacraments of Healing: A Rite-Based Approach* (Chicago: Liturgy Training Publications, 2015), 18–21.

149. Ibid., 23.

150. Chapter 2, "Language of the Liturgy," in ibid., 22–40.

151. John C. Kasza, *Understanding Sacramental Healing: Anointing and Viaticum* (Chicago: Hillenbrand Books, 2007), 13–14.

152. Chapter 8, "The Church as Sacramental Healer," in ibid., 176–187.

153. Corinna Delkeskamp-Hayes, "Christian Credentials for Roman Catholic Health Care: Medicine versus the Healing Mission of the Church," *Christian Bioethics* 7 (2001): 117–150, 119–120.

154. Harakas, "The Eastern Orthodox Tradition," 156.

155. Ferngren, *Medicine and Health Care in Early Christianity*, 124–125.

156. Demakis, "Historical Precedents for Syngeria," 17.

157. Porterfield, *Healing in the History of Christianity*, 53.

158. Anna M. Silvas, *The Asketikon of St. Basil the Great* (Oxford: Oxford University Press, 2005); and *The Rule of St. Basil in Latin and English: A Revised Critical Edition*, trans. Anna M. Silvas (Collegeville, MN: Liturgical Press, 2013).

159. A video series, "Pilgrimages of Europe" (Palm Plus Producties B.V., 1995; reissued by Janson Media, 2004), provides travelogue-style accounts of Croagh Patrick, Iona, Les Saintes Maries de la Mer, Lourdes, Amsterdam, Fátima, El Rocio, Santiago de Compostela, Kalwaria Zebrzydowska, Scherpenheuvel, Kevelaer, and Medjugorje.

160. Maurice Ryan, "Fátima, Lourdes, and Medjugorje: A Challenge for Religious Educators," *Religious Education* 98 (1993): 564–575.

161. Ibid., 571.

162. Bernard Francois, Esther M. Sternberg, and Elizabeth Fee, "The Lourdes Medical Cures Revisited," *Journal of the History of Medicine and Allied Health Sciences* 69 (2014): 135–162.

163. Ibid.

164. Ibid., 160.

165. Ibid., 137.

166. Will Gesler, "Lourdes: Healing in a Place of Pilgrimage," *Health and Place* 2 (1996): 95–105, 101.

167. Joel Robbins, "The Globalization of Pentecostal and Charismatic Christianity," *Annual Review of Anthropology* 33 (2004): 117–143.

168. At Chimayó sanctuary in New Mexico, while priests have collected testimonials of healing for decades, the Catholic Church shows little interest in pursuing claims (Brett Hendrickson, *The Healing Power of the Santuario de Chimayó: America's Miraculous Church* (New York: New York University Press, 2017)).

169. Vuk Stambolovic, "Medical Heresy—The View of a Heretic," *Social Science and Medicine* 43 (1996): 601–604; and Kevin Dew, "Apostasy to Orthodoxy: Debates before a Commission of Inquiry into Chiropractic," *Sociology of Health and Illness* 22 (2000): 310–330.

170. See Hickey, *Mind Cure*.

171. Franz Anton Mesmer, *Mesmerism: A Translation of the Original Scientific and Medical Writings of F. A. Mesmer*, trans. and comp. George Bloch (Los Altos, CA: W. Kaufman, 1980).

172. Ralph Waldo Emerson, *Nature* (Boston: James Munroe and Company, 1836).

173. Horatio W. Dresser, *Health and the Inner Life: An Analytical and Historical Study of Spiritual Healing Theories, with an Account of the Life and Teachings of P. P. Quimby* (New York: G. P. Putnam's Sons, 1906).

174. Mumtaz A. Siddiqui, Nirav J. Mehta, and Ijaz A. Khan, "Paracelsus: The Hippocrates of the Renaissance," *Journal of Medical Biography* 11, 2 (2003):78–80.

175. Martin Lamm, *Swedenborg: The Development of His Thought*, trans. Tomas Spiers and Anders Hallengren (1915; West Chester, PA: Swedenborg Foundation, 2000).

176. H. C. Erik Midelfort, *Exorcism and Enlightenment: Johann Joseph Gassner and the Demons of Eighteenth-Century Germany* (New Haven, CT: Yale University Press, 2005), esp. the material in chapter 3, "Healing," 59–86.

177. Helena Blavatsky, *Isis Unveiled: A Master-Key to the Mysteries of Ancient and Modern Science and Theosophy* (1877; Pasadena, CA: Theosophical University Press, 1988). See also Peter Washington, *Madame Blavatsky's Baboon: A History of the Mystics, Mediums, and Misfits Who Brought Spiritualism to America* (New York: Schocken Books, 1995).

178. Eddy, *Science and Health with Key to the Scriptures*. See also Walter I. Wardwell, "Christian Science Healing," *Journal for the Scientific Study of Religion* 4 (1965): 175–181.

179. Julius A. Dresser, *The True History of Mental Science: The Facts concerning the Discovery of Mental Healing*, rev. by Horatio W. Dresser (1887; Boston: George H. Ellis, 1899).

180. Deidre Michell, "New Thinking, New Thought, New Age: The Theology and Influence of Emma Curtis Hopkins (1849–1925)," *Counterpoints* 2, 1 (2002): 6–18.

181. One significant history of New Thought failed to mention Hopkins: Alfred Whitney Griswold, "New Thought: A Cult of Success," *American Journal of Sociology* 40 (1934): 309–318, took a sarcastic tone, reducing New Thought to "a new get-rich-quick scheme" (314), overlooking its identity as a healing movement and the role of Hopkins.

182. Horatio W. Dresser, "Preface," in *A History of the New Thought Movement* (New York: Thomas Y. Crowell, 1919), iii–ix, quotation iii.

183. Seen in limited treatment afforded New Thought in American religious history texts: e.g., Sydney E. Ahlstrom, *A Religious History of the American People*, 2nd ed. (New Haven, CT: Yale University Press, 2004), 1026–1029; and Edwin S. Gaustad and Leigh Schmidt, *The Religious History of America: The Heart of the American Story from Colonial Times to Today*, rev. ed. (New York: HarperSanFrancisco, 2002), 228–229.

184. Porterfield, *Healing in the History of Christianity*, esp. 174–180.

185. P. P. Quimby, *The Quimby Manuscripts*, ed. Horatio W. Dress (New York: Thomas Y. Crowell, 1921), 58.

186. Ibid.

187. Ibid.

188. Ibid., 58–59.

189. Catherine L. Albanese, "Physic and Metaphysic in Nineteenth-Century America: Medical Sectarians and Religious Healing," *Church History* 55 (1986): 489–501, quotations 498.

190. Amanda Porterfield, "Native American Shamanism and the American Mind-Cure Movement: A Comparative Study of Religious Healing," *Horizons* 11 (1984): 276–289.

191. Eddy, "Preface," in *Science and Health with Key to the Scriptures*, vii–xii, quotation viii.

192. Porterfield, *Healing in the History of Christianity*, 179.

193. Eddy, "Preface," quotation x.

194. Ibid.

195. Eddy, "Prayer," in *Science and Health with Key to the Scriptures*, 1–17, 11.

196. Emma Curtis Hopkins, *Scientific Christian Medical Practice: The Original Text* (1888; Charleston, SC: CreateSpace, 2014), 8.

197. Ibid., 85.

198. Ibid., 86.

199. Ibid., 118.

200. William James, *The Varieties of Religious Experience: A Study in Human Nature* (1902; New York: Mentor, 1958), 87.

201. See chapter 4, "Prophets," in Lynn Bridgers, *Contemporary Varieties of Religious Experience: James' Classic Study in Light of Resiliency, Temperament, and Trauma* (Lanham, MD: Rowman and Littlefield, 2005), 67–99.

202. Ibid., 76–111.

203. Ibid., 83.

204. Ibid., 112–139.

205. Ibid., 89.

206. Ibid., 77–79.

207. Holmes, *The Science of Mind*.

208. Malinda E. Cramer, *Divine Science and Healing* (1890; Denver: Colorado College of Divine Science, 1923).

209. Fillmore, *Jesus Christ Heals*.

210. Ellen M. Umansky, *From Christian Science to Jewish Science: Spiritual Healing and American Jews* (New York: Oxford University Press, 2005).

211. Elwood Worcester, Samuel McComb, and Isador H. Coriat, *Religion and Medicine: The Moral Control of Nervous Disorders* (New York: Moffat, Yard and Company, 1908).

212. Hickey, *Mind Cure*.

213. H. K. Challoner, *The Path of Healing* (Wheaton, IL: Quest Books, 1972); H. Tudor Edmunds and Associates, eds., *Some Unrecognized Factors in Medicine* (1934; Wheaton, IL: Quest, 1976); Rudolf Steiner, *Fundamentals of Anthroposophical Medicine* (Spring Valley, NY: Mercury Press, 1986); and Michael Evans and Iain Rodger, *Anthroposophical Medicine: Healing for Body, Soul, and Spirit* (London: Thorson, 1992).

214. Alice Bailey, *Esoteric Healing* (New York: Lucis, 1953), 256.

215. Hickey, *Mind Cure*.

216. W. F. Evans, *The Mental Cure, Illustrating the Influence of the Mind on the Body* (Boston: H. H. and T. W. Carter, 1869); *Mental Medicine: A Theoretical and Practical Treatise on Medical Psychology* (Boston: Carter and Petree, 1873); and *The Primitive Mind-Cure: The Nature and Power of Faith; or, Elementary Lessons in Christian Philosophy and Transcendental Medicine* (Boston: H. H. Carter and Co., 1885).

217. Christian D. Larson, *The Mind Cure* (Los Angeles: New Literature, 1912); and *Healing Yourself* (New York: Thomas Y. Crowell, 1918).

218. Stanley M. Burgess and Eduard M. van der Maas, eds., *The New International Dictionary of Pentecostal and Charismatic Movements*, rev. and exp. ed. (Grand Rapids: Zondervan, 2003). See especially F. Martin, "Healing, Gift of," 694–698; and R. A. N. Kydd, "Healing in the Christian Church," 698–711.

219. Jeff Levin, "Energy Healers: Who They Are and What They Do," *EXPLORE: The Journal of Science and Healing* 7 (2011): 13–26.

220. J. Gordon Melton makes the same connection in "Toward a Typology of the Megachurch," in *Handbook of Global Contemporary Christianity: Megachurches*, ed. Stephen Hunt (Leiden, Netherlands: Brill, in press).

221. Constance E. Cumbey, *A Planned Deception: The Staging of a New Age "Messiah"* (East Detroit, MI: Pointe Publishers, 1985).

222. Louise Hay, *Heal Your Body: The Mental Causes for Physical Illness and the Metaphysical Way to Overcome Them*, exp. rev. ed. (Carson, CA: Hay House, 1988).

223. Ibid., quotations 22.

224. C. Norman Shealy and Carolyn M. Myss, *The Creation of Health: Merging Traditional Medicine with Intuitive Diagnosis* (Walpole, NH: Stillpoint Publishing, 1988).

225. This same point is emphasized in John S. Haller, *Swedenborg, Mesmer, and the Mind/Body Connection: The Roots of Complementary Medicine* (West Chester, PA: Swedenborg Foundation Press, 2010).

226. Dresser, *A History of the New Thought Movement*, 18.

227. William E. Stempsey, "Institutional Identity and Roman Catholic Hospitals," *Christian Bioethics* 7 (2001): 3–14.

228. Risse, *Mending Bodies, Saving Souls*.

229. Levin, "Partnerships between the Faith-Based and Medical Sectors," 345.

230. Numbers and Sawyer, "Medicine and Christianity in the Modern World."

231. Ibid., 148–149.

232. Elizabeth B. Deutsch, "Expanding Conscience, Shrinking Care: The Crisis in Access to Reproductive Care and the Affordable Care Act's Nondiscrimination Mandate," *Yale Law Journal* 124 (2015): 2470–2514.

233. If considering the many Roman Catholic healthcare systems operated by religious orders as separate institutions. If instead treated as a single entity, then the Adventist Health System would qualify as the largest Protestant healthcare system.

234. "Our Mission and Values," Adventist Health System. https://www.adventisthealthsystem.com/page.php?section=about&page=mission.

235. "History," Adventist Health System. https://www.adventisthealthsystem.com/page.php?section=about&page=history.

236. Harold G. Koenig, Kathleen Perno, and Ted Hamilton, "Integrating Spirituality into Outpatient Practice in the Adventist Health System," *Southern Medical Journal* 110 (2017): 1–7.

237. Ibid., 1.

238. Harold G. Koenig, Kathleen Perno, and Ted Hamilton, "The Spiritual History in Outpatient Practice: Attitudes and Practices of Health Professionals in the Adventist Health System," *BMC Medical Education* 17 (2017): 102. doi: 10.1186/s12909-017-0938-8.

239. Ronald L. Numbers and David R. Larson, "The Adventist Tradition," in Numbers and Amundsen, *Caring and Curing*, 447–467.

240. Ronald L. Numbers, *Prophetess of Health: A Study of Ellen G. White*, 3rd ed. (Grand Rapids: Eerdmans, 2008).

241. Ibid., 461.

242. Erie Chapman, *Radical Loving Care: Building the Healing Hospital in America* (Nashville: Baptist Healing Hospital Trust, 2005), 4.

243. Patch Adams, with Maureen Mylander, *Gesundheit!: Bringing Good Health to You, the Medical System, and Society through Physician Service, Complementary Therapies, Humor, and Joy* (Rochester, VT: Healing Arts Press, 1993).

244. Patch Adams, "When Healing Is More Than Simply Clowning Around," *JAMA* 279 (1998): 401.

245. Patch Adams, "Medicine as a Vehicle for Social Change," *Journal of Alternative and Complementary Medicine* 11 (2008): 578–582.

246. Judith Lynn Failer, "Jewish Giving by Doing: *Tikkun Ha-Olam*," in *Religious Giving: For the Love of God*, ed. David H. Smith (Bloomington: Indiana University Press, 2010), 49–64.

247. Robert A. Katz, "Paging Dr. Shylock!: Jewish Hospitals and the Prudent Reinvestment of Jewish Philanthropy," in Smith, *Religious Giving*, 162–184.

248. "The Jewish Hospital Mission Statement," The Jewish Hospital–Mercy Health, https://www.mercy.com/cincinnati/locations/hospitals/the-jewish-hospital.

249. Stephen Lutz, "The History of Hospice and Palliative Care," *Current Problems in Cancer* 35 (2011): 304–309.

250. Shirley du Boulay with Marianne Rankin, *Cicely Saunders: The Founder of the Modern Hospice Movement*, updated and exp. ed. (London: SPCK, 2007), 120.

251. Maurice Lamm, *The Jewish Way in Death and Mourning*, rev. and exp. ed. (Middle Village, NY: Jonathan David Publishers, 2000).

252. Ibid., quotations 31.

253. Reinhard Bonnke, *Raised from the Dead: The Miracle That Brings Promise to America* (New Kensington, PA: Whitaker House, 2014). Evangelicals have been cautious about endorsing such phenomena, but are not exclusively opposed (see Chris Armstrong, "Do Nigerian Miracle Ministries Discredit the Faith?," *Christianity Today* (May 2004), http://www.christianitytoday.com/ct/2004/mayweb-only/5-17-53.0.html).

254. Francis MacNutt, *Healing* (New York: Bantam Books, 1974).

255. Antônio Flávio Pierucci and Reginaldo Prandi, "Religious Diversity in Brazil: Numbers and Perspectives in a Sociological Evaluation, *International Sociology* 15, 4 (2000): 629–639.

256. Heather Cumming and Karen Leffler, *John of God: The Brazilian Healer Who's Touched the Lives of Millions* (New York: Atria Books, 2007).

257. Julie Motz, *Hands of Life: Use Your Body's Own Energy Medicine for Healing, Recovery, and Transformation* (New York: Bantam Books, 1998).

Chapter 3

1. Schweitzer, *Out of My Life and Thought*; and Brabazon, *Albert Schweitzer*.

2. Gunnar Jahn, "Award Ceremony Speech," *The Nobel Peace Prize 1952* (December 5, 2018), https://www.nobelprize.org/prizes/peace/1952/ceremony-speech/.

3. During his lifetime, hagiography of Schweitzer was ubiquitous. In 1947 *LIFE* magazine called him "The Greatest Man in the World," at a time when Gandhi, Churchill, and Einstein were still alive.

4. Marvin Meyer and Kurt Begel, eds., *Reverence for Life: The Ethics of Albert Schweitzer for the Twenty-First Century* (Syracuse, NY: Syracuse University Press, 2002).

5. Lachlan Forrow, "Foreword to the 60th Anniversary Edition," in Schweitzer, *Out of My Life and Thought*, vii–xii, quotation ix.

6. Schweitzer, *Out of My Life and Thought*, 157.

7. Ibid., 91.

8. Ibid., 114.

9. Ibid., 92.

10. Ibid.

11. Manuel M. Davenport, "The Moral Paternalism of Albert Schweitzer," *Ethics* 84 (1974): 116–127.

12. Gerald McKnight, *Verdict on Schweitzer: The Man behind the Legend of Lambaréné* (New York: John Day Co., 1964); and Bertrand Taithe and Katherine Davis, "'Heroes of Charity?' Between Memory and Hagiography: Colonial Medical Heroes in the Era of Decolonisation," *Journal of Imperial and Commonwealth History* 42 (2014): 912–935.

13. Peter Worsley, "Albert Schweitzer and the Liberal Conscience," *New Reasoner* 58, 3 (1957): 39–54.

14. A. G. Rud, "Icon, Scoundrel, Prophet, Paradigm?: A Recovery Project for Schools," in *Albert Schweitzer's Legacy for Education* (New York: Palgrave Macmillan, 2011), 107–120.

15. Cornel du Toit, "Post-Colonialism and the Deconstruction of Moral Imperialism: The Case of Albert Schweitzer and His Ethics of Reverence for Life," in *The Legacies of Albert Schweitzer Reconsidered*, ed. Izak Spangenberg and Christina Landman (Durbanville, South Africa: AOSIS, 2017), 3–41, 19.

16. Ruth Harris, "The Allure of Albert Schweitzer," *History of European Ideas* 40 (2014): 804–825, 813.

17. Joanne Miyang Cho, "Provincializing Albert Schweitzer's Ethical Colonialism in Africa," *European Legacy* 16 (2011): 71–86, 71.

18. Said Amir Arjomand, "Thinking Globally about Islam," in *The Oxford Handbook of Global Religions*, ed. Mark Juergensmeyer (New York: Oxford University Press, 2006), 401–418, 401.

19. Janet Westberg with Jill Westberg McNamara, *Gentle Rebel: The Life and Work of Granger Westberg, Pioneer in Whole Person Care* (Memphis, TN: Church Health, 2015), 260–263; and Sybil D. Smith, "From the Westberg Project to the New Millennium," in *Parish Nursing: A Handbook for the New Millennium*, ed. Sybil D. Smith (New York: Haworth Pastoral Press, 2003), 55–75.

20. Leslie Van Dover and Jane Bacon Pfeiffer, "Spiritual Care in Christian Parish Nursing," *Journal of Advanced Nursing* 57 (2007): 213–221.

21. Westberg with McNamara, *Gentle Rebel*.

22. Matthew 28:19 (RSV).

23. Carlos F. Cardoza-Orlandi and Justo L. González, *To All Nations from All Nations: A History of the Christian Missionary Movement* (Nashville: Abingdon Press, 2013).

24. Ibid., 5.

25. Ibid., 1.

26. Kenneth Scott Latourette, *A History of the Expansion of Christianity*, 7 vols. (New York: Harper and Brothers, 1937–1945).

27. Dan Cohn-Sherbok, *The Crucified Jew: Twenty Centuries of Christian Anti-Semitism* (Grand Rapids: Eerdmans, 1992).

28. Rodney Stark, *God's Battalions: The Case for the Crusades* (New York: HarperOne, 2009).

29. David Hardiman, "Introduction," in *Healing Bodies, Saving Souls: Medical Missions in Asia and Africa*, ed. David Hardiman (Amsterdam: Rodopi, 2006), 5–57.

30. Ibid., 344–350.

31. Ibid., 5.

32. Ibid.

33. Ibid., 11.

34. Ibid., 8.

35. Nancy Rose Hunt, *A Colonial Lexicon: Of Birth Ritual, Medicalization and Mobility in the Congo* (Durham, NC: Duke University Press, 1999).

36. Richard Gottheil and Meyer Kaserling, "Inquisition (Called Also Sanctum Officium or Holy Office)," *The Jewish Encyclopedia: A Descriptive Record of the History, Religion, Literature, and Customs of the Jewish People from the Earliest Times to the Present Day*, vol. 6, ed. Isidore Singer (New York: Funk & Wagnalls, 1904), 587–603.

37. Megan Vaughan, *Curing Their Ills: Colonial Power and African Illness* (Cambridge: Polity Press, 1991).

38. Hardiman, "Introduction," 6.

39. Ibid., 25.

40. Ibid., 5.

41. Ibid., 48.

42. Ibid., 16.

43. These numbers are cited in ibid, 16.

44. Eliza J. Gillett Bridgman, ed., *The Pioneer of American Missions in China: The Life and Labors of Elijah Coleman Bridgman* (New York: Anson D. F. Randolph, 1864).

45. Hardiman, *Healing Bodies, Saving Souls*; Alex McKay, "Towards a History of Medical Mission," *Medical History* 51 (2007): 547–551; and Charles M. Good, "Pioneer Medical Missions in Colonial Africa," *Social Science and Medicine* 32 (1991): 1–10.

46. Michael C. Lazich, "Seeking Souls through the Eyes of the Blind: The Birth of the Medical Missionary Society in Nineteenth-Century China," in Hardiman, *Healing Bodies, Saving Souls*, 59–86.

47. Christoffer H. Grundmann, "Mission and Healing in Historical Perspective," *International Bulletin of Missionary Research* 32 (2008): 185–188.

48. Susan R. Holman, *Beholden: Religion, Global Health, and Human Rights* (New York: Oxford University Press, 2015).

49. Christoffer Grundmann, "Healing and Medical Missions," in *Dictionary of Mission: Theology, History, Perspectives*, ed. Karl Müller, Theo Sundermeier, Stephen B. Bevans, and Richard H. Bliese (Eugene, OR: Wipf and Stock, 1999), 184–187, 184.

50. Ibid.

51. "About Us: Releasing Children from Poverty in Jesus' Name," Compassion International (2018), https://www.compassion.com/about/about-us.htm.

52. Alistair T. R. Sim and Mark Peters, "Compassion International: Holistic Child Development through Sponsorship and Church Partnership," in *Child Sponsorship: Exploring Pathways to a Brighter Future*, ed. Brad Watson and Matthew Clarke (London: Palgrave Macmillan, 2014), 163–190.

53. Bruce Wydick, Paul Glewwe, and Laine Rutledge, "Does International Child Sponsorship Work?: A Six-Country Study of Impacts on Adult Life Outcomes," *Journal of Political Economy* 121 (2013): 393–436.

54. International Medical Relief (2018), http://www.internationalmedicalrelief.org/.

55. Elizabeth Ferris, "Faith-Based and Secular Humanitarian Organizations," *International Review of the Red Cross* 87 (2005): 311–325, 315.

56. To find out more, use the search function at "Missions Opportunities," Baylor Missions, https://www.baylor.edu/missions/index.php?id=867916.

57. Melissa K. Melby, Lawrence C. Loh, Jessica Evert, Christopher Prater, Henry Lin, and Omar A. Khan, "Beyond Medical 'Missions' to Impact-Driven Short-Term Experiences in Global Health (STEGHs): Ethical Principles to Optimize Community Benefit and Learner Experience," *Academic Medicine* 91 (2016): 633–638.

58. Ibid., esp. 635.

59. Kevin J. Sykes, "Short-Term Medical Service Trips: A Systematic Review of the Evidence," *American Journal of Public Health* 104, 7 (2014): e38–e48, 38.

60. Catholic Health Association of the United States, *Short-Term Medical Mission Trips: Phase I Research Findings: Practices & Perspectives of U.S. Partners, 2014* (St. Louis, MO: Catholic Health Association of the United States, 2014), 6–7.

61. Ibid.

62. James B. Nickoloff, ed., *Gustavo Gutiérrez: Essential Writings* (Minneapolis: Fortress Press, 1996), 104.

63. Laura M. Montgomery, "Short-Term Medical Missions: Enhancing or Eroding Health?," *Missiology* 21 (1993): 333–341

64. Sykes, "Short-Term Medical Service Trips."

65. Jesse Maki, Munirih Qualls, Benjamin White, Sharon Kleefield, and Robert Crone, "Health Impact Assessment and Short-Term Medical Missions: A Methods Study to Evaluate Quality of Care," *BMC Health Services Research* 8 (2008): 121, doi.org/10.1186/1472-6963-8-121.

66. Janice Hawkins, "Potential Pitfalls of Short-Term Medical Missions," *Journal of Christian Nursing* 30, 4 (2013): E1–E6.

67. Kelly Stuart and Camille Grippon, "Implementing Recommendations for Short-Term Medical Missions," *Health Progress* 97, 5 (2016): 37–41.

68. Christoffer Grundmann, "The Role of Medical Missions in the Missionary Enterprise: A Historical and Missiological Survey," *Missions Studies* 2 (1985): 39–48.

69. Rachel A. Bishop and James A. Litch, "Medical Tourism Can Do Harm," *British Medical Journal* 320 (2000): 1017.

70. Christian C. Dupuis, "Humanitarian Missions in the Third World: A Polite Dissent," *Plastic and Reconstructive Surgery* 113 (2004): 433–435, 433.

71. E.g., Christoffer H. Grundmann, "The Contribution of Medical Missions: The Intercultural Transfer of Standards and Values," *Academic Medicine* 66 (1991): 731–733.

72. Melby et al., "Beyond Medical 'Missions' to Impact-Driven Short-Term Experiences in Global Health (STEGHs)."

73. Gerard Jansen, "The Tradition of Medical Missions in the Maelstrom of the International Health Arena," *Missiology* 27 (1999): 377–392.

74. Gerard Jansen, "Medical Missiology: An Undeveloped Discipline without Disciples. A Retrospective View," *Exchange* 24 (1995): 222–246.

75. Gerard Jansen, "Christian Ministry of Healing on Its Way to the Year 2000: An Archaeology of Medical Missions," *Missiology* 23 (1995): 295–307.

76. Maki et al., "Health Impact Assessment and Short-Term Medical Missions."

77. Alexandra L. C. Martiniuk, "Brain Gains: A Literature Review of Medical Missions to Low and Middle-Income Countries," *BMC Health Services Research* 12 (2012): 134, doi.org/10.1186/1472-6963-12-134.

78. Michael N. Dohn and Anita L. Dohn, "Quality of Care on Short-Term Medical Missions: Experience with a Standardized Patient Record and Related Issues," *Missiology* 31 (2003): 417–429.

79. Shahid R. Aziz, Vincent B. Zaccardi, and Sung-Kiang Chuang, "Survey of Residents Who Have Participated in Humanitarian Medical Missions," *Journal of Oral and Maxillofacial Surgery* 70 (2012): e147–e157.

80. Robert Riviello, Michael S. Lipnick, and Doruk Ozgediz, "Medical Missions, Surgical Education, and Capacity Building," *Journal of the American College of Surgeons* 213 (2011): 572.

81. Alex Campbell, Maura Sullivan, Randy Sherman, and William Magee, "The Medical Mission and Modern Cultural Competency Training," *Journal of the American College of Surgeons* 212 (2011): 124–129.

82. Operation Smile (2018), https://www.operationsmile.org/.

83. Nicole S. Berry, "Did We Do Good?: NGOs, Conflicts of Interest, and the Evaluation of Short-Term Medical Missions in Sololá, Guatemala," *Social Science and Medicine* 120 (2014): 344–351.

84. Garrett Logan Matlick, "Short-Term Medical Missions: Toward an Ethical Approach," *American Journal of Nursing* 118, 4 (2018): 11.

85. G. Richard Holt, "Ethical Conduct of Humanitarian Medical Missions. I. Informed Consent," *Archives of Facial Plastic Surgery* 14 (2012): 215–217.

86. G. Richard Holt, "Ethical Conduct of Humanitarian Medical Missions. II. Use of Photographic Images," *Archives Facial Plastic Surgery* 14 (2012): 295–296.

87. David R. Welling, James M. Ryan, David G. Burris, and Norman M. Rich, "The Seven Sins of Humanitarian Medicine," *World Journal of Surgery* 34 (2010): 466–470, 467.

88. Ya-Wen Chiu, Yi-Hao Weng, Chih-Fu Chen, Chun-Yuh Yang, Hung-Yi Choiu, and Ming-Liang Lee, "A Comparative Study of Taiwan's Short-Term Medical Missions to the South Pacific and Central America," *BMC International Health and Human Rights* 12 (2012): 37, doi.org/10.1186/1472-698X-12-37.

89. "Abayudaya Health & Development Project," Be'chol Lashon: In Every Tongue (2018), http://www.bechollashon.org/projects/abayudaya/projects.php.

90. See the section on "Gerut" in Wayne Dosick, *Living Judaism: The Complete Guide to Jewish Tradition, Belief, and Practice* (New York: HarperSanFrancisco, 1995), 65–71.

91. Diane Tobin, Gary A. Tobin, and Scott Rubin, *In Every Tongue: The Racial and Ethnic Diversity of the Jewish People* (San Francisco: Institute for Jewish and Community Research, 2005).

92. "The Gerson L'Chaim Prize for Outstanding Christian Medical Missionary Service," African Mission Healthcare (June 27, 2016), http://www.amhf.us/gersons.

93. African Mission Healthcare, http://www.amhf.us/amhf.

94. Katharine Webster, "The Case against Swami Rama of the Himalayas," *Yoga Journal* 95 (2001): 59–69.

95. Overton McGeehee, "Ex-Followers Say Swami Demanded Sexual Favors," *Richmond Times Dispatch* (August 2, 1991)..

96. "Case 1984-02: The Rajneeshees, August–September 1984," in W. Seth Carus, *Bioterrorism and Biocrimes: The Illicit Use of Biological Agents since 1900* (Washington, DC: Center for Counterproliferation Research, National Defense University, 2001), 50–58, https://fas.org/irp/threat/cbw/carus.pdf.

97. Cadge, *Paging God*, 23.

98. Ibid.

99. W. R. Monfalcone, "General Hospital Chaplaincy," in *Dictionary of Pastoral Care and Counseling*, ed. Rodney J. Hunter (Nashville: Abingdon Press, 1990), 456–457; and Richard Coble, "Modern Hospital Chaplaincy: Negotiations," in *The Chaplain's Presence and Medical Power: Rethinking Loss in the Hospital System* (Lanham, MD: Lexington Books, 2018), 19–49.

100. Richard C. Cabot, "A Plea for a Clinical Year in the Course of Theological Study," in *Adventures in the Borderlands of Ethics* (New York: Harper and Brothers, 1926), 1–22 (reprinted from the September 1925 issue of the periodical *Survey Graphic*).

101. Donald C. Beatty, "Reflections on the Early Beginnings of the Clinical Training Movement," *Pastoral Psychology* 16 (1965): 27–30.

102. A. T. Boison, "Theological Education via the Clinic," *Religious Education* 25 (1930): 235–239.

103. Cadge, *Paging God*, 24.

104. Ibid.

105. George F. Handzo, Walter J. Smith, John Twiname, Carolyn Twiname, and Will Maitland Weiss, "The HealthCare Chaplaincy, Inc., New York, New York," *Journal of Health Care Chaplaincy* 9 (1999): 29–42.

106. "About ACPE," ACPE, https://www.acpe.edu/ACPE/About_ACPE/ACPE/About_ACPE/About_ACPE.aspx?hkey=8bda1439-a609-475c-83ba-d86c9ca8e7e4.

107. Association of Professional Chaplains (2018), http://www.professionalchaplains.org/index.asp.

108. "Professional Standards," Association of Professional Chaplains (2018), http://www.professionalchaplains.org/content.asp?pl=198&contentid=198.

109. "BCCI Certification," Board of Chaplaincy Certification (2016), http://bcci. professionalchaplains.org/content.asp?pl=25&contentid=25.

110. National Association of Catholic Chaplains (2018), https://www.nacc.org/.

111. Neshama: Association of Jewish Chaplains (2018), http://jewishchaplain.net/. See also Dayle A. Friedman, *Jewish Pastoral Care: A Practical Handbook from Traditional and Contemporary Sources*, 2nd ed. (Woodstock, VT: Jewish Lights, 2005).

112. "About," Spiritual Care Association (2018), https://spiritualcareassociation.org/ about.html.

113. Seward Hiltner, *Religion and Health* (New York: Macmillan, 1947).

114. Wayne E. Oates, *Religious Factors in Mental Illness* (New York: Association Press, 1955).

115. Wendy Cadge, "Healthcare Chaplaincy as a Companion Profession: Historical Developments," *Journal of Healthcare Chaplaincy* (2018), online prepublication, doi.org/10.1080/08854726.2018.1463617.

116. Ibid., 2.

117. Raymond de Vries, Nancy Berlinger, and Wendy Cadge, "Lost in Translation: The Chaplain's Role in Health Care," *Hastings Center Report* 38 (2008): 23–27, 23.

118. Cadge, *Paging God*, 29.

119. Ibid., 31–32.

120. Ibid., 36.

121. CPE certification has been received by Protestant, Catholic, and Orthodox Christians; Jews; Muslims; Buddhists; and Native Americans. See "About ACPE," ACPE.

122. Cadge, *Paging God*, 48.

123. "About ACPE," ACPE.

124. Handzo et al., "The HealthCare Chaplaincy, Inc., New York, New York."

125. George Handzo, "The Process of Spiritual/Pastoral Care: A General Theory for Providing Spiritual/Pastoral Care Using Palliative Care as a Paradigm," in *Professional Spiritual and Pastoral Care: A Practical Clergy and Chaplain's Handbook*, ed. Stephen B. Roberts (Woodstock, VT: Skylight Paths, 2012), 21–41, 24.

126. Ibid., quotation 25, emphasis added.

127. Ibid.

128. George Fitchett and Andrea L. Canada, "The Role of Religion/Spirituality in Coping with Cancer: Evidence, Assessment, and Intervention," in *Psycho-oncology*, 2nd edition, ed. Jimmie C. Holland (New York: Oxford University Press, 2010), 440–446.

129. Handzo, "The Process of Spiritual/Pastoral Care," 25–26.

130. Ibid., 33.

131. E.g., Tim Ford and Alexander Tartaglia, "The Development, Status, and Future of Healthcare Chaplaincy," *Southern Medical Journal* 99 (2006): 675–679.

132. Larry VandeCreek and Laurel Burton, eds., "Professional Chaplaincy: Its Role and Importance in Healthcare," *Journal of Pastoral Care* 55 (2001): 81–97.

133. VandeCreek notes that chaplains are overlooked in the academic literature for their contributions to healthcare (Larry VandeCreek, "Professional Chaplaincy: An Absent Profession?," *Journal of Pastoral Care and Counseling* 53 (1999): 417–432).

134. VandeCreek and Burton, "Professional Chaplaincy: Its Role and Importance in Healthcare," 88.

135. Wendy Cadge, Jeremy Freese, and Nicholas Christakos, "The Provision of Hospital Chaplaincy in the United States: A National Overview," *Southern Medical Journal* 101 (2008): 626–630.

136. Similar results from a survey of CEOs of licensed healthcare institutions: Kevin J. Flannelly, George F. Handzo, and Andrew J. Weaver, "Factors Affecting HealthCare Chaplaincy in the United States," *Journal of Pastoral Care and Counseling* 58 (2004): 127–130.

137. Cadge et al., "The Provision of Hospital Chaplaincy in the United States."

138. Ibid., 629.

139. Fiona Timmins, Silvia Caldeira, Maryanne Murphy, Nicolas Pujol, Greg Sheaf, Elizabeth Weathers, Jaqueline Whelan, and Bernadette Flanagan, "The Role of the Healthcare Chaplain: A Literature Review," *Journal of Healthcare Chaplaincy* 24 (2018): 87–106.

140. A. R. Gatrad, E. Brown, and A. Sheikh, "Developing Multi-Faith Chaplaincy," *Archives of Disease in Childhood* 89 (2004): 504–505.

141. Margaret J. Orton, "Transforming Chaplaincy: The Emergence of a Healthcare Pastoral Care for a Post-Modern World," *Journal of Healthcare Chaplaincy* 15 (2008): 114–131; and Ewan Kelly, "The Development of Healthcare Chaplaincy," *Expository Times* 123 (2012): 469–478.

142. Jason A. Nieuwsma, Robyn D. Walser, and Steven C. Hayes, eds., *ACT for Clergy and Pastoral Counselors: Using Acceptance and Commitment Therapy to Bridge Psychological and Spiritual Care* (Oakland, CA: Context Press, 2016).

143. Jason A. Nieuwsma, George L. Jackson, Mark B. DeKraai, Denise J. Bulling, William C. Cantrell, Jeffrey E. Rhodes, Mark J. Bates, Keith Ethridge, Marian E. Lane, Wendy N. Tenhula, Sonja V. Batten, and Keith G. Meador, "Collaborating across the Departments of Veterans Affairs and Defense to Integrate Mental Health and Chaplaincy Services," *Journal of General Internal Medicine* 29, Suppl. 4 (2014): 885–894.

144. Jason A. Nieuwsma, Jeffrey E. Rhodes, George L. Jackson, William C. Cantrell, Marian E. Lane, Mark J. Bates, Mark B. Dekraai, Denise J. Bulling, Keith Ethridge, Kent D. Drescher, George Fitchett, Wendy N. Tenhula, Glen Milstein, Robert M. Bray, and Keith G. Meador, "Chaplaincy and Mental Health in the Department of Veterans Affairs and Department of Defense," *Journal of Health Care Chaplaincy* 19 (2013): 3–21, 7.

145. Jason A. Nieuwsma and Keith G. Meador, *VA/DoD Integrated Mental Health Strategy: The Intersection of Chaplaincy and Mental Health Care in VA and DoD: Expanded Report on Strategic Action #23* (Washington, DC: Department of Veterans Affairs, n.d.), https://www.mirecc.va.gov/mentalhealthandchaplaincy/Docs_and_Images/Expanded%20IMHS%20SA23%20Mental%20Health%20and%20Chaplaincy%20Report.pdf.

146. Jeff Levin, "Why Religion Matters for Health: An Epidemiologist's Perspective," VA Mental Health and Chaplaincy Forum, Department of Veterans Affairs, Washington, DC, September 1, 2011.

147. George Fitchett, "Envisioning a Research-Informed Chaplaincy," VA Mental Health and Chaplaincy Forum, Department of Veterans Affairs, Washington, DC, September 1, 2011.

148. Gary E. Berg, Norman Fonss, Arthur J. Reed, and Larry VandeCreek, "The Impact of Religious Faith and Practice on Patients Suffering from a Major Affective Disorder: A Cost Analysis," *Journal of Pastoral Care* 49 (1995): 359–363.

149. Larry VandeCreek, "Research in the Pastoral Care Department," in *Chaplaincy Services in Contemporary Health Care*, ed. Laurel Arthur Burton (Chicago: College of Chaplains, 1992).

150. Larry VandeCreek, *A Research Primer for Pastoral Care and Counseling* (Decatur, GA: Journal of Pastoral Care Publications, 1988).

151. George Fitchett, Kelsey B. White, and Kathryn Lyndes, eds., *Evidence-Based Healthcare Chaplaincy: A Research Reader* (London: Jessica Kingsley, 2018).

152. Larry VandeCreek, ed., *Professional Chaplaincy and Clinical Pastoral Education Should Become More Scientific: Yes and No* (New York: Haworth Press, 2002).

153. Larry Burton, "Chaplaincy *Is* Becoming More 'Scientific.' What's the Problem?," *Journal of Health Care Chaplaincy* 12 (2002): 43–51; and David B. McCurdy, "But What Are We Trying to Prove?," *Journal of Health Care Chaplaincy* 12 (2002): 151–163.

154. Andrew J. Weaver, Kevin J. Flannelly, and Chaplain Clarence Liu, "Chaplaincy Research: Its Value, Its Quality, and Its Future," *Journal of Health Care Chaplaincy* 14 (2008): 3–19.

155. Handzo, "The Process of Spiritual/Pastoral Care," 38.

156. Thomas St. James O'Connor, "The Search for Truth: The Case for Evidence-Based Chaplaincy," *Journal of Health Care Chaplaincy* 13 (2002): 185–194.

157. Michele Shields, Allison Kestenbaum, and Laura B. Dunn, "Spiritual AIM and the Work of the Chaplain: A Model for Assessing Spiritual Needs and Outcomes in Relationship," *Palliative and Supportive Care* 13 (2015): 75–89.

158. Linda Emmanuel, George F. Handzo, George Grant, Kevin Massey, Angelika Zollfrank, Diana Wilke, Richard Powell, Walter Smith, and Kenneth Pargament, "Workings of the Human Spirit in Palliative Care Situations: A Consensus Model from the Chaplaincy Research Consortium," *BMC Palliative Care* 14 (2015): 29, https://doi.org/10.1186/s12904-015-0005-3.

159. George F. Handzo, Mark Cobb, Cheryl Holmes, Ewan Kelly, and Shane Sinclair, "Outcomes for Professional Health Care Chaplaincy: An International Call to Action," *Journal of Health Care Chaplaincy* 20 (2014): 43–53.

160. Katherine R. B. Jankowski, George F. Handzo, and Kevin J. Flannelly, "Testing the Efficacy of Chaplaincy Care," *Journal of Health Care Chaplaincy* 17 (2011): 100–125.

161. Deborah B. Marin, Vanshdeep Sharma, Eugene Sosunov, Natalia Egorova, Rafael Goldstein, and George F. Handzo, "Relationship between Chaplain Visits and Patient Satisfaction," *Journal of Health Care Chaplaincy* 21 (2015): 14–24.

162. Kevin J. Flannelly, "Expanding and Improving Chaplaincy Research," *Journal of Health Care Chaplaincy* 16 (2010): 77–78.

163. Kevin J. Flannelly, Andrew J. Weaver, Walter J. Smith, and George F. Handzo, "Psychologists and Health Care Chaplains Doing Research Together," *Journal of Psychology and Christianity* 22 (2003): 327–332.

164. Nieuwsma et al., "Chaplaincy and Mental Health in the Department of Veterans Affairs and Department of Defense."

165. Larry VandeCreek, Eileen Gorey, Karolynn Siegel, Sharon Brown, and Rhoda Torperzer, "How Many Chaplains per 1000 Inpatients?: Benchmarks of Healthcare Chaplaincy Departments," *Journal of Pastoral Care and Counseling* 55 (2001): 289–301.

166. George Fitchett and Steve Nolan, eds., *Spiritual Care in Practice: Case Studies in Healthcare Chaplaincy* (London: Jessica Kingsley, 2015).

167. George Fitchett, "Introduction," in Fitchett and Nolan, *Spiritual Care in Practice*, 11–24, esp. 13–14.

168. Ibid., 12–13.

169. George Fitchett and Steve Nolan, eds., *Case Studies in Spiritual Care: Healthcare Chaplaincy Assessments, Interventions, and Outcomes* (London: Jessica Kingsley, 2018); and Fitchett and Nolan, *Spiritual Care in Practice*.

170. George Fitchett, "Recent Progress in Chaplaincy-Related Research," *Journal of Pastoral Care and Counseling* 71 (2017): 163–175; and George Fitchett, Jason A. Nieuwsma, Mark J. Bates, Jeffrey E. Rhodes, and Keith G. Meador, "Evidence-Based Chaplaincy Care: Attitudes and Practices in Diverse Healthcare Chaplain Samples," *Journal of Health Care Chaplaincy* 20 (2014): 144–160.

171. Renske Kruizinga, Michael Scherer-Rath, Hans J.B.A.M. Schilderman, Christina M. Puchalski, Hanneke H.W.M. van Laarhoven, "Toward a Fully Fledged Integration of Spiritual Care and Medical Care," *Journal of Pain and Symptom Management* 55 (2018): 1035–1040.

172. "Transforming Chaplaincy," Transforming Chaplaincy (2018), http://www.transformchaplaincy.org/projects/transforming-chaplaincy/#.

173. Ibid.

174. Kevin Massey, "Surfing through a Sea Change: The Coming Transformation of Chaplaincy Training," *Reflective Practice: Formation and Supervision in Ministry* 34 (2014): 144–152.

175. David B. Larson, Ann A. Hohmann, Larry G. Kessler, Keith G. Meador, Jeffrey H. Boyd, and Elisabeth McSherry, "The Couch and the Cloth: The Need for Linkage," *Hospital and Community Psychiatry* 39 (1988): 1064–1069.

176. Ibid., 1068.

177. Ibid.

178. Ibid., 1068.

179. Ibid.

180. Andrew J. Weaver, Kevin J. Flannelly, Laura T. Flannelly, and Julia E. Oppenheimer, "Collaboration between Clergy and Mental Health Professionals: A Review of Professional Health Care Journals from 1980 through 1999," *Counseling and Values* 47 (2003): 162–171.

181. Larson et al, "The Couch and the Cloth."

182. Curtis W. Hart, "Present at the Creation: The Clinical Pastoral Movement and the Origins of the Dialogue between Religion and Psychiatry," *Journal of Religion and Health* 49 (2010): 536–546.

183. Frank B. Minirth and Walter Byrd, *Christian Psychiatry* (Old Tappan, NJ: F. H. Revell Co., 1990).

184. Christopher G. Harding, "The Emergence of 'Christian Psychiatry' in Post-Independence India," *Edinburgh Papers in South Asian Studies* 24 (2011): 1–17.

185. "Mission & Vision," Christian Medical and Dental Associations (2018), https://cmda.org/mission-and-vision/.

186. Marc Galanter, David Larson, and Elizabeth Rubenstone, "Christian Psychiatry: The Impact of Evangelical Belief on Clinical Practice," *American Journal of Psychiatry* 148 (1991): 90–95.

187. Paul D. Meier, Frank B. Minirth, Frank B. Wichern, and Donald E. Ratcliff, *Introduction to Psychology and Counseling: Christian Perspectives and Applications*, 2nd ed. (Grand Rapids: Baker Book House, 1991).

188. Smears of Christian psychotherapy are not uncommon, often with unfactual claims about qualifications of practitioners, content of care, and religious beliefs of therapists and patients (e.g., Edmund D. Cohen, "And Now—Psychiatric Wards for Born-Again Christians Only," *Free Inquiry* 13, 3 (1993): 25–30).

189. "A Brief History of the CPA," Catholic Psychotherapy Association, https://www.catholicpsychotherapy.org/Our-History.

190. "Our Mission," Catholic Psychotherapy Association, https://www.catholicpsychotherapy.org/mission.

191. Andrew R. Heinze, "The Americanization of *Mussar*: Abraham Twerski's Twelve Steps," *Judaism* 48 (1999): 450–469.

192. Robert Booth, "Master of Mindfulness, Jon Kabat-Zinn: 'People Are Losing Their Minds. That Is What We Need to Wake Up To,'" *The Guardian* (October 22, 2017), https://www.theguardian.com/lifeandstyle/2017/oct/22/mindfulness-jon-kabat-zinn-depression-trump-grenfell.

193. E.g., Kenneth I. Pargament, of Bowling Green State University; David H. Rosmarin, of Harvard University; David Pelcovitz, of Yeshiva University; and Kate Miriam Loewenthal, of the University of London.

194. Kate Miriam Loewenthal, "Strictly Orthodox Jews and Their Relations with Psychotherapy and Psychiatry," *World Cultural Psychiatry Research Review* 1 (2006): 128–132.

195. Jeffrey J. Kripal, *Esalen: America and the Religion of No Religion* (Chicago: University of Chicago Press, 2007).

196. Saxby Pridmore and Mohamed Iqbal Pasha, "Psychiatry and Islam," *Australasian Psychiatry* 12 (2004): 380–385.

197. Arthur J. Deikman, "Sufism and Psychiatry," *Journal of Nervous and Mental Disease* 165 (1977): 318–329; and S. Haque Nizamie, Mohammed Zia Ul Haq Katshu, and N. A. Uvais, "Sufism and Mental Health," *Indian Journal of Psychiatry* 55, Suppl. 2 (2013): S215–S223.

198. Ajit Avashthi, Natasha Kate, and Sandeep Grover, "Indianization of Psychiatry Using Indian Mental Concepts," *Indian Journal of Psychiatry* 55, Supp. 2 (2013): S136–S144.

199. Graham Meadows, "Buddhism and Psychiatry: Confluence and Conflict," *Australasian Psychiatry* 11 (2003): 16–20.

200. Gurvinder Kalra, Kamaldeep S. Bhui, and Dinesh Bhugra, "Sikhism, Spirituality and Psychiatry," *Asian Journal of Psychiatry* 5 (2012): 339–343.

201. Manilal Gada, "Jaina Religion and Psychiatry," *Mens Sana Monographs* 13 (2015): 70–81.

202. Yalin Zhang, Derson Young, Sing Lee, Lingjiang Li, Honggen Zhang, Zeping Xiao, Wei Hao, Yongmin Feng, Hongxiang Zhou, and Doris F. Chang, "Chinese Taoist Cognitive Psychotherapy in the Treatment of Generalized Anxiety Disorder in Contemporary China," *Transcultural Psychiatry* 39 (2002): 115–129.

203. Wen-Shing Tseng, "The Concept of Personality in Confucian Thought," *Psychiatry* 36 (1973): 191–202.

204. Padmasiri de Silva, *An Introduction to Buddhist Psychology and Counseling: Pathways of Mindfulness-Based Therapies*, 5th ed. (New York: Palgrave Macmillan, 2014).

205. Jon Kabat-Zinn, "Mindfulness-Based Interventions in Context: Past, Present, and Future," *Clinical Psychology* 10 (2003): 144–156, 145.

206. Nazila Isgandarova, "*Muraqaba* as a Mindfulness-Based Therapy in Islamic Psychotherapy," *Journal of Religion and Health* (2018), online prepublication, doi: 10.1007/s10943-018-0695-y; and Gretty M. Mirdal, "Mevlana Jalāl-ad-Dīn Rumi and Mindfulness," *Journal of Religion and Health* 51 (2012): 1202–1215.

207. Mira Niculescu, "Going Online and Taking the Plane. From San Francisco to Jerusalem. The Physical and Electronic Networks of 'Jewish Mindfulness,'" *Online: Heidelberg Journal of Religions on the Internet* 8 (2015): 98–114.

208. Adam Valerio, "Owning Mindfulness: A Bibliometric Analysis of Mindfulness Literature Trends within and outside of Buddhist Contexts," *Contemporary Buddhism* 17 (2016): 157–183.

209. Jeff Levin, "Transcendent Experience and Health: Concepts, Cases, and Sociological Themes," in *Toward a Sociological Theory of Religion and Health*, ed. Anthony J. Blasi (Leiden, Netherlands: Brill, 2011), 69–93; and Jeff Levin and Lea Steele, "The Transcendent Experience: Conceptual, Theoretical, and Epidemiologic Perspectives," *EXPLORE: The Journal of Science and Healing* 1 (2005): 89–101.

210. Levin and Steele, "The Transcendent Experience," 89.

211. Ibid.

212. Levin, "Transcendent Experience and Health."

213. Kathleen D. Noble, "Psychological Health and the Experience of Transcendence," *Counseling Psychologist* 15 (1987): 601–614; and Paul Gelderloos, Hubert J. M. Hermans, Henry H. Alscröm, and Rita Jacoby, "Transcendence and Psychological Health: Studies with Long-Term Participants of the Transcendental Meditation and TM-Sidhi Program," *Journal of Psychology* 124 (1990): 177–197.

214. An early review: Greg Bogart, "The Use of Meditation in Psychotherapy: A Review of the Literature," *American Journal of Psychotherapy* 45 (1991): 383–412.

215. Tyler J. VanderWeele, "On the Promotion of Human Flourishing," *Proceedings of the National Academy of Sciences* 114 (2017): 8148–8156.

Chapter 4

1. Westberg with McNamara, *Gentle Rebel*, 171. See esp. chapter 15, "Creating a Church Clinic," 171–182.

2. Ibid., quotations 179.

3. Ibid., 172. From a 1969 convocation address titled "The Church Should Reenter the Health Field: A Proposal for Neighborhood Church-Clinics and a New Medical Specialist—The Clergy Physician."

4. Westberg with McNamara, *Gentle Rebel*, 174–179.

5. Ibid., 175.

6. Granger F. Westberg, "Churches Are Joining the Health Care Team," *Urban Health* 13, 9 (1984): 34–36.

7. Westberg with McNamara, *Gentle Rebel*, esp. chapter 16, "A 30-Year Dream," 183–190, and chapter 17, "As a Matter of Faith," 191–198.

8. John W. Hatch and Curtis Jackson, "North Carolina Baptist Church Program," *Urban Health* 10 (1981): 61–62.

9. "IHP Programs," Interfaith Health Program (2018), http://ihpemory.org/ihp-programs/.

10. Melissa Bopp and Elizabeth A. Fallon, "Health and Wellness Programming in Faith-Based Organizations: A Description of a Nationwide Sample," *Health Promotion Practice* 14 (2013): 122–131.

11. Marci Kramish Campbell, Marlyn Allicock Hudson, Ken Resnicow, Natasha Blakeney, Amy Paxton, and Monica Baskin, "Church-Based Health Promotion Interventions: Evidence and Lessons Learned," *Annual Review of Public Health* 28 (2007): 213–234.

12. M. Anita Holmes and John Hatch, "Health Promotion and African-American Baptist Churches in North Carolina," *North Carolina Medical Journal* 68 (2007): 376.

13. Thomas J. Ward Jr., *Out in the Rural: A Mississippi Health Center and Its War on Poverty* (New York: Oxford University Press, 2017). Hatch's key role is detailed in chapter 2, "Community Organizing," 37–63.

14. "Collection Title: John W. Hatch Papers, 1967–1995," The Southern Historical Collection at the Louis Round Wilson Special Collections Library, UNC University Libraries (2008), https://finding-aids.lib.unc.edu/04801/.

15. Jeffrey S. Levin, "The Role of the Black Church in Community Medicine," *Journal of the National Medical Association* 76 (1984): 477–483, 481.

16. M. Anita Holmes, "Health Disparities, the Faith Agenda, and Health Promotion/ Disease Prevention: The General Baptist State Convention of North Carolina Model," *North Carolina Medical Journal* 65 (2004): 373–376.

17. Eugenia Eng and John W. Hatch, "Networking between Agencies and Black Churches: The Lay Health Advisor Model," *Prevention in Human Services* 10 (1991): 123–146.

18. Eugenia Eng, John Hatch, and Anne Callan, "Institutionalizing Social Support through the Church and into the Community," *Health Education Quarterly* 12 (1985): 81–92, 81.

19. "About Us," Center for Health and Healing, http://www.c4hh.org/aboutus.html.

20. "Faith and Health Initiative," Center for Health and Healing, http://www.c4hh.org/ healthinitiative.html.

21. John W. Hatch and Kay A. Lovelace, "Involving the Southern Rural Church and Students of the Health Professions in Health Education," *Public Health Reports* 95 (1980): 23–25.

22. Larry S. Chapman, "Spiritual Health: A Component Missing from Health Promotion," *American Journal of Health Promotion* 1 (1986): 38–41.

23. Ibid., 40.

24. Levin, "Faith-Based Initiatives in Health Promotion."

25. Ibid.

26. Ibid., 141.

27. Levin, "Partnerships between the Faith-Based and Medical Sectors," esp. 346.

28. Campbell et al., "Church-Based Health Promotion Interventions," 215.

29. Ibid.

30. Benjamin E. Mays and Joseph W. Nicholson, *The Negro's Church* (New York: Institute of Social and Religious Research, 1933).

31. E. Franklin Frazier, *The Negro Church in America* (1963) / C. Eric Lincoln, *The Black Church since Frazier* (1970; New York: Schocken Books, 1974).

32. Cheryl T. Gilkes, "The Black Church as a Therapeutic Community: Suggested Areas for Research into the Black Religious Experience," *Journal of the Interdenominational Theological Center* 8 (1980): 29–44.

33. Mary B. McRae, Patricia M. Carey, and Roxanna Anderson-Scott, "Black Churches as Therapeutic Systems: A Group Process Perspective," *Health Education Behavior* 25 (1998): 778–789.

34. Frederick C. Harris, "Black Churches and Civic Traditions: Outreach, Activism, and the Politics of Public Funding of Faith-Based Ministries," in *Can Charitable Choice Work?: Covering Religion's Impact on Urban Affairs and Social Services*, ed. Andrew Walsh (Hartford, CT: Leonard E. Greenberg Center for the Study of Religion in Public Life, 2001), 140–156.

35. Levin, "The Role of the Black Church in Community Medicine."

36. Ibid.

37. Jeffrey S. Levin, "Roles for the Black Pastor in Preventive Medicine," *Pastoral Psychology* 35 (1986): 94–103.

38. Lisa R. Yanek, Diane M. Becker, Taryn F. Moy, Joel Gittelsohn, and Dyann Matson Koffman, "Project Joy: Faith-Based Cardiovascular Health Promotion for African

American Women," *Public Health Reports* 116, Suppl. 1 (2001): 68–81; and Phoebe Butler-Ajibade, William Booth, and Cynthia Burwell, "Partnering with the Black Church: Recipe for Promoting Heart Health in the Stroke Belt," *ABNF Journal* 223 (2012): 34–37.

39. Lisa L. Agate, D'Mrtri Cato-Watson, Jolene M. Mullins, Gloria S. Scott, Vanice Rolle, Donna Markland, and David L. Roach, "Churches United to Stop HIV (CUSH): A Faith-Based HIV Prevention Initiative," *Journal of the National Medical Association* 97, Suppl. 7 (2005): 60S–63S.

40. Kelley Newlin, Susan MacLeod Dyess, Emily Allard, Susan Chase, and Gail D'Eramo Melkus, "A Methodological Review of Faith-Based Health Promotion Literature: Advancing the Science to Expand Delivery of Diabetes Education to Black Americans," *Journal of Religion and Health* 51 (2012): 1075–1097.

41. Susan Markens, Sarah A. Fox, Bonnie Taub, and Mary Lou Gilbert, "Role of Black Churches in Health Promotion Programs: Lessons from the Los Angeles Mammography Promotion in Churches Program," *American Journal of Public Health* 92 (2002): 805–810.

42. Meghan Baruth, Sara Wilcox, Marilyn Laken, Melissa Bopp, and Ruth Saunders, "Implementation of a Faith-Based Physical Activity Intervention: Insights from Church Health Directors," *Journal of Community Health* 33 (2008): 304–312.

43. Greer Sullivan, Justin Hunt, Tiffany F. Haynes, Keneshia Bryant, Ann M. Cheney, Jeffrey M. Pyne, Christina Reaves, Steve Sullivan, Caleb Lewis, Bonita Barnes, Michael Barnes, Cliff Hudson, Susan Jegley, Bridgette Larkin, Shane Russell, Penny White, LaNissa Gilmore, Sterling Claypoole, Rev. Johnny Smith, and Ruth Richison, "Building Partnerships with Rural Arkansas Faith Communities to Promote Veterans' Mental Health: Lessons Learned," *Progress in Community Health Partnerships* 8 (2014): 11–19.

44. Lena Butler-Flowers, *Public Health Education in the African American Community: The Role of the Black Church in Eliminating Health Disparities* (Pittsburgh, PA: RoseDog Books, 2013), 47.

45. Markens et al., "Role of Black Churches in Health Promotion Programs," 805.

46. Dorine J. Brand and Reginald J. Alston, "The Brand's PREACH Model: Predicting Readiness to Engage African American Churches in Health," *Health Promotion Practice* 18 (2017): 763–771; and "The Brand's PREACH Survey: A Capacity Assessment Tool for Predicting Readiness to Engage African American Churches in Health," *Journal of Religion and Health* 57 (2018): 1246–1255.

47. Carol R. Freedman-Doan, Leanna Fortunato, Erin J. Henshaw, and Jacqueline M. Titus, "Faith-Based Sex Education Programs: What They Look Like and Who Uses Them," *Journal of Religion and Health* 52 (2013): 247–262.

48. Angela Wallace and Barbara C. Campbell, "A Supplementary Education Model Rooted in an Academic, Community, and Faith-Based Coalition: Closing the Education and Health Gaps," in *Toward Equity in Health: A New Global Approach to Health Disparities*, ed. Barbara C. Wallace (New York: Springer, 2008), 491–506.

49. Teresa Cutts, "The Memphis Model: ARHAP Theory Comes to Ground in the Congregational Health Network," in *When Religion and Health Align: Mobilising Religious Health Assets for Transformation*, ed. James R. Cochrane, Barbara Schmid, and Teresa Cutts (Dorpspruit, South Africa: Cluster Publications, 2011), 193–209.

50. James R. Cochrane, "Religion, Public Health, and Church for the 21st Century," *International Review of Mission* 95 (2006): 59–72; and Miriam Kiser, Deborah L. Jones, and Gary R. Gunderson, "Faith and Health: Leadership Aligning Assets to Transform Communities," *International Review of Mission* 95 (2006): 50–58.

51. Cutts, "The Memphis Model," 195.

52. Ibid., 207.

53. Teresa Cutts, Gary Gunderson, Dean Carter, Melanie Childers, Phillip Long, Lisa Marisiddaiah, Helen Milleson, Dennis Stamper, Annika Archie, Jeremy Moseley, Emily Viverette, and Bobby Baker, "From the Memphis Model to the North Carolina Way: Lessons Learned from Emerging Health System and Faith Community Partnerships," *North Carolina Medical Journal* 78 (2017): 267–272.

54. G. Scott Morris, "Holistic Health Care for the Medically Uninsured: The Church Health Center of Memphis," *Ethnicity and Disease* 25 (2015): 507–510.

55. Teresa Cutts and Joy D. Sharp, "The Memphis Model: Faith and Health System Collaboration," Presentation at Faith-Health Collaboration to Improve Community and Population Health: A Workshop, National Academy of Sciences Roundtable on Population Health Improvement, March 22, 2018, Raleigh, North Carolina, http://www.nationalacademies.org/hmd/~/media/Files/Activity%20 Files/PublicHealth/PopulationHealthImprovementRT/18-MAR-22/4BCutts%20 %20Sharp.pdf.

56. Cutts et al., "From the Memphis Model to the North Carolina Way."

57. Mara Vanderslice, "Faith Filled & Healthy Communities: The Memphis Congregational Health Network," The White House blog (June 21, 2011), https://obamawhitehouse.archives.gov/blog/2011/06/21/faith-filled-healthy-communities-memphis-congregational-health-network.

58. Holman, *Beholden*, esp. chapter 5, "Between Cape Town and Memphis: Religious Health Assets," 125–161.

59. John Kretzmann and John McKnight, "Assets-Based Community Development," *National Civic Review* 85, 4 (1996): 23–29.

60. Sidney L. Kark and Guy W. Steuart, eds., *A Practice of Social Medicine: A South African Team's Experiences in Different African Communities* (Edinburgh: E. and S. Livingston, 1962).

61. Sidney L. Kark and John Cassel, "The Pholela Health Centre: A Progress Report," *South African Medical Journal* 26, 6 (1952): 101–104.

62. S. M. Tollman, "The Pholela Health Centre—The Origins of Community-Oriented Primary Care (COPC)," *South African Medical Journal* 84 (1994): 653–658.

63. Michel A. Ibrahim, Berton H. Kaplan, Ralph C. Patrick, Cecil Slome, Herman A. Tyroler, and Robert N. Wilson, "The Legacy of John C. Cassel," *American Journal of Epidemiology* 112 (1980): 1–7.

64. Allan B. Steckler, Barbara A. Israel, Leonard Dawson, and Eugenia Eng, guest eds., "Community Health Development: An Anthology of the Works of Guy W. Steuart," *Health Education Quarterly* 20, Suppl. 1 (1993): S1–S146.

65. Allan B. Steckler, Leonard Dawson, Barbara A. Israel, and Eugenia Eng, "Community Health Development: An Overview of the Works of Guy W. Steuart," *Health Education Quarterly* 20, Suppl. 1 (1993): S3–S20.

66. Ward, *Out in the Rural*, esp. chapter 1, "From South Africa to Mississippi," 11–35.

67. Cutts et al., "From the Memphis Model to the North Carolina Way."

68. Ibid.; Gary R. Gunderson, "Faith and the Health of Complex Human Populations," 14th Annual David B. Larson Memorial Lecture on Religion and Health, Duke University School of Medicine, March 3, 2016, Durham, North Carolina.

69. United Methodist Health Ministry Fund, https://healthfund.org/a/.

70. Judy A. Johnston, Kurt Konda, and Elizabeth Ablah, "Building Capacity among Laity: A Faith-Based Health Ministry Initiative," *Journal of Religion and Health* 57 (2018): 1276–1284.

71. Michele Prince and Adina Bodenstein, *A Program Assessment: Exploration of the Field of Judaism, Health, and Healing through Program Review and Key Stakeholder Interviews: A Report by the Kalsman Institute on Judaism and Health* (Los Angeles: Hebrew Union College–Jewish Institute of Religion, 2010).

72. Susan Rosenthal, *Jewish Health Programs: Best Practices Sampler, 2008*, UJA-Federation (April 2008), http://huc.edu/sites/default/files/Kalsman/NCJH%20healing%20best%20practicespdffinal%202008.pdf.

73. Byron Johnson and William H. Wubbenhorst, *Incorporating Faith and Works within a Healthcare Network: Baylor Scott & White's Office of Mission and Ministry* (Waco, TX: Baylor Institute for Studies of Religion, 2017), 4.

74. Ibid., 17.

75. "Faith Health Waco . . . The Good Samaritan Network" (unpublished document) (Waco, TX: Waco Regional Baptist Association, n.d.).

76. Ibid.

77. Byron R. Johnson, *Objective Hope: Assessing the Effectiveness of Faith-Based Organizations: A Review of the Literature* (Philadelphia: Center for Research on Religion and Urban Civil Society, 2002). An earlier review: Mary Sutherland and Charles D. Hale, "Community Health Promotion: The Church as Partner," *Journal of Primary Prevention* 16 (1995): 201–216.

78. Bopp and Fallon, "Health and Wellness Programming in Faith-Based Organizations," 127.

79. Mark J. DeHaven, Irby B. Hunter, Laura Wilder, James W. Walton, and Jarrett Berry, "Health Programs in Faith-Based Organizations: Are They Effective?," *American Journal of Public Health* 94 (2004): 1030–1036.

80. Ibid., 1033.

81. Richard A. Windsor, *Evaluation of Health Promotion and Disease Prevention Programs: Improving Population Health through Evidence-Based Practice*, 2nd ed. (New York: Oxford University Press, 2015).

82. E.g., Jane Peterson, Jan R. Atwood, and Bernice Yates, "Key Elements for Church-Based Health Promotion Programs: Outcome-Based Literature Review," *Public Health Nursing* 19 (2002): 401–411; DeHaven et al., "Health Programs in Faith-Based Organizations"; Michelle Crozier Kegler, Mimi Kiser, and Sarah M. Hall, "Evaluation Findings from the Institute for Public Health and Faith Collaborations," *Public Health Reports* 122 (2007): 793–802; and Michael E. Rowland and Lolita Chappel-Aiken, "Faith-Based Partnerships Promoting Health," *New Directions for Adult and Continuing Education* 133 (2012): 23–33.

83. Peterson et al., "Key Elements for Church-Based Health Promotion Programs," quotations 404.

84. Ibid.

85. Ibid.

86. Campbell et al., "Church-Based Health Promotion Interventions."

87. Bopp and Fallon, "Health and Wellness Programming in Faith-Based Organizations," 123.

88. John J. Chin, Joanne Mantell, Linda Weiss, Mamatha Bhagavan, and Xiaoting Luo, "Chinese and South Asian Religious Institutions and HIV Prevention in New York City," *AIDS Education and Prevention* 17 (2005): 484–502.

89. "About," Himalayan Institute (2018), https://www.himalayaninstitute.org/about/ . See also Edward M. Bruner, "My Life in an Ashram," *Qualitative Inquiry* 2 (1996): 300–319.

90. Priscilla A. Barnes and Amy B. Curtis, "A National Examination of Partnerships among Local Health Department and Faith Communities in the United States," *Journal of Public Health Management Practice* 15 (2009): 253–263.

91. E.g., Michelle C. Kegler, Sarah M. Hall, and Mimi Kiser, "Facilitators, Challenges, and Collaborative Activities in Faith and Health Partnerships to Address Health Disparities," *Health Education and Behavior* 37 (2010): 665–679; and Susan J. Zahner and Susan M. Corrado, "Local Health Department Partnership with Faith-Based Organization," *Journal of Public Health Management Practice* 10 (2004): 258–265.

92. Priscilla Barnes, Teresa Cutts, Stephanie Dickinson, Hao Guo, Danielle Squires, Sean Bowman, and Gary Gunderson, "Methods for Managing and Analyzing Electronic Medical Records: A Formative Examination of a Hospital-Congregation-Based Intervention," *Population Health Management* 17 (2014): 279–286.

93. Moses V. Goldmon and James T. Roberson Jr., "Churches, Academic Institutions, and Public Health: Partnerships to Eliminate Health Disparities," *North Carolina Medical Journal* 65 (2004): 368–372.

94. Ibid., 368.

95. Ibid., 370.

96. Kegler et al., "Facilitators, Challenges, and Collaborative Activities in Faith and Health Partnerships to Address Health Disparities."

97. Ibid.

98. Ibid., 674.

99. Kegler et al., "Evaluation Findings from the Institute for Public Health and Faith Collaboration."

100. Ellen Idler and Allan Kellehear, "Religion in Public Health-Care Institutions: U.S. and U.K. Perspectives," *Journal for the Scientific Study of Religion* 56 (2017): 234–240.

101. Ibid., 235.

102. Ibid., 239.

103. Richard G. Bennett and W. Daniel Hale, *Building Healthy Communities through Medical-Religious Partnerships*, 2nd ed. (Baltimore: Johns Hopkins University Press, 2009).

104. Ibid., 2.

105. Ibid.

106. Gary R. Gunderson and James R. Cochrane, *Religion and the Health of the Public: Shifting the Paradigm* (New York: Palgrave Macmillan, 2012).

107. Ibid., 46.

108. Ibid, 46.

109. Ibid.

110. "Religious Health Assets: What Religion Brings to Health of the Public," in Gunderson and Cochrane, *Religion and the Health of the Public*, 41–58.

111. Ibid., quotations 53.

112. Ibid., 54.

113. Ibid., 49.

114. Ibid., 48.

115. Vilma T. Falck and Lea Steele, "Promoting the Health of Aging Adults in the Community," *Journal of Community Health* 19 (1994): 389–393.

116. Ibid., 392.

117. Let's Help, http://www.letshelpinc.org/.

118. Joel S. Meister and Jill Guernsey de Zapien, "Bringing Health Policy Issues Front and Center in the Community: Expanding the Role of Community Health Coalitions," *Preventing Chronic Disease* 2, 1 (2005): 1–7.

119. Elbert C. Cole, "Lay Ministries with Older Adults," in *Ministry with the Aging: Designs, Challenges, Foundations*, ed. William M. Clements (San Francisco: Harper and Row, 1981), 250–265.

120. Jeff Levin, "SCA 2002 General Survey: Summary Report," Annual Conference, Shepherd's Centers of America, Lake Junaluska, North Carolina, October 20–23, 2002.

121. "Adventures in Wellness," Shepherd's Centers of America (2017), https://www.shepherdcenters.org/adventures-in-wellness-1.

122. "Mission Statement," Mission Waco (2017), http://missionwaco.org/mission-waco/
.

123. "Programs," Mission Waco (2017), http://missionwaco.org/programs/.

124. "Develop," Mission Waco (2017), http://missionwaco.org/develop/.

125. Linda M. Chatters, Christopher G. Ellison, and Jeffrey S. Levin, guest eds., "Public Health and Health Education in Faith Communities" (special issue), *Health Education and Behavior* 25, 6 (1998): 685–809.

126. Linda M. Chatters, Christopher G. Ellison, and Jeffrey S. Levin, "Public Health and Health Education in Faith Communities," *Health Education and Behavior* 25 (1998): 689–699, 689.

127. John M. Wallace Jr. and Tyrone A. Forman, "Religion's Role in Promoting Health and Reducing Risk among American Youth," *Health Education and Behavior* 25 (1998): 721–741.

128. Sarah A. Fox, Kathryn Pitkin, Christopher Paul, Sally Carson, and Naihua Duan, "Breast Cancer Screening Adherence: Does Church Attendance Matter?," *Health Education and Behavior* 25 (2018): 742–758.

129. Harold W. Neighbors, Marc A. Musick, and David R. Williams, "The African American Minister as a Source of Help for Serious Personal Crises: Bridge or Barrier to Mental Health Care?," *Health Education and Behavior* 25 (1998): 759–777.

130. Antonia (Anne) van Loon, "The Development of Faith Community Nursing Programs as a Response to Changing Australian Health Policy," *Health Education and Behavior* 25 (1998): 790–799.

131. Chatters et al., "Public Health and Health Education in Faith Communities," 692.

132. Ellen L. Idler, Jeff Levin, Tyler J. VanderWeele, and Anwar Khan, guest eds., "Partnerships in Religion and Public Health: From Local to Global" (special issue), *American Journal of Public Health* 109, 3 (2019).

133. Ellen L. Idler, Jeff Levin, Tyler J. VanderWeele, and Anwar Khan, "Partnerships between Public Health Agencies and Faith Communities," *American Journal of Public Health* 109 (2019): 346–347, 347.

134. Paul Jellinek, "Faith in Action: Building Capacity for Interfaith Volunteer Caregiving," *Health Affairs* 20 (2001): 273–278.

135. Ibid., 273. See also Paul Jellinek, Terri Gibbs Appel, and Terrance Keenan, "Faith in Action," in *To Improve Health and Health Care 1998–1999: The Robert Wood Johnson Foundation Anthology,* ed. Stephen L. Isaacs and James R. Knickman (San Francisco: Jossey-Bass, 1998), 131–144.

136. *Faith in Action: An RWJF National Program,* Robert Wood Johnson Foundation (May 21, 2009), https://www.rwjf.org/content/dam/farm/reports/program_results_reports/2009/rwjf69788.

137. Ibid., 40–42.

138. Barry Checkoway, "Six Strategies of Community Change," *Community Development Journal* 30 (1995): 2–20, 4.

139. Jade L. Dell and Steven Whitman, "A History of the Movement to Address Health Disparities," in *Urban Health: Combating Disparities with Local Data,* ed. Steven Whitman, Ami M. Shah, and Maureen R. Benjamin (New York: Oxford University Press, 2011), 8–30, 18.

140. C. David Jenkins, "New Horizons for Psychosomatic Medicine," *Psychosomatic Medicine* 47 (1985): 3–25.

141. Jeff Levin, "Engaging the Faith Community for Public Health Advocacy: An Agenda for the Surgeon General," *Journal of Religion and Health* 52 (2013): 368–385, 374.

142. Daniel S. Goldberg, "In Support of a Broad Model of Public Health: Disparities, Social Epidemiology, and Public Health Causation," *Public Health Ethics* 2 (2009): 70–83.

143. Ana V. Diez Roux, "Conceptual Approaches to the Study of Health Disparities," *Annual Review of Public Health* 33 (2012): 41–58.

144. Gary R. Gunderson, "Backing onto Sacred Ground," *Public Health Reports* 115 (2000): 257–261, 258.

145. Ibid.

146. David Satcher, "Opening Address," *CDC/ATSDR Forum: Engaging Faith Communities as Partners in Improving Community Health*, CDC Public Health Practice Program Office (Atlanta: Centers for Disease Control and Prevention, 1999), 2–3, 3.

147. Gunderson, "Backing onto Sacred Ground."

Chapter 5

1. Randolph C. Byrd, "Positive Therapeutic Effects of Intercessory Prayer in a Coronary Care Unit Population," *Southern Medical Journal* 81 (1988): 826–829.

2. Ibid., 827–828.

3. Ibid., 829.

4. Wendy Cadge, "Possibilities and Limits of Medical Science: Debates over Double-Blind Clinical Trials of Intercessory Prayer," *Zygon* 47 (2012): 43–64.

5. Sloan, *Blind Faith*.

6. Larry VandeCreek, ed., *Scientific Perspectives on Intercessory Prayer: An Exchange between Larry Dossey, M.D. and Health Care Chaplains* (New York: Haworth Pastoral Press, 1998).

7. When told of the Byrd study prior to publication, surgeon William Nolen, noted critic of faith healers, replied, "It sounds like this study will stand up to scrutiny. . . . Maybe we doctors ought to be writing on our order sheets, 'Pray three times a day.' If it works, it works" (quoted in Howard Wolinsky, "Prayers Do Aid Sick, Study Finds," *Chicago Sun Times* (January 26, 1986)). The most notable advocate for this research has been Larry Dossey (see *Healing Words: The Power of Prayer and the Practice of Medicine* (New York: HarperSanFrancisco, 1993)).

8. Steven Kreisman, "Letter to the Editor: Religion and Medicine," *Southern Medical Journal* 81 (1988): 1598.

9. Ibid.

10. "Editor's Note," *Southern Medical Journal* 81 (1988): 1598.

11. Osler, "The Faith That Heals."

12. Paulsen, "Religious Healing."

13. Larry Dossey and David J. Hufford, "Are Prayer Experiments Legitimate?: Twenty Criticisms," *EXPLORE: The Journal of Science and Healing* 1 (2005): 109–117; and Jeff Levin, "Scientists and Healers: Toward Collaborative Research Partnerships," *EXPLORE: The Journal of Science and Healing* 4 (2008): 302–310.

14. Larry Dossey, *Prayer Is Good Medicine: How to Reap the Healing Benefits of Prayer* (New York: HarperSanFrancisco, 1996), 4.

15. Spindrift, *The Spindrift Papers: Exploring Prayer and Healing through the Experimental Test, 1975–1993* (N.p.: Spindrift, 1993).

16. Ibid., 15.

17. Ibid.

18. Ibid., xii.

19. Bill Sweet, *A Journey into Prayer: Pioneers of Prayer in the Laboratory, Agents of Science or Satan?* (N.p.: Xlibris, 2004).

20. William S. Harris, Manohar Gowda, Jerry W. Kolb, Christopher Strychacz, James L. Vacek, Philip G. Jones, Alan Forker, James H. O'Keefe, and Ben D. McCallister, "A Randomized, Controlled Trial of the Effects of Remote, Intercessory Prayer on Outcomes in Patients Admitted to the Coronary Care Unit," *Archives of Internal Medicine* 159 (1999): 2273–2278.

21. Fred Sicher, Elisabeth Targ, Dan Moore II, and Helene S. Smith, "A Randomized Double-Blind Study of the Effect of Distant Healing in a Population with Advanced AIDS," *Western Journal of Medicine* 169 (1998): 356–363.

22. Dossey, *Healing Words*.

23. Daniel J. Benor, *Spiritual Healing: Scientific Validation of a Healing Revolution* (Southfield, MI: Vision Publications, 2001).

24. Ibid., 187–376.

25. Ibid., 371–376.

26. Richard Wiseman and Marilyn J. Schlitz, "Experimenter Effects and the Remote Detection of Staring," *Journal of Parapsychology* 61 (1997): 197–207; and Marilyn Schlitz, Richard Wiseman, Caroline Watt, and Dean Radin, "Of Two Minds: Sceptic-Proponent Collaboration within Parapsychology," *British Journal of Psychology* 97 (2006): 313–322.

27. Leonard Leibovici, "Effects of Remote, Retroactive Intercessory Prayer on Outcomes in Patients with Bloodstream Infection: Randomised Controlled Trial," *British Medical Journal* 323 (2001): 1450–1451; and Brian Olshansky and Larry Dossey, "Retroactive Prayer: A Preposterous Hypothesis?," *British Medical Journal* 327 (2003): 1465–1468.

28. Rollin McCraty, Mike Atkinson, Dana Tomasino, and William A. Tiller, "The Electricity of Touch: Detection and Measurement of Cardiac Energy Exchange between People," in *Brain and Values: Is a Biological Science of Values Possible?*, ed. Karl H. Pribham (Mahwah, NJ: Lawrence Erlbaum Associates, 1998), 359–379.

29. Stefan Schmidt, "Direct Mental Interactions with Living Systems (DMILS)," in Wayne B. Jonas and Cindy C. Crawford, eds., *Healing, Intention, and Energy Medicine: Science, Research Methods, and Clinical Implications* (Edinburgh: Churchill Livingstone, 2003), 23–38.

30. Drew Leder, "'Spooky Actions at a Distance': Physics, Psi, and Distant Healing," *Journal of Alternative and Complementary Medicine* 11 (2005): 923–930.

31. Larry Dossey, *One Mind: How Our Individual Mind Is Part of a Greater Consciousness and Why It Matters* (Carlsbad, CA: Hay House, 2013); Dean Radin, *Entangled Minds: Extrasensory Experiences in a Quantum Reality* (New York: Paraview, 2006); and Cheryl L. Fracasso, Kaleb R. Smith, and Stanley Krippner, eds., "Special Issue: Health, Healing & Consciousness," *NeuroQuantology* 14, 2 (2016): 149–446.

32. Jonas and Crawford, *Healing, Intention, and Energy Medicine*.

33. Paul N. Duckro and Philip R. Magaletta, "The Effect of Prayer on Physical Health: Experimental Evidence," *Journal of Religion and Health* 33 (1994): 211–219; and Michael E. McCullough, "Prayer and Health: Conceptual Issues, Research Review, and Research Agenda," *Journal of Psychology and Theology* 23 (1995): 15–29.

34. Jeffrey S. Levin, "How Prayer Heals: A Theoretical Model," *Alternative Therapies in Health and Medicine* 2, 1 (1996): 66–73.

35. Ibid.; "Appendix 4: Healing and the Mind: A Summing Up," in Dossey, *Healing Words*, 249–253; and M. J. Breslin and Christopher A. Lewis, "Theoretical Models of the Nature of Prayer and Health: A Review," *Mental Health, Religion and Culture* 11 (2008): 9–21.

36. Herbert Benson, Jeffrey A. Dusek, Jane B. Sherwood, Peter Lam, Charles W. Bethea, William Carpenter, Sidney Levitsky, Peter C. Hill, Donald W. Clem Jr., Manoj K. Jain, David Drumel, Stephen J. Kopecky, Paul S. Mueller, Dean Marek, Sue Rollins, and Patricia L. Hibbard, "Study of the Therapeutic Effects of Intercessory Prayer (STEP) in Cardiac Bypass Patients: A Multicenter Randomized Trial of Uncertainty and Certainty of Receiving Intercessory Prayer," *American Heart Journal* 151 (2006): 934–942.

37. Mitchell W. Krucoff, Suzanne W. Crater, and Kerry L. Lee, "From Efficacy to Safety Concerns: A STEP Forward or a Step Back for Clinical Research and Intercessory Prayer?: The Study of Therapeutic Effects of Intercessory Prayer (STEP)," *American Heart Journal* 151 (2006): 762–764.

38. Larry Dossey, "Healing Research: What We Know and Don't Know," *EXPLORE: The Journal of Science and Healing* 4 (2008): 341–352, 346.

39. Mitchell W. Krucoff, Suzanne W. Crater, Cindy L. Green, Arthur C. Maas, Jon E. Seskevich, James D. Lane, Karen A. Loeffler, Kenneth Morris, Thomas M. Bashore, and Harold G. Koenig, "Integrative Noetic Therapies as Adjuncts to Percutaneous Intervention during Unstable Coronary Cyndromes: Monitoring and Actualization of Noetic Training (MANTRA) Feasibility Pilot," *American Heart Journal* 142 (2001): 760–769; and Mitchell W. Krucoff, Suzanne W. Crater, Dianne Gallup, James C. Blankenship, Michael Cuffe, Mimi Guarneri, Richard A. Krieger, Vib R. Kshettry, Kenneth Morris, Mehmet Oz, August Pichard, Michael H. Sketch Jr., Harold G. Koenig, Daniel Mark, and Kerry L. Lee, "Music, Imagery, Touch, and Prayer as Adjuncts to Interventional Cardiac Care: The Monitoring and Actualisation of Noetic Trainings (MANTRA) II Randomised Study," *The Lancet* 366 (2005): P211–P217.

40. Benor, *Spiritual Healing*.

41. Sloan, *Blind Faith*; and Dossey, "Healing Research."

42. Christopher A. Roe, Charmaine Sonnex, and Elizabeth C. Roxburgh, "Two Meta-Analyses of Noncontact Healing Studies," *EXPLORE: The Journal of Science and Healing* 11 (2015): 11–23. Another meta-analysis of human studies: Marilyn Schlitz and William Braud, "Distant Intentionality and Healing: Assessing the Evidence," *Alternative Therapies in Health and Medicine* 3, 6 (1997): 62–73.

43. Dossey, "Healing Research," 24.

44. Miquel Porta, *A Dictionary of Epidemiology*, 6th ed. (New York: Oxford University Press, 2014), 218.

45. Jeff Levin, "The Epidemiology of Religion," in *Religion and the Social Sciences: Basic and Applied Research Perspectives*, ed. Jeff Levin (West Conshohocken, PA: Templeton Press, 2018), 259–286.

46. Jeffrey S. Levin, "Religion and Health: Is There an Association, Is It Valid, and Is It Causal?," *Social Science and Medicine* 38 (1994): 1475–1482.

47. Thomas W. Graham, Berton H. Kaplan, Joan C. Cornoni-Huntley, Sherman A. James, Caroline Becker, Curtis G. Hames, and Siegfried Heyden, "Frequency of Church Attendance and Blood Pressure Elevation," *Journal of Behavioral Medicine* 1 (1978): 37–43.

48. Berton H. Kaplan, "A Note on Religious Beliefs and Coronary Heart Disease," *Journal of the South Carolina Medical Association* 15, 5, Suppl. (1976): 60–64.

49. Ibid., 64.

50. Jeffrey S. Levin and Preston L. Schiller, "Is There a Religious Factor in Health?," *Journal of Religion and Health* 26 (1987): 9–36.

51. George K. Jarvis and Herbert C. Northcott, "Religious Differences in Morbidity and Mortality," *Social Science and Medicine* 25 (1987): 813–824.

52. Ellen L. Idler, "Religious Involvement and the Health of the Elderly: Some Hypotheses and an Initial Test," *Social Forces* 66 (1987): 226–238.

53. Jeffrey S. Levin and Harold Y. Vanderpool, "Religious Factors in Physical Health and the Prevention of Illness," in *Religion and Prevention in Mental Health: Research, Vision, and Action*, ed. Kenneth I. Pargament, Kenneth I. Maton, and Robert E. Hess (New York: Haworth Press, 1992), 83–103, 84.

54. John Shaw Billings, "Vital Statistics of the Jews," *North American Review* 153 (1891): 70–84.

55. Benjamin Travers, "Observations on the Local Disease Termed Malignant: Being a Sequel to the Paper Published in Vol. XV of the Society's Transactions, Part III," *Medico-Chirurgical Transactions* 17 (1832): 300–422.

56. Levin and Schiller, "Is There a Religious Factor in Health?," 25n12.

57. E. L. Kennaway, "The Racial and Social Incidence of Cancer of the Uterus," *British Journal of Cancer* 2 (1948): 177–212.

58. E.g., George W. Comstock and Kay B. Partridge, "Church Attendance and Health," *Journal of Chronic Diseases* 25 (1972): 665–672. Comstock published nearly a dozen such studies.

59. Jeffrey S. Levin and Harold Y. Vanderpool, "Is Frequent Religious Attendance *Really* Conducive to Better Health?: Toward an Epidemiology of Religion," *Social Science and Medicine* 24 (1987): 589–600.

60. A product of this grant was the first edited academic book on the subject: Jeffrey S. Levin, ed., *Religion and Aging and Health: Theoretical Foundations and Methodological Frontiers* (Thousand Oaks, CA: Sage, 1994).

61. Summarized in Robert Joseph Taylor, Linda M. Chatters, and Jeffrey S. Levin, *Religion in the Lives of African Americans: Social, Psychological, and Health Perspectives* (Thousand Oaks, CA: Sage, 2004).

62. A research summary: Dale A. Matthews, David B. Larson, and Constance Barry, *The Faith Factor: An Annotated Bibliography of Clinical Research on Spiritual Subjects,* vol. 1 (Rockville, MD: National Institute for Healthcare Research, 1993). A consensus report: David B. Larson, James Swyers, and Michael E. McCullough, eds., *Scientific Research on Spirituality and Health: A Report Based on the Scientific Progress in Spirituality Conferences* (Rockville, MD: National Institute for

Healthcare Research, 1998). A continuing education curriculum: David B. Larson and Susan S. Larson, *The Forgotten Factor in Physical and Mental Health: What Does the Research Show?: An Independent Study Seminar* (N.p.: David and Susan Larson, 1994).

63. Conference on Methodological Approaches to the Study of Religion, Health, and Aging. Sponsored by the National Institute on Aging and the Fetzer Institute, National Institutes of Health, Bethesda, Maryland, March 16–17, 1995.

64. National Institute on Aging / Fetzer Institute, *Multidimensional Measurement of Religiousness/Spirituality for Use in Health Research* (Kalamazoo, MI: John E. Fetzer Institute, 1999).

65. Ellen L. Idler, Marc A. Musick, Christopher G. Ellison, Linda K. George, Neal Krause, Marcia G. Ory, Kenneth I. Pargament, Lynda H. Powell, Lynn G. Underwood, and David R. Williams, "Measuring Multiple Dimensions of Religion and Spirituality for Health Research: Conceptual Background and Findings from the 1998 General Social Survey," *Research on Aging* 25 (2003): 327–365.

66. E.g., Linda M. Chatters, "Religion and Health: Public Health Research and Practice," *Annual Review of Public Health* 21 (2000): 335–367.

67. E.g., Neal Krause and R. David Hayward, "Religion, Health, and Aging," in *Handbook of Aging and the Social Sciences,* 8th ed., ed. Linda K. George and Kenneth F. Ferraro (Boston: Elsevier, 2016), 251–270.

68. E.g., Jeffrey S. Levin, Linda M. Chatters, Christopher G. Ellison, and Robert Joseph Taylor, "Religious Involvement, Health Outcomes, and Public Health Practice," *Current Issues in Public Health* 2 (1996): 220–225.

69. Sara C. Charles, "Religion and Health: *Handbook of Religion and Health*" (Book review), *JAMA* 286 (2001): 465–466, 465.

70. Levin, "The Epidemiology of Religion," 265–269. These numbers are based on my cumulation of entries in Koenig's bibliographies. He might come up with different totals.

71. William J. Strawbridge, Richard D. Cohen, Sarah J. Shema, and George A. Kaplan, "Frequent Attendance at Religious Services and Mortality over 28 Years," *American Journal of Public Health* 87 (1997): 957–961; Comstock and Partridge, "Church Attendance and Health"; Graham et al., "Frequency of Church Attendance and Blood Pressure Elevation"; and James House, Cynthia Robbins, and Helen L. Metzner, "The Association of Social Relationships and Activities with Mortality: Prospective Evidence from the Tecumseh Community Health Study," *American Journal of Epidemiology* 116 (1982): 123–140.

72. Notably Kyriakos S. Markides, Robert Joseph Taylor, Ellen L. Idler, David R. Williams, Christopher G. Ellison, Kenneth F. Ferraro, Diane R. Brown, Neal Krause, and Linda K. George.

73. Ellen L. Idler and Yael Benyamini, "Self-Rated Health and Mortality: A Review of Twenty-Seven Community Studies," *Journal of Health and Social Behavior* 38 (1997): 21–37.

74. Jeffrey S. Levin, "How Religion Influences Morbidity and Health: Reflections on Natural History, Salutogenesis, and Host Resistance," *Social Science and Medicine* 43 (1996): 849–864, esp. 854–857.

75. Florence A. Summerlin, comp., *Religion and Mental Health: A Bibliography*, DHHS Pub. No. (ADM) 80-964 (Washington, DC: U.S. Government Printing Office, 1980).

76. Leo Srole and Thomas Langner, "Religious Origin," in Leo Srole, Thomas S. Langner, Stanley T. Michael, Marvin K. Opler, and Thomas A. C. Rennie, *Mental Health in the Metropolis: The Midtown Manhattan Study* (New York: McGraw-Hill, 1962), 300–324.

77. E.g., Harold G. Koenig, Judith C. Hays, Linda K. George, Dan G. Blazer, David B. Larson, and Lawrence R. Landerman, "Modeling the Cross-Sectional Relationships between Religion, Physical Health, Social Support, and Depressive Symptoms," *American Journal of Geriatric Psychiatry* 5 (1997): 131–144.

78. E.g., P. P. Yeung and S. Greenwald, "Jewish Americans and Mental Health: Results of the NIMH Epidemiologic Catchment Area Study," *Social Psychiatry and Psychiatric Epidemiology* 27 (1992): 292–297.

79. Robert A. Witter, William A. Stock, Morris A. Okun, and Marilyn J. Haring, "Religion and Subjective Well-Being in Adulthood: A Quantitative Synthesis," *Review of Religious Research* 26 (1985): 332–342; Harold G. Koenig, comp., *Research on Religion and Aging: An Annotated Bibliography* (Westport, CT: Greenwood Press, 1995); Jeffrey S. Levin, "Religious Research in Gerontology, 1980–1994: A Systematic Review," *Journal of Religious Gerontology* 10, 3 (1997): 3–31; Ellen L. Idler, "Religion and Aging," in *Handbook of Aging and the Social Sciences,* 6th ed., ed. Robert H. Binstock and Linda K. George (San Diego: Academic Press / Elsevier, 2006), 277–300.

80. George, "Religion and Social Gerontology," in Levin, *Religion and the Social Sciences,* 209–234; and Vincent J. Fecher, *Religion & Aging: An Annotated Bibliography* (San Antonio, TX: Trinity University Press, 1982).

81. E.g., David O. Moberg, "The Christian Religion and Personal Adjustment in Old Age," *American Sociological Review* 18 (1953): 87–90.

82. E. Mansell Pattison, "Psychiatry and Religion circa 1978: Analysis of a Decade, Part I," *Pastoral Psychology* 27 (1978): 8–25; and "Psychiatry and Religion circa 1978: Analysis of a Decade, Part II," *Pastoral Psychology* 27 (1978): 119–141.

83. Victor D. Sanua, "Religion, Mental Health, and Personality: A Review of Empirical Studies," *American Journal of Psychiatry* 125 (1969): 1203–1213.

84. David B. Larson and William Wilson, "Religious Life of Alcoholics," *Southern Medical Journal* 73 (1980): 723–727; Louis A. Cancellaro, David B. Larson, and William Wilson, "Religious Life of Narcotic Addicts," *Southern Medical Journal* 75 (1982): 1166–1168; William Wilson, David B. Larson, and Paul D. Meier, "Religious Life of Schizophrenics," *Southern Medical Journal* 76 (1983): 1096–1100; and Leigh C. Bishop, David B. Larson, and William Wilson, "Religious Life of Individuals with Affective Disorders," *Southern Medical Journal* 80 (1987): 1083–1086.

85. Allen E. Bergin, "Religiosity and Mental Health: A Critical Reevaluation and Meta-Analysis," *Professional Psychology: Research and Practice* 14 (1983): 170–184.

86. David B. Larson, E. Mansell Pattison, Dan G. Blazer, Abdul R. Omran, and Berton H. Kaplan, "Systematic Analysis of Research on Religious Variables in Four Major

Psychiatric Journals, 1978–1982," *American Journal of Psychiatry* 143 (1986): 329–334; David B. Larson, Kimberly A. Sherrill, John S. Lyons, Frederic C. Craigie Jr., Samuel B. Thielman, Mary A. Greenwold, and Susan S. Larson, "Associations between Dimensions of Religious Commitment and Mental Health Reported in the *American Journal of Psychiatry* and *Archives of General Psychiatry*: 1978–1989," *American Journal of Psychiatry* 149 (1992): 557–559; and John Gartner, David B. Larson, and George D. Allen, "Religious Commitment and Mental Health: A Review of the Empirical Literature," *Journal of Psychology and Theology* 19 (1991): 6–25.

87. Koenig, *Research on Religion and Aging.*
88. Levin, "Religious Research in Gerontology."
89. Harold G. Koenig and David B. Larson, "Religion and Mental Health: Evidence for an Association," *International Review of Psychiatry* 13 (2001): 67–78, 67.
90. Ibid., 75.
91. Taylor et al., *Religion in the Lives of African Americans*; and Jeff Levin, Linda M. Chatters, and Robert Joseph Taylor, "Religion, Health, and Medicine in African Americans: Implications for Physicians," *Journal of the National Medical Association* 97 (2005): 237–249.
92. Jeff Levin, "'And Let Us Make Us a Name': Reflections on the Future of the Religion and Health Field," *Journal of Religion and Health* 48 (2009): 125–145.
93. Jeff Levin, "Etiology Recapitulates Ontology: Reflections on Restoring the Spiritual Dimension to Models of the Determinants of Health," *Subtle Energies and Energy Medicine* 12 (2001): 17–37, 28.
94. Disability studies include longitudinal evidence that religious participation contributes to maintenance of physical functioning, especially in older adults (e.g., Ellen L. Idler and Stanislav V. Kasl, "Religion among Disabled and Nondisabled Persons II: Attendance at Religious Services as a Predictor of the Course of Disability," *Journal of Gerontology: Psychological Sciences* 52 (1997): S306–S316).
95. Ellen L. Idler, ed., *Religion as a Social Determinant of Public Health* (New York: Oxford University Press, 2014). See also Pekka Martikainen, Mel Bartley, and Eero Lahelma, "Psychosocial Determinants of Health in Social Epidemiology," *International Journal of Epidemiology* 31 (2002): 1091–1093.
96. Jeff Levin, "Prayer, Love, and Transcendence: An Epidemiologic Perspective," in *Religious Influences on Health and Well-Being in the Elderly*, ed. K. Warner-Schaie, Neal Krause, and Alan Booth (New York: Springer, 2004), 69–95.
97. Levin, "The Discourse on Faith and Medicine," 267.
98. Harold G. Koenig, *The Healing Power of Faith: Science Explores Medicine's Last Great Frontier* (New York: Simon and Schuster, 1999).
99. Harold G. Koenig, "Religion and Depression in Older Medical Inpatients," *American Journal of Geriatric Psychiatry* 15 (2007): 282–291.
100. Harold G. Koenig, Linda K. George, and Bercedis L. Peterson, "Religiosity and Remission in Medically Ill Older Patients," *American Journal of Psychiatry* 155 (1998): 536–542.
101. Levin, "The Epidemiology of Religion," 277.

102. Kenneth I. Pargament, ed., *APA Handbook of Psychology, Religion, and Spirituality,* vol. 1: *Context, Theory, and Research* and *APA Handbook of Psychology, Religion, and Spirituality,* vol. 2: *An Applied Psychology of Religion and Spirituality* (Washington, DC: American Psychological Association, 2013); and Raymond F. Paloutzian and Crystal L. Park, eds., *Handbook of the Psychology of Religion and Spirituality* (New York: Guilford, 2005).

103. Kenneth I. Pargament and Julie J. Exline, "The Psychology of Religion: The State of an Evolving Field," in Levin, *Religion and the Social Sciences,* 17–37.

104. Edward Shafranske, "Religious Beliefs, Affiliations, and Practices of Clinical Psychologists," in *Religion and the Clinical Practice of Psychology,* ed. Edward Shafranske (Washington, DC: American Psychological Association, 1996), 149–162.

105. E.g., Crystal L. Park, "Religiousness/Spirituality and Health: A Meaning Systems Perspective," *Journal of Behavioral Medicine* 30 (2007): 319–328.

106. E.g., Linda M. Chatters, Kai McKeever Bullard, Robert Joseph Taylor, Amanda Toler Woodward, Harold W. Neighbors, and James S. Jackson, "Religious Participation and DSM-IV Disorders among Older African Americans: Findings from the National Survey of American Life (NSAL)," *American Journal of Geriatric Psychiatry* 16 (2008): 957–965; and Michael E. McCullough and David B. Larson, "Religion and Depression: A Review of the Literature," *Twin Research* 2 (1999): 126–136.

107. E.g., David G. Myers, "The Funds, Friends, and Faith of Happy People," *American Psychologist* 55 (2000): 56–67; Robert Emmons, Chi Cheung, and Keivan Tehrani, "Assessing Spirituality through Personal Goals: Implications for Research on Religion and Subjective Well-Being," *Social Indicators Research* 45 (1998): 391–422; and Susan H. McFadden, "Religion and Well-Being in Aging Persons in an Aging Society," *Journal of Social Issues* 51 (1995): 161–175.

108. Raymond F. Paloutzian, Rodger K. Bufford, and Ashley J. Wildman, "Spiritual Well-Being Scale: Mental and Physical Health Relationships," in *Oxford Textbook of Spirituality in Healthcare,* ed. Mark Cobb, Christina M. Puchalski, and Bruce Rumbold (New York: Oxford University Press, 2012), 353–358.

109. Lisa Miller, Ravi Bansal, and Priya Wickramaratne, "Neuroanatomical Correlates of Religiosity and Spirituality: A Study in Adults at High and Low Familial Risk for Depression," *JAMA Psychiatry* 71 (2014): 128–135.

110. Peter Fenwick, "The Neurophysiology of Religious Experience," in *Psychosis and Spirituality: Exploring the New Frontier,* ed. Isabel Clarke (Philadelphia: Whurr, 2001), 15–26.

111. Kenneth I. Pargament, *The Psychology of Religion and Coping: Theory, Research, Practice* (New York: Guilford Press, 1997).

112. David H. Rosmarin, Devora Greer Shabtai, Steven Pirutinsky, and Kenneth I. Pargament, "Jewish Religious Coping and Trust in God: A Review of the Empirical Literature," in *Judaism and Health: A Handbook of Practical, Professional, and Scholarly Resources,* ed. Jeff Levin and Michele F. Prince (Woodstock, VT: Jewish Lights, 2013), 265–281, 377–382.

113. David H. Rosmarin, Kenneth I. Pargament, Steven Pirutinsky, and Annette Mahoney, "A Randomized Controlled Evaluation of a Spiritually Integrated Treatment for Subclinical Anxiety in the Jewish Community, Delivered via the Internet," *Journal of Anxiety* 24 (2010): 799–808.

114. David H. Rosmarin, Joseph S. Bigda-Peyton, Sarah J. Kertz, Nasya Smith, Scott L. Rauch, and Thröstur Björgvinsson, "A Test of Faith in God and Treatment: The Relationship of Belief in God to Psychiatric Treatment Outcome," *Journal of Affective Disorders* 146 (2013): 441–446.

115. David H. Rosmarin, *Spirituality, Religion, Cognitive-Behavioral Therapy: A Guide for Clinicians* (New York: Guilford Press, 2018).

116. Pargament, *APA Handbook of Psychology, Religion, and Spirituality*.

117. Ronald Max Andersen, "National Health Surveys and the Behavioral Model of Health Services Use," *Medical Care* 46 (2008): 647–653.

118. Cheryl A. Maurana, Robert L. Eichhorn, and Lynn E. Lonnquist, *The Use of Health Services: Indices and Correlates—A Research Bibliography 1981*, NCHSR Pub. No. 82-65 (Washington, DC: U.S. Government Printing Office, 1983).

119. Preston L. Schiller and Jeffrey S. Levin, "Is There a Religious Factor in Health Care Utilization?: A Review," *Social Science and Medicine* 27 (1988): 1369–1379.

120. Albert L. Johnson, C. David Jenkins, Ralph Patrick, and Travis J Northcutt Jr., "Epidemiology of Polio Vaccine Acceptance: A Social and Psychological Analysis," *Florida State Board of Health Monographs* 3 (1962): 90–98.

121. Maurana et al., *The Use of Health Services*, 7.

122. Ibid., 15.

123. Schiller and Levin, "Is There a Religious Factor in Health Care Utilization?," 1371.

124. Ronald Andersen and John F. Newman, "Societal and Individual Determinants of Medical Care Utilization in the United States," *Millbank Memorial Fund Quarterly* 51 (1973): 95–124.

125. David Mechanic, *Public Expectations and Health Care: Essays on the Changing Organization of Health Services* (New York: John Wiley and Sons, 1972), 206–208.

126. Avedis Donabedian, *Aspects of Medical Care Administration: Specifying Requirements for Health Care* (Cambridge, MA: Harvard University Press, 1973), 422–425.

127. David B. Larson, Ann A. Hohmann, Larry G. Kessler, Keith G. Meador, Jeffrey H. Boyd, and Elisabeth McSherry, "The Couch and the Cloth: The Need for Linkage," *Hospital and Community Psychiatry* 39 (1988): 1064–1069.

128. Koenig et al., *Handbook of Religion and Health*, 397–434.

129. Ibid., 574–576.

130. Harold G. Koenig, Linda K. George, Patricia Titus, and Keith G. Meador, "Religion, Spirituality, and Acute Care Hospitalization and Long-Term Care Use by Older Patients," *Archives of Internal Medicine* 164 (2004): 1579–1585.

131. Harold G. Koenig and David B. Larson, "Use of Hospital Services, Religious Attendance, and Religious Affiliation," *Southern Medical Journal* 91 (1998): 925–932.

132. Jeff Levin, Robert Joseph Taylor, and Linda M. Chatters, "Prevalence and Sociodemographic Correlates of Spiritual Healer Use: Findings from the National Survey of American Life," *Complementary Therapies in Medicine* 19 (2011): 63–70.

133. Ibid., 63.

134. Ibid., 69.

135. Jeff Levin, "Prevalence and Religious Predictors of Healing Prayer Use in the USA: Findings from the Baylor Religion Survey," *Journal of Religion and Health* 55 (2016): 1136–1158.

136. Quoted in "Most Americans Pray for Healing; More Than One Fourth Have Practiced 'Laying On of Hands,' Baylor University Study Finds," Baylor Media Communications (April 18, 2016), https://www.baylor.edu/mediacommunications/news.php?action=story&story=167956.

137. Stanley H. King and Daniel H. Funkenstein, "Religious Practice and Cardiovascular Reactions during Stress," *Journal of Abnormal Social Psychology* 55 (1957): 135–137.

138. Walter W. Surwillo and Douglas Hobson, "Brain Electrical Activity during Prayer," *Psychological Reports* 43 (1978): 135–143.

139. Ibid., 135.

140. Herbert Benson, *The Relaxation Response* (New York: William Morrow and Co., 1975).

141. Herbert Benson, John F. Beary, and Mark Carol, "The Relaxation Response," *Psychiatry* 37 (1974): 37–46, 37.

142. Ibid.

143. Herbert Benson with Marg Stark, *Timeless Healing: The Power and Biology of Belief* (New York: Fireside, 1996).

144. Michael Murphy and Steven Donovan, *The Physical and Psychological Effects of Meditation: A Review of Contemporary Research with a Comprehensive Bibliography, 1931–1996*, ed. Eugene Taylor (Sausalito, CA: Institute of Noetic Sciences, 1997).

145. "IONS Meditation Bibliography (1997–2013)," https://noetic.org/meditation-bibliography.

146. David S. Holmes, "Meditation and Somatic Arousal Reduction: A Review of the Experimental Evidence," *American Psychologist* 39 (1984): 1–10.

147. James Funderburk, *Science Studies Yoga: A Review of Physiological Data* (Glenview, IL: Himalayan International Institute of Yoga Science and Philosophy, 1977).

148. Brendan O'Regan and Caryle Hirshberg, *Spontaneous Remission: An Annotated Bibliography* (Sausalito, CA: Institute of Noetic Sciences, 1993).

149. Ibid., 2.

150. Ibid., quotations 3.

151. Jeff Levin, "Spiritual Determinants of Health and Healing: An Epidemiologic Perspective on Salutogenic Mechanisms," *Alternative Therapies in Health and Medicine* 9 (2003): 48–57, 53.

152. Jeff Levin, "Preface," in Koenig et al., *Handbook of Religion and Health,* 2nd ed., xiii–xv.

153. Hyungjun Suh, Terrence D. Hill, and Harold G. Koenig, "Religious Attendance and Biological Risk: A National Longitudinal Study of Older Adults," *Journal of Religion and Health* 58 (2019): 1188–1202.

154. Robert Ader, ed., *Psychoneuroimmunology,* 4th ed., Amsterdam: Elsevier/Academic Press, 2007). Popular works include Candace B. Pert, *Molecules of Emotion: The Science behind Mind-Body Medicine* (New York: Touchstone, 1997); and Esther M. Sternberg, *The Balance Within: The Science Connecting Health and Emotions* (New York: W. H. Freeman and Co., 2001).

155. Seymour Reichlin, "Neuroendocrine-Immune Interactions," *New England Journal of Medicine* 329 (1993): 1246–1253.

156. Levin, "How Faith Heals," esp. 87–89.

157. Sternberg, *The Balance Within,* 168–169.

158. Koenig et al., *Handbook of Religion and Health,* 276–291; and Koenig et al., *Handbook of Religion and Health,* 2nd ed., 394–438.

159. Harold G. Koenig, Harvey Jay Cohen, Linda K. George, Judith C. Hays, David B. Larson, and Dan G. Blazer, "Attendance at Religious Services, Interleukin-6, and Other Biological Parameters of Immune Function in Older Adults," *International Journal of Psychiatry in Medicine* 27 (1997): 233–250.

160. Harold G. Koenig and Harvey Jay Cohen, *The Link Between Religion and Health: Psychoneuroimmunology and the Faith Factor* (New York: Oxford University Press, 2002).

161. Jeff Levin, Linda M. Chatters, and Robert Joseph Taylor, "Religious Factors in Health and Medical Care among Older Adults," *Southern Medical Journal* 99 (2006): 1168–1169.

162. Jeff Levin, "Health," in *Vocabulary for the Study of Religion,* vol. 2: *F–O,* ed. Robert A. Segal and Kocku von Stuckrad (Leiden, Netherlands: Brill, 2015), 142–146, 145, emphasis added.

163. Jeff Levin, "Religion and Mental Health: Theory and Research," *International Journal of Applied Psychoanalytic Studies* 7 (2010): 102–115, 108.

164. Jeff Levin and Linda M. Chatters, "Religion, Aging, and Health: Historical Perspectives, Current Trends, and Future Directions," *Journal of Religion, Spirituality and Aging* 20 (2008): 153–172; and Jeff Levin, "Religion, Health, and Happiness: An Epidemiologist's Perspective," in *Homo Religiosus: Exploring the Roots of Religion and Religious Freedom in Human Experience,* ed. Timothy Samuel Shah and Jack Friedman (New York: Cambridge University Press, 2018), 177–194.

165. Levin and Schiller, "Is There a Religious Factor in Health?," and Jarvis and Northcott, "Religious Differences in Morbidity and Mortality."

166. E.g., Strawbridge et al., "Frequent Attendance at Religious Services and Mortality over 28 Years."

167. Michael E. McCullough, William T. Hoyt, David B. Larson, Harold G. Koenig, and Carl Thoresen, "Religious Involvement and Mortality: A Meta-Analytic Review," *Health Psychology* 19 (2000): 211–222.

168. Cited in Levin, "The Epidemiology of Religion," 267.

169. Harold G. Koenig, Bruce Nelson, Sally F. Shaw, Salil Saxena, and Harvey Jay Cohen, "Religious Involvement and Telomere Length in Women Family Caregivers," *Journal of Nervous and Mental Disease* 204 (2016): 36–42; Terrence D. Hill, Christopher G. Ellison, Amy M. Burdette, John Taylor, and Katherine L. Friedman,

"Dimensions of Religious Involvement and Leukocyte Telomere Length," *Social Science and Medicine* 163 (2016): 168–175; and Mahmoud Shaheen Al Ahwal, Fateh Al Zaben, Mohammad Gamal Sehlo, Doaa Ahmed Khalifa, and Harold G. Koenig, "Religiosity and Telomere Length in Colorectal Cancer Patients in Saudi Arabia," *Journal of Religion and Health* 57 (2018): 672–682.

170. Masood A. Shammas, "Telomeres, Lifestyle, Cancer, and Aging," *Current Opinion in Clinical Nutrition and Metabolic Care* 14 (2011): 28–34.

171. Tyler J. VanderWeele and Alexandra E. Shields, "Religiosity and Telomere Length: One Step Forward, One Step Back," *Social Science and Medicine* 163 (2016): 176–178.

172. Ibid.

173. A. Phillip Owens, Nathan Robbins, Keith Saum, Shannon M. Jones, Akiva W. Kirschner, Jessica G. Woo, Connie McCoy, Samuel Slone, Marc E. Rothenberg, Elaine M. Urbina, Michael Tranter, and Jack Rubinstein, "Tefillin Use Induces Remote Ischemic Preconditioning Pathways in Healthy Males," *American Journal of Physiology—Heart and Circulatory Physiology* (2018), doi: 10.1152/ajpheart.00347.2018.

174. E.g., Levin, "Energy Healers"; and Jeff Levin and Laura Mead, "Bioenergy Healing: A Theoretical Model and Case Series," *EXPLORE: The Journal of Science and Healing* 4 (2008): 201–209.

175. Jeff Levin, "What is 'Healing'?: Reflections on Diagnostic Criteria, Nosology, and Etiology," *EXPLORE: The Journal of Science and Healing* 13 (2017): 244–256; and "A Response," *EXPLORE: The Journal of Science and Healing* 13 (2007): 271–273.

176. John A. Astin, Elaine Harkness, and Edzard Ernst, "The Efficacy of 'Distant Healing': A Systematic Review of Randomized Trials," *Annals of Internal Medicine* 132 (2000): 903–910.

177. Taxonomies and typologies exist that define *energy healing* and parse conceptual distinctions among energy healers (e.g., Lawrence LeShan, *The Medium, the Mystic, and the Physicist: Toward a General Theory of the Paranormal* (1966; New York: Helios Press, 2003)).

178. Benor, *Spiritual Healing*; and David Aldridge, *Spirituality, Healing and Medicine: Return to the Silence* (London: Jessica Kingsley Publishers, 2000).

179. Larry Dossey, "But Is It Energy?: Reflections on Consciousness, Healing, and the New Paradigm," *Subtle Energies* 3 (1992): 69–82.

180. Questions have been raised about the legitimacy of studies by Daniel Wirth, and some journals have withdrawn his publications (see Jerry Solfvin, Eric Leskowitz, and Daniel J. Benor, "Questions concerning the Work of Daniel Wirth" [Letter], *Journal of Alternative and Complementary Medicine* 11 (2005): 949–950). For the age-old phenomenon of fake faith healers, see James Randi, "Peter Popoff and His Wonderful Machine," in *The Faith Healers*, new, updated ed. (Amherst, NY: Prometheus Books, 1989), 139–182.

181. The question taken up in Levin, *God, Faith, and Health*.

182. Ibid., 10–11.

183. Kenneth Vaux, "Religion and Health," *Preventive Medicine* 5 (1976): 522–536.

184. Idler, "Religious Involvement and the Health of the Elderly"; and Christopher G. Ellison, "Religion, the Life Stress Paradigm, and the Study of Depression," in *Religion in Aging and Health: Theoretical Foundations and Methodological Frontiers*, ed. Jeffrey S. Levin (Thousand Oaks, CA: Sage, 1994), 78–121.

185. Daniel McIntosh and Bernard Spilka, "Religion and Physical Health: The Role of Personal Faith and Control Beliefs," *Research on the Social Scientific Study of Religion* 2 (1990): 167–194; Everett L. Worthington Jr., Jack W. Berry, and Les Parrott III, "Unforgiveness, Forgiveness, Religion, and Health," in *Faith and Health: Psychological Perspectives*, ed. Thomas G. Plante and Allen C. Sherman (New York: Guilford, 2001), 107–138; and Doug Oman and Carl E. Thoresen, "'Does Religion Cause Health?': Differing Interpretations and Diverse Meanings," *Journal of Health Psychology* 7 (2002): 365–380.

186. Christopher G. Ellison and Jeffrey S. Levin, "The Religion-Health Connection: Evidence, Theory, and Future Directions," *Health Education and Behavior* 25 (1998): 700–720; and Linda K. George, David B. Larson, and Christopher G. Ellison, "Explaining the Relationships between Religious Involvement and Health," *Psychological Inquiry* 13 (2002): 190–200.

187. Jeffrey S. Levin and Harold Y. Vanderpool, "Is Religion Therapeutically Significant for Hypertension?," *Social Science and Medicine* 29 (1989): 69–78; later expanded in Levin, "How Religion Influences Morbidity and Health."

188. One study controlled for most of the mechanisms in the Levin and Vanderpool model, yet a statistically significant effect remained. What accounts for this remnant effect remains a mystery (Anthony Walsh, "Religion and Hypertension: Testing Alternative Explanations among Immigrants," *Behavioral Medicine* 24 (1998): 122–130).

189. Jeff Levin, Linda M. Chatters, and Robert Joseph Taylor, "Theory in Religion, Aging, and Health: An Overview," *Journal of Religion and Health* 50 (2011): 389–406.

190. Steve Paulson, Allan Kellehear, Jeffrey J. Kripal, and Lani Leary, "Confronting Mortality: Faith and Meaning across Cultures," *Annals of the New York Academy of Sciences* 1330 (2014): 58–74.

191. Linda L. Barnes and Susan S. Sered, eds., *Religion and Healing in America* (New York: Oxford University Press, 2005).

192. Levin, "Transcendent Experience and Health."

193. Robert C. Atchley, *Spirituality and Aging* (Baltimore: Johns Hopkins University Press, 2009); Harry R. Moody and David Carroll, *The Five Stages of the Soul: Charting the Spiritual Passages That Shape Our Lives* (New York: Anchor Books, 1997); W. Andrew Achenbaum, "Aging in Grace: The Spiritual Journey of Henri Nouwen," *Journal of Aging and Identity* 6 (2001): 183–198; and Thomas R. Cole, "On the Possibilities of Spirituality and Religious Humanism in Gerontology," in *Aging, Spirituality, and Religion: A Handbook*, vol. 2, ed. Melvin A. Kimble and Susan H. McFadden (Minneapolis: Fortress Press, 2003), 434–448.

194. E.g., L. Eugene Thomas, "Dialogues with Three Religious Renunciates and Reflections on Wisdom and Maturity," *International Journal of Aging and Human Development* 32 (1991): 211–227.

195. Ibid.

196. Ibid., quotation 225, emphasis added.

197. Joan Engebretson and Diane Wind Wardell, "Energy-Based Modalities," *Nursing Clinics of North America* 42 (2007): 243–259. A later article introduces their taxonomy of spiritual experiences, developed for studies of healing: Joan Engebretson and Diane Wind Wardell, "Energy Therapies: Focus on Spirituality," *EXPLORE: The Journal of Science and Healing* 8 (2012): 353–359.

198. Joel James Shuman and Keith G. Meador, *Heal Thyself: Spirituality, Medicine, and the Distortion of Christianity* (New York: Oxford University Press, 2008).

199. Ibid., 44.

200. Levin, "How Faith Heals," 92.

201. Neal Krause, "Religion and Health: Making Sense of a Disheveled Literature," *Journal of Religion and Health* 50 (2011): 20–35.

202. Jeff Levin and Keith G. Meador, eds., *Healing to All Their Flesh: Jewish and Christian Perspectives on Spirituality, Theology, and Health* (West Conshohocken, PA: Templeton Press, 2002).

203. Victor Frankl, *Man's Search for Meaning*, rev. and updated ed. (1959; New York: Washington Square Press, 1984), 141–142.

204. Dossey, *Healing Words*, 253.

Chapter 6

1. Frederick C. Elliott, *The Birth of the Texas Medical Center: A Personal Account*, ed. William Henry Kellar (College Station: Texas A&M University Press, 2004).

2. See the historical material at http://www.tmc.edu/.

3. Elliott, *The Birth of the Texas Medical Center*, 154.

4. Quoted in ibid, 199.

5. Westberg with McNamara, *Gentle Rebel*.

6. Cathey Graham Nickell, *Uniting Faith, Medicine and Healthcare: A 57-Year History of the Institute for Spirituality and Health at the Texas Medical Center* (La Vergne, TX: Lightning Source, 2012).

7. "Granger Westberg First Dean at Institute of Religion," *Pastoral Psychology* 15 (1964): 50.

8. Westberg with McNamara, *Gentle Rebel*, 273.

9. Nickell, *Uniting Faith, Medicine and Healthcare*, 28.

10. Kenneth L. Vaux, "Tomorrow's Education in Medicine and Ministry," *Journal of Religion and Health* 9 (1970): 285–291.

11. Nickell, *Uniting Faith, Medicine and Healthcare*, 23–29.

12. Westberg with McNamara, *Gentle Rebel*; and Nickell, *Uniting Faith, Medicine and Healthcare*.

13. Westberg with McNamara, *Gentle Rebel*, 155–156.

14. Nickell, *Uniting Faith, Medicine and Healthcare*, 34.

15. Kenneth L. Vaux, *This Mortal Coil: The Meaning of Health and Disease* (New York: Harper and Row, 1978).

16. Albert R. Jonsen, Andrew L. Jameton, and Abbyann Lynch, "Medical Ethics, History of: North America in the Twentieth Century," in *Encyclopedia of Bioethics,* vol. 3 (New York: Free Press, 1978), 992–1004, 1000.

17. Nickell, *Uniting Faith, Medicine and Healthcare,* 61–67.

18. Ibid., 40.

19. A Festschrift in Brody's honor: Mark J. Cherry and Ana Smith Iltis, eds., *Pluralistic Casuistry: Balancing Moral Arguments, Economic Realities, and Political Theory* (Dordrecht, Netherlands: Springer, 2007).

20. Program on Religion and Population Health (PRPH), Institute for Studies of Religion, Baylor University, http://www.baylorisr.org/programs-research/program-on-religion-and-population-health-prph/.

21. See William T. Butler's five-volume *Arming for Battle against Disease through Education, Research, and Patient Care at Baylor College of Medicine,* esp. book 2: *Independence* (Houston: Baylor College of Medicine, 2011).

22. Vicki Samuels Levy, "If You Build It, They Will Heal," *Jewish Herald Voice* (October 24, 2013), http://jhvonline.com/if-you-build-it-they-will-heal-p16054-89.htm.

23. In 1977 the Salk Institute's Roger Guillemin shared the Nobel Prize for Physiology or Medicine for research conducted earlier in his career in the Jewish Building ("Guillemin Recruitment Results in Nobel Prize," in Butler, *Arming for Battle against Disease through Education, Research, and Patient Care at Baylor College of Medicine,* book 1: *Rebirth in Houston,* 233–236).

24. Levy, "If You Build It, They Will Heal."

25. Daniel T. Kim, Farr A. Curlin, Kelly M. Wolenberg, and Daniel Sulmasy, "Back to the Future: The AMA and Religion, 1961–1974," *Academic Medicine* 89 (2014): 1603–1609; and Daniel Kim, Farr Curlin, Kelly Wolenberg, and Daniel Sulmasy, "Religion in Organized Medicine: The AMA's Committee and Department of Medicine and Religion, 1961–1974," *Perspectives in Biology and Medicine* 57 (2014): 393–414.

26. Kim et al, "Back to the Future," 1605.

27. Ibid.

28. Ibid., 1605.

29. Westberg with McNamara, *Gentle Rebel,* 156.

30. Kim et al., "Religion in Organized Medicine," 406–411.

31. Kim et al., "Back to the Future," and "Religion in Organized Medicine."

32. "Curriculum Vitae," in *Faith, Medicine, and Science: A Festschrift in Honor of Dr. David B. Larson,* ed. Jeff Levin and Harold G. Koenig (New York: Haworth Pastoral Press, 2005), 241–307.

33. Atwood D. Gaines, "The Twice-Born: 'Christian Psychiatry' and Christian Psychiatrists," *Culture, Medicine and Psychiatry* 6 (1982): 305–324.

34. See "Curriculum Vitae," in *Faith, Medicine, and Science.*

35. Khalid Khan, Regina Kunz, Jos Kleijnen, and Gerd Antes, *Systematic Reviews to Support Evidence-Based Medicine,* 2nd ed. (London: Hodder and Stoughton, 2011).

36. Levin and Koenig, *Faith, Medicine, and Science,* 18.

37. As revealed by a PubMed search on "systematic review." See also Mike Clarke and Iain Chalmers, "Reflections on the History of Systematic Reviews," *BMJ Evidence Based Medicine* 23 (2018): 121–122.

38. Mark Petticrew and Helen Roberts, *Systematic Reviews in the Social Sciences: A Practical Guide* (Malden, MA: Blackwell, 2006).

39. Khan et al., *Systematic Reviews to Support Evidence-Based Medicine*.

40. E.g., David B. Larson, John S. Lyons, Ann A. Hohmann, Robert S. Beardsley, Wendy M. Huckeba, Peter V. Rabins, and Barry D. Lebowitz, "A Systematic Review of Nursing Home Research in Three Psychiatric Journals: 1966–1985," *International Journal of Geriatric Psychiatry* 4, 3 (1989): 129–134.

41. David B. Larson, "Have Faith: Religion Can Heal Mental Ills," *Insight* (March 6, 1995), 18–20.

42. David B. Larson, panel moderator, "Religion and Mental Health," 117th Annual Meeting of the American Public Health Association, Chicago, Illinois, October 22–26, 1989.

43. Stephen G. Post, *Is Ultimate Reality Unlimited Love?* (West Conshohocken, PA: Templeton Press, 2014). See also John Marks Templeton, *Worldwide Laws of Life: 200 Eternal Spiritual Principles* (Philadelphia: Templeton Foundation Press, 1997).

44. Robert L. Hermann, *Sir John Templeton: Supporting Scientific Research for Spiritual Discoveries*, rev. ed. (Radnor, PA: Templeton Foundation Press, 2004).

45. Spiritual Dimensions in Clinical Research, sponsored by NIHR and JTF, Leesburg, Virginia, April 20–23, 1995; Religious, Social, and Environmental Factors That Influence Disease States, AAAS Annual Meeting, Baltimore, Maryland, February 11, 1996; and Spiritual Intervention in Clinical Practice, sponsored by NIHR and JTF, Leesburg, Virginia, April 18–21, 1996.

46. Matthews et al., *The Faith Factor*; Larson et al., *Scientific Research on Spirituality and Health*; and Larson and Larson, *The Forgotten Factor in Physical and Mental Health*.

47. Dale Matthews with Connie Clark, *The Faith Factor: Proof of the Healing Power of Prayer* (New York: Viking, 1998).

48. Ibid., 274.

49. Hermann, *Sir John Templeton*, 60.

50. Ibid., 59–62.

51. Christina M. Puchalski and David B. Larson, "Developing Curricula in Spirituality and Medicine," *Academic Medicine* 73 (1998): 970–974. See also "Medical Story: More Grants for Doctors to Understand Spirituality," *Religion News Service* (August 28, 1996), https://religionnews.com/1996/08/28/medical-story-more-grants-to-help-doctors-understand-spirituality/; and "Awards Recognize Residencies for Incorporating Spirituality," *Psychiatric News* (May 1, 1998), http://psychnews.org/pnews/98-05-01/award.html.

52. Quoted in B. Denise Hawkins, "In the Spirit of Healing; Morehouse Medical Professors Win Grant to Teach the Medicinal Power of Spirituality," *Black Issues in Higher Education* (October 16, 1997), https://www.questia.com/read/1G1-20211542/in-the-spirit-of-healing-morehouse-medical-professors.

53. "Awards Recognize Residencies for Incorporating Spirituality."

54. Mentioned by John Templeton, in Levin and Koenig, *Faith, Medicine and Science*, 65.
55. Ibid., 65.
56. Harold G. Koenig, Elizabeth G. Hooten, Erin Lindsay-Calkins, and Keith G. Meador, "Spirituality in Medical School Curricula: Findings from a National Survey," *International Journal of Psychiatry in Medicine* 40 (2010): 391–398.
57. Ibid.
58. Center for Spirituality, Theology and Health, Duke University (2014), https://spiritualityandhealth.duke.edu/.
59. Ibid.
60. Harold Koenig with Gregg Lewis, *The Healing Connection: A World-Renowned Medical Scientist Discovers the Powerful Link between Christian Faith and Health* (Nashville: Word, 2000).
61. Duke Summer Research Workshops, Center for Spirituality, Theology and Health, Duke University (2014), https://spiritualityandhealth.duke.edu/index.php/education/workshops.
62. Koenig, *The Healing Power of Faith*.
63. Levin and Koenig, *Faith, Medicine, and Science*.
64. Jeff Levin and Harold G. Koenig, "Faith Matters: Reflections on the Life and Work of Dr. David B. Larson," in Levin and Koenig, *Faith, Medicine, and Science*, 3–25, esp. 11.
65. Theology, Medicine, and Culture, Duke Divinity School (2015), https://tmc.divinity.duke.edu/.
66. Ellen Idler and Mimi Kiser, "Religion and Public Health at Emory University," in *Why Religion and Spirituality Matter for Public Health: Evidence, Implications, and Resources*, ed. Doug Oman (Cham, Switzerland: Springer Nature, 2018), 357–370.
67. Interfaith Health Program, Emory University (2014), http://www.interfaithhealth.emory.edu/.
68. E.g., Thomas A. Droege, "Congregations as Communities of Health and Healing," *Journal of Religion and Health* 49 (1995): 117–129.
69. "About IHP," Interfaith Health Program, Emory University (2018), http://ihpemory.org/ihp-what-we-do/.
70. "IHP Reports," Interfaith Health Program, Emory University (2018), http://ihpemory.org/publications/ihp-reports/.
71. Kegler et al., "Evaluation Findings from the Institute for Public Health and Faith Collaborations," and Kegler et al., "Facilitators, Challenges, and Collaborative Activities in Faith and Health Partnerships to Address Health Disparities."
72. "The Institute for Public Health & Faith Collaborations," Interfaith Health Program, Emory University (2018), http://ihpemory.org/ihp-programs/the-institute-for-public-health-faith-collaborations/.
73. Religion and Public Health Collaborative, Emory University (2018), http://www.rphcemory.org/.
74. Idler, *Religion as a Social Determinant of Health*.
75. Christina M. Puchalski and Betty Ferrell, *Making Health Care Whole: Integrating Spirituality into Patient Care* (West Conshohocken, PA: Templeton Press, 2010). See also https://smhs.gwu.edu/gwish/.

76. Puchalski and Larson, "Developing Curricula in Spirituality and Medicine"; and Christina M. Puchalski, David B. Larson, and Francis G. Lu, "Spirituality Courses in Psychiatry Residency Programs," *Psychiatric Annals* 30 (2000): 543–548.

77. Christina M. Puchalski, Robert J. Vitillo, and Najmeh Jafari, "Global Network for Spirituality and Health (GNSAH): Seeking More Compassionate Health Systems," *Journal for the Study of Spirituality* 6 (2016): 106–112.

78. Aparna Sajja and Christina M. Puchalski, "Training Physicians as Healers," *AMA Journal of Ethics* 20 (2018): E655–E663.

79. Jeffrey S. Levin, David B. Larson, and Christina M. Puchalski, "Religion and Spirituality in Medicine: Research and Education," *JAMA* 278 (1997): 792–793.

80. Mark Cobb, Christina M. Puchalski, and Bruce Rumbold, *Oxford Textbook of Spirituality in Healthcare* (New York: Oxford University Press, 2012).

81. Allen H. Neims, Monika Ardelt, Shaya R. Isenberg, and Louis A. Ritz, "The Center for Spirituality and Health at the University of Florida," *Spirituality in Higher Education Newsletter* 4, 2 (2008): 1–8. See also Center for Spirituality and Health, University of Florida (2006), http://www.ufspiritualityandhealth.org/.

82. "Mission," Center for Spirituality and Health, University of Florida (2006), http://www.ufspiritualityandhealth.org/mission/.

83. Jeff Levin, "God, Faith, and Health: Epidemiologic Reflections on Spirituality," University of Florida Center for Spirituality and Health, Gainesville, Florida, March 20, 2003.

84. Program on Medicine and Religion, University of Chicago (2018), https://pmr.uchicago.edu/.

85. Ibid.

86. Aasim I. Padela, "Islamic Medical Ethics: A Primer," *Bioethics* 21 (2007): 169–178.

87. Quoted from https://pmr.uchicago.edu/.

88. Initiative on Health, Religion, and Spirituality, Harvard University (2018), https://projects.iq.harvard.edu/rshm.

89. Tyler J. VanderWeele, Michael J. Balboni, and Tracy A. Balboni, "The Initiative on Health, Religion and Spirituality at Harvard: From Research to Education," in Oman, *Why Religion and Spirituality Matter for Public Health*, 371–382.

90. "Research Programs," Initiative on Health, Religion, and Spirituality, Harvard University (2018), https://projects.iq.harvard.edu/rshm/research-programs.

91. E.g., Tyler J. VanderWeele, Tracy A. Balboni, and Howard K. Koh, "Health and Spirituality," *JAMA* 318 (2017): 519–520.

92. "Religion, Health and Medicine Program," SRC: Science, Religion, and Culture, Harvard Divinity School, Harvard University (2018), https://src.hds.harvard.edu/pages/religion-health-medicine-program.

93. An early review of program websites: Mona Stevermer, "Spirituality and Health Care: Internet Resources," *Medical Reference Services Quarterly* 23, 2 (2004): 57–71.

94. Earl E. Bakken Center for Spirituality and Healing, University of Minnesota (2018), https://www.csh.umn.edu/.

95. Mary Jo Kreitzer, "Spirituality and Well-Being: Focusing on What Matters," *Western Journal of Nursing Research* 34 (2012): 707–711.

96. Quoted from "Spirituality and Health at MUSC," Department of Family Medicine, Medical University of South Carolina (June 11, 2008), https://web.archive.org/web/20130111012006/http://www.musc.edu/dfm/Spirituality/Spirituality.htm.

97. Dana E. King, *Faith, Spirituality, and Medicine: Toward the Making of the Healing Practitioner* (New York: Haworth Pastoral Press, 2000).

98. King coauthored the second edition of the *Handbook of Religion and Health.*

99. Center for the Study of Health, Religion and Spirituality, Indiana State University (2013), https://web.archive.org/web/20130616001949/http://www.unboundedpossibilities.com:80/center-for-the-study-of-health-religion-and-spirituality.aspx.

100. Christine Kennedy and Sharon E. Cheston, "Spiritual Distress at Life's End: Finding Meaning in the Maelstrom," *Journal of Pastoral Care and Counseling* 57 (2003): 131–141.

101. Thomas M. Haney, "The Role of Religion in a Catholic Law School: A Century of Experience at Loyola University Chicago," *Social Justice Paper* 14 (2014): 126, https://ecommons.luc.edu/cgi/viewcontent.cgi?article=1013&context=social_justice.

102. Kalsman Institute on Judaism and Health, Hebrew Union College–Jewish Institute of Religion, http://kalsman.huc.edu/.

103. Centre for Spirituality, Health and Disability, The School of Divinity, History and Philosophy, University of Aberdeen (December 11, 2019), https://www.abdn.ac.uk/sdhp/centre-for-spirituality-health-and-disability-182.php.

104. John Swinton, *Becoming Friends of Time: Disability, Timefullness, and Gentle Discipleship* (Waco, TX: Baylor University Press, 2016).

105. The Scientific and Medical Network (2019), https://explore.scimednet.org/.

106. "About the United States Spiritist Medical Association SMA-US," SMA-US (2018), http://www.sma-us.org/.

107. AME Internacional (2018), http://www.ameinternational.org/site/en/.

108. Mark Hart, "Review of Spirituality and Healing in Medicine Symposium," *Caregiver Journal* 12, 3 (1996): 32–34.

109. "Annual Meeting of the Society for Spirituality, Theology & Health," Center for Spirituality, Theology and Health, Duke University (2014), https://spiritualityandhealth.duke.edu/index.php/education/annual-meeting.

110. "About Us," Conference on Medicine & Religion, http://www.medicineandreligion.com/about-us.html.

111. Quoted from ibid.

112. Kenneth E. Appel, "Academy of Religion and Mental Health: Past and Future," *Journal of Religion and Health* 4 (1965): 207–216.

113. The first volume: Academy of Religion and Mental Health, *Religion, Science, and Mental Health: Proceedings of the First Academy Symposium on Inter-Discipline Responsibility for Mental Health—A Religious and Scientific Concern—1957* (New York: New York University Press, 1959). Several volumes were published over the next decade.

114. "Blanton-Peale Timeline," Blanton-Peale Institute and Counseling Center (2018), https://www.blantonpeale.org/timeline.html.

115. Bruce Buursma, "Medical Ethics and Religion," *Chicago Tribune* (May 4, 1986), http://www.chicagotribune.com/news/ct-xpm-1986-05-04-8602010151-story. html.

116. "Our Mission," Park Ridge Center for Health, Faith, and Ethics (2003), https://web. archive.org/web/20110707150247/http://www.parkridgecenter.org/Page700.html.

117. The initial volume: Marty and Vaux, *Health/Medicine and the Faith Traditions*.

118. Monographs were commissioned for the Catholic, Anglican, Methodist, Lutheran, Reformed, Eastern Orthodox, Anabaptist, Evangelical, Latter-Day Saints, Christian Science, Jewish, Islamic, Hindu, and Native American traditions.

119. Puchalski and Larson, "Developing Curricula in Spirituality and Medicine," 971.

120. Auguste H. Fortin and Katherine Gergen Barnett, "Medical School Curricula in Spirituality and Medicine," *JAMA* 291 (2004): 2883.

121. Koenig et al., "Spirituality in Medical School Curricula." At that time, comparable numbers for the United Kingdom were nearly 60% (David Neely and Eunice J. Minford, "Current Status of Teaching on Spirituality in UK Medical Schools," *Medical Education* 42 (2008): 176–182).

122. Fortin and Barnett, "Medical School Curricula in Spirituality and Medicine."

123. Harold G. Koenig, "Taking a Spiritual History," *JAMA* 291 (2004): 2881–2882.

124. Puchalski and Larson, "Developing Curricula in Spirituality and Medicine."

125. Levin et al., "Religion and Spirituality in Medicine," 792.

126. Puchalski et al., "Spirituality Course in Psychiatry Residency Programs."

127. Keith G. Meador and Harold G. Koenig, "Spirituality and Religion in Psychiatric Practice: Parameters and Implications," *Psychiatric Annals* 30 (2000): 549–555.

128. "Faith and Medicine: Exploring Religious Faith and Spirituality as Part of Good Medicine," Albert Einstein College of Medicine (August 30, 2011), http://www. einstein.yu.edu/features/stories/699/exploring-religious-faith-and-spirituality-as-part-of-good-medicine/.

129. Beverly D. Taylor, Ayanna V. Buckner, Carla Durham Walker, and Daniel S. Blumenthal, "Faith-Based Partnerships in Graduate Medical Education: The Experience of the Morehouse School of Medicine Public Health / Preventive Medicine Residency Program," *American Journal of Preventive Medicine* 41 (2011): S283–S289.

130. "Competency Cluster #10: Proficiency in the Appropriate Use of Religion/Spirituality in Clinical Practice," in "Training Competencies," Loma Linda University School of Medicine (2018), https://medicine.llu.edu/clinical-psychology-internship/academics/ training-competencies.

131. David Neely and Eunice J. Minford, "Current Status of Teaching on Spirituality in UK Medical Schools," *Medical Education* 42 (2008): 176–182.

132. Giancarlo Lucchetti, Alessandra Lamas Granero Lucchetti, Daniele Corcioli Mendes Espinha, Leandro Romani de Oliveira, José Roberto Leite, and Harold G. Koenig, "Spirituality and Health in the Curricula of Medical Schools in Brazil," *BMC Medical Education* 12 (2012): 78, doi: 10.1186/1472-6920-12-78.

133. Lisa Marr, J. Andrew Billings, and David E. Weissman, "Spirituality Training for Palliative Care Fellows," *Journal of Palliative Medicine* 10 (2007): 169–177.

134. Wendy M. Greenstreet, "Teaching Spirituality in Nursing: A Literature Review," *Nurse Education Today* 19 (1999): 649–658.

135. Meredith Wallace, Suzanne Campbell, Sheila C. Grossman, Joyce M. Shea, Jean W. Lange, and Theresa T. Quell, "Integrating Spirituality into Undergraduate Nursing Curricula," *International Journal of Nursing Education Scholarship* 5, 1 (2008): Article 10, https://www-degruyter-com.proxy.lib.duke.edu/downloadpdf/j/ijnes.2008.5.issue-1/ijnes.2008.5.1.1443/ijnes.2008.5.1.1443.pdf.

136. E.g., a report from Turkey: Meryem Yilmaz and Hesna Gurler, "The Efficacy of Integrating Spirituality into Undergraduate Nursing Curricula," *Nursing Ethics* 21 (2014): 929–945.

137. Wallace et al., "Integrating Spirituality into Undergraduate Nursing Curricula."

138. Lynn Clark Callister, A. Elaine Bond, Gerry Matusmura, and Sandra Mangum, "Threading Spirituality throughout Nursing Education," *Holistic Nursing Practice* 18 (2004): 160–166.

139. Wallace et al., "Integrating Spirituality into Undergraduate Nursing Curricula."

140. Thomas R. Cole, Nathan S. Carlin, and Ronald A. Carson, *Medical Humanities: An Introduction* (New York: Cambridge University Press, 2015), esp. part IV, "Religion and Medicine," 291–372.

141. "About Us," Center for Medical Ethics and Health Policy, Baylor College of Medicine (2018), https://www.bcm.edu/centers/medical-ethics-and-health-policy/about-us.

142. American Society for Bioethics and Humanities (2018), asbh.org/.

143. Sarah L. Berry, Erin Gentry Lamb, and Therese Jones, *Health Humanities Baccalaureate Programs in the United States* (Hiram, OH: Hiram College, 2017), http://www.hiram.edu/wp-content/uploads/2017/09/HHBP2017.pdf.

144. Erin Gentry Lamb and Sarah Berry, "Snapshots of Baccalaureate Health Humanities Programs," *Journal of Medical Humanities* 38 (2017): 511–534.

145. Linda L. Barnes and Inés Talamantez, *Teaching Religion and Healing* (New York: Oxford University Press, 2006).

146. Oman, *Why Religion and Spirituality Matter for Public Health*.

147. Doug Oman, "An Evidence-Based Course at U.C. Berkeley on Religious and Spiritual Factors in Public Health," in Oman, *Why Religion and Spirituality Matter for Public Health*, 383–395.

148. Christine M. A. Gebel, Katelyn N. G. Long, and Michael A. Grodin, "The Boston University Experience: Religion, Ethics, and Public Health," in Oman, *Why Religion and Spirituality Matter for Public Health*, 397–408.

149. Linda M. Chatters, "Faith Matters: 'HBHE 710: Religion, Spirituality, and Health' at the University of Michigan," in Oman, *Why Religion and Spirituality Matter for Public Health*, 409–420.

150. Nancy E. Epstein, "Incorporating Religion and Spirituality into Teaching and Practice: The Drexel School of Public Health Experience," in Oman, *Why Religion and Spirituality Matter for Public Health*, 421–433.

151. Kathryn Lyndes, Wendy Cadge, and George Fitchett, "Online Teaching of Public Health and Spirituality at University of Illinois: Chaplains for the Twenty-First Century," in Oman, *Why Religion and Spirituality Matter for Public Health*, 435–444.

152. Levin, "Engaging the Faith Community for Public Health Advocacy."
153. Levin, "'And Let Us Make Us a Name.'"
154. Brian M. Berman and David B. Larson, *Alternative Medicine: Expanding Medical Horizons: A Report to the National Institutes of Health on Alternative Medical Systems and Practices in the United States*, NIH Pub. No. 94-066 (Washington, DC: U.S. Government Printing Office, 1995).
155. Jeanne Achterberg, Larry Dossey, James S. Gordon, Carol Hegedus, Marian W. Hermann, and Roger Nelson, "Mind-Body Interventions," in Berman and Larson, 3–43.
156. Websites and mission statements for major academic centers are found at Academic Consortium for Integrative Medicine and Health (2018), https://imconsortium.org/.
157. Marilyn Schlitz and Tina Amorok with Marc S. Micozzi, eds., *Consciousness and Healing: Integral Approaches to Mind-Body Medicine* (St. Louis: Elsevier Churchill Livingstone, 2005).
158. Jonas and Crawford, *Healing, Intention, and Energy Medicine*.
159. Christian Medical and Dental Association (2018), https://cmda.org/.
160. A network of professional associations for physicians, each sponsored by a local medical society, Jewish federation, or medical school. Each is independent with its own schedule of events, including educational lectures.
161. IMANA: Islamic Medical Association of North America, https://imana.org/.
162. Christian Medical Fellowship (2018), https://www.cmf.org.uk/.
163. Nurses Christian Fellowship, InterVarsity Christian Fellowship/USA (2018), https://ncf-jcn.org/.
164. American Holistic Nurses Association (2018), https://www.ahna.org/.
165. Catholic Student Ministry at the Texas Medical Center (2018), https://tmc-catholic.org/.
166. Chabad at the Medical Center (2018), https://www.chabadtmc.org/.
167. Jacquline Sarver, "Footpath of Faith," *The Houston Review* 2,1 (2010): 20–25.
168. Duke Summer Research Workshops.
169. "Trainees," Initiative on Health, Religion, and Spirituality, Harvard University (2018), https://projects.iq.harvard.edu/rshm/people/trainees.
170. E.g., Cassandra Vieten and Shelley Scammell, *Spiritual and Religious Competencies in Clinical Practice: Guidelines for Psychotherapists and Mental Health Professionals* (Oakland, CA: New Harbinger Publications, 2015).
171. Michael Balboni and John Peteet, eds., *Spirituality and Religion Within the Culture of Medicine: From Evidence to Practice* (New York: Oxford University Press, 2017).
172. E.g., Philip R. Muskin and Anna L. Dickerman, eds., *Study Guide for the Psychiatry Board Examination* (Arlington, VA: American Psychiatric Association, 2016) contains dozens of mentions of religion, religiousness, or spirituality, including a chapter on the topic (135–136).

Chapter 7

1. Alvin Toffler, *Future Shock* (New York: Random House, 1970).
2. Marilyn Ferguson, *The Aquarian Conspiracy: Personal and Social Transformation in the 1980s* (Los Angeles: Jeremy Tarcher, 1980).
3. Norman Cousins, "Anatomy of an Illness (as Perceived by the Patient)," *New England Journal of Medicine* 295 (1976): 1458–1463, expanded into *Anatomy of an Illness as Perceived by the Patient: Reflections on Healing and Regeneration* (New York: Norton, 1979).
4. George L. Engel, "The Need for a New Medical Model: A Challenge for Biomedicine," *Science* 196 (1977): 129–136.
5. Soma Hewa and Robert W. Hetherington, "Specialists without Spirit: Limitations of the Mechanistic Biomedical Model," *Theoretical Medicine* 16 (1995): 129–139.
6. Albert R. Jonsen, *The Birth of Bioethics* (New York: Oxford University Press, 1998), quotations 11.
7. Ibid., 12.
8. Ibid., 13.
9. Ibid., 3.
10. See Van Renssalaer Potter, "Bioethics, the Science of Survival," *Perspectives in Biology and Medicine* 14 (1970): 127–153, and his *Bioethics: Bridge to the Future* (Englewood Cliffs, NJ: Prentice-Hall, 1971). He later preferred the term *global bioethics* (Henk A. M. J. ten Have, "Potter's Notion of Bioethics," *Kennedy Institute of Ethics Journal* 22 (2012): 59–82).
11. Thomas Percival, *Medical Ethics; or, a Code of Institutes and Precepts, Adapted to the Professional Conduct of Physicians and Surgeons* (London: S. Russell, 1803).
12. Jonsen, *The Birth of Bioethics*, esp. chapter 2, "The Theologians: Rediscovering the Tradition," 34–64, and chapter 3, "The Philosophers: Clarifying the Concepts," 65–89.
13. Albert R. Jonsen, *A Short History of Medical Ethics* (New York: Oxford University Press, 2000).
14. Jonsen, *The Birth of Bioethics*, esp. chapter 1, "Great Issues of Conscience: Medical Ethics before Bioethics," 3–33; and Chapter 4, "Commissioning Bioethics: The Government in Bioethics, 1974–1983," 90–122.
15. Farr A. Curlin, "Religion and Spirituality in Medical Ethics," in Balboni and Peteet, *Spirituality and Religion within the Culture of Medicine*, 179–194, 179.
16. Jonsen, *The Birth of Bioethics*, 352.
17. Immanuel Jakobovits, *Jewish Medical Ethics: A Comparative and Historical Study of the Jewish Religious Attitude to Medicine and Its Practice* (New York: Bloch, 1959).
18. Alan Brill, "Immanuel Jakobovits and the Birth of Jewish Medical Ethics," in *Halakhic Realities: Collected Essays on Brain Death*, ed. Zev Farber (New Milford, CT: Maggid Books, 2015), 327–348.
19. Immanuel Jakobovits, "Jewish Medical Ethics" [Letter], *British Medical Journal* 2, 5203 (1960): 946, 946.

20. Immanuel Jakobovits, "Jewish Medical Ethics—A Brief Overview," *Journal of Medical Ethics* 9 (1983): 109–112; and "Ethical Problems regarding the Termination of Life," in *Jewish Values in Bioethics*, ed. Levi Meier (New York: Human Sciences Press, 1986), 84–95. See also Yoel Jakobovits, "Lord Immanuel Jakobovits (1921–)," in *Pioneers of Jewish Medical Ethics*, ed. Fred Rosner (Northvale, NJ: Jason Aronson, 1997), 127–164.

21. Brill, "Immanuel Jacobovits and the Birth of Jewish Medical Ethics."

22. Jakobovits, *Jewish Medical Ethics*, esp. the introduction (xxxi–xlii) and first chapter (1–23).

23. Moshe Feinstein, *Responsa of Rav Moshe Feinstein,* vol. 1: *Care of the Critically Ill,* trans. and annotated by Moshe Dovid Tendler (Hoboken, NJ: KTAV, 1995), a compilation of material from Feinstein's *Iggeros Moshe*, a 7-volume Hebrew-language collection of his *t'shuvot.*

24. Avraham Steinberg, "Rabbi Shlomo Zalman Auerbach (1910–1995)," in Rosner, *Pioneers in Jewish Medical Ethics*, 99–126.

25. Avraham Steinberg, "Rabbi Eliezer Yehudah Waldenberg (1920–)," in Rosner, *Pioneers in Jewish Medical Ethics*, 165–201.

26. Brill, "Immanuel Jacobovits and the Birth of Jewish Medical Ethics," 329.

27. Ibid.

28. Jonsen, *The Birth of Bioethics*, 41–55.

29. Vaux, *This Mortal Coil.*.

30. Allen D. Verhey, ed., *Religion and Medical Ethics: Looking Back, Looking Forward* (Grand Rapids: Eerdmans, 1996).

31. Harmon L. Smith, "Medical Ethics in the Primary Care Setting," *Social Science and Medicine* 25 (1987): 705–709.

32. Stanley Hauerwas, *Suffering Presence: Theological Reflections on Medicine, the Mentally Handicapped, and the Church* (Notre Dame, IN: University of Notre Dame Press, 1986), and Hauerwas, *God, Medicine, and Suffering* (Grand Rapids: Eerdmans, 1990). See also Stanley Hauerwas, "Suffering Presence: Twenty-Five Years Later," in Levin and Meador, *Healing to All Their Flesh*, 242–258.

33. Gilbert Meilaender, *Bioethics: A Primer for Christians*, 3rd ed. (Grand Rapids: Eerdmans, 2013).

34. Edmund D. Pellegrino and David C. Thomasma, *The Christian Virtues in Medical Practice* (Washington, DC: Georgetown University Press, 1996), and Pellegrino and Thomasma, *Helping and Healing: Religious Commitment in Health Care* (Washington, DC: Georgetown University Press, 1997).

35. Swinton, *Becoming Friends of Time*. See also John Swinton, ed., *Critical Reflections on Stanley Hauerwas' Theology of Disability: Disabling Society, Enabling Theology* (Binghamton, NY: Haworth Pastoral Press, 2004).

36. Stephen G. Post, ed., *Encyclopedia of Bioethics*, 3rd ed. (New York: Macmillan Reference USA, 2004).

37. Albert R. Jonsen, "A History of Religion and Bioethics," in *Handbook of Bioethics and Religion*, ed. David E. Guinn (New York: Oxford University Press, 2006), 103–136.

38. Ibid., 23.

39. Ibid., 34.

40. David H. Smith, "Religion and the Roots of the Bioethics Revival," in Verhey, *Religion and Medical Ethics*, 9–18; and Leroy Walters, "Religion and the Renaissance of Medical Ethics in the United States: 1965–1975," in *Theology and Bioethics*, ed. Earl E. Shelp (Dordrecht, Netherlands: Springer Science + Business Media, 1985), 3–16.

41. Fred Rosner, "Lord Immanuel Jakobovits: Grandfather of Jewish Medical Ethics," *Israel Medical Association Journal* 3 (2001): 304–310.

42. Paul F. Camenisch, ed., *Religious Methods and Resources in Bioethics* (Dordrecht, Netherlands: Kluwer Academic Publishers, 1994).

43. John H. Evans, "Who Legitimately Speaks for Religion in Public Bioethics?," in Guinn, *Handbook of Religion and Bioethics*, 61–79, 61.

44. Albert R. Jonsen, "The Confessor as Experienced Physician: Casuistry and Clinical Ethics," in Guinn, *Handbook of Religion and Bioethics*, 165–180, and James F. Childress, "Ethical Theories, Principles, and Casuistry in Bioethics: An Interpretation and Defense of Principlism," in Guinn, *Handbook of Religion and Bioethics*, 181–201.

45. Mark Kuczewski, "Casuistry and Principlism: The Convergence of Method in Biomedical Ethics," *Theoretical Medicine and Bioethics* 19 (1998): 509–524; Carson Strong, "Specified Principlism: What Is It, and Does It Really Resolve Cases Better Than Casuistry?," *Journal of Medicine and Philosophy* 25 (2000): 323–341; and Paul Cudney, "What Really Separates Casuistry from Principlism in Biomedical Ethics," *Theoretical Medicine and Bioethics* 35 (2014): 205–229.

46. Aaron L. Mackler, *Introduction to Jewish and Catholic Bioethics: A Comparative Analysis* (Washington, DC: Georgetown University Press, 2003); and Edmund D. Pellegrino and Alan I. Faden, eds., *Jewish and Catholic Bioethics: An Ecumenical Dialogue* (Washington, DC: Georgetown University Press, 1999).

47. Peggy Morgan and Clive A. Lawton, eds., *Ethical Issues in Six Religious Traditions*, 2nd ed. (Edinburgh: Edinburgh University Press, 2007), summarizes the views of Hinduism, Buddhism, Sikhism, Judaism, Christianity, and Islam.

48. Francis W. Peabody, "The Care of the Patient," *JAMA* 88 (1927): 877–882.

49. Paul Weindling, "The Origins of Informed Consent: The International Scientific Commission on Medical War Crimes, and the Nuremberg Code," *Bulletin of the History of Medicine* 75 (2001): 37–71; Michael A. Grodin and George J. Annas, "Legacies of Nuremberg: Medical Ethics and Human Rights," *JAMA* 276 (1996): 1682–1683; and George J. Annas and Michael A. Grodin, "The Nuremberg Code," in *The Oxford Textbook of Clinical Research Ethics*, ed. Ezekiel J. Emanuel, Christine Grady, Robert A. Crouch, Reider K. Lie, Franklin G. Miller, and David Wendler (New York: Oxford University Press, 2008), 136–140.

50. "The Theologians: Rediscovering the Tradition," chapter 2 in Emanuel et al., *The Oxford Textbook of Clinical Research Ethics*, 34–64.

51. "The Philosophers: Clarifying the Concepts," chapter 3 in Emanuel et al., *The Oxford Textbook of Clinical Research Ethics*, 65–89.

52. "Bioethics as a Discipline," chapter 10 in Emanuel et al., *The Oxford Textbook of Clinical Research Ethics*, 325–351.

53. Bioethics has been termed a "second-order discipline," an interdisciplinary field bringing together scholars from other professions, disciplines, and fields (Loretta M. Kopelman, "The Growth of Bioethics as a Second-Order Discipline," in *The Development of Bioethics in the United States*, ed. Jeremy R. Garrett, Fabrice Jotterand, and D. Christopher Ralston, eds. (Dordrecht, Netherlands: Springer Science + Business Media, 2013), 137–159).

54. H. Tristram Engelhardt Jr., *The Foundations of Bioethics*, second ed. (New York: Oxford University Press, 1996), quotation vii.

55. Ibid., 11.

56. Ibid., 3.

57. Ibid., 36.

58. Ibid.

59. K. Danner Clouser and Bernard Gert, "A Critique of Principlism," *Journal of Medicine and Philosophy* 15 (1990): 219–236.

60. Engelhardt, *The Foundations of Bioethics*, 124–125.

61. Lisa Sowle Cahill, "Theologians and Bioethics: Some History and a Proposal," in *On Moral Medicine: Theological Perspectives in Medical Ethics*, ed. M. Therese Lysaught and Joseph J. Kotna, with Stephen E. Lammers and Allen Verhey (Grand Rapids: Eerdmans, 2012), 60–76 (excerpted from the author's *Theological Bioethics: Participation, Justice, and Change* (Washington, DC: Georgetown University Press, 2005)).

62. A summary of its work is found in Stephen G. Post, "Interacting with Other Worlds: A Review of Books from the Park Ridge Center" [Book Review], *Medical Humanities Review* 42, 2 (1990): 45–54.

63. The Kennedy Institute of Ethics, Georgetown University, https://kennedyinstitute. georgetown.edu/.

64. The Hastings Center, https://www.thehastingscenter.org/.

65. Daniel Callahan, "Bioethics as a Discipline," *Hastings Center Studies* 1, 1 (1973): 66–73.

66. See the special supplement on "Theology, Religious Traditions, and Bioethics," in *Hastings Center Report* 20, 4, Suppl. (1990): 1–24; and Warren T. Reich, "Revisiting the Launching of the Kennedy Institute: Re-Visioning the Origins of Bioethics," *Kennedy Institute of Ethics Journal* 6 (1996): 323–327.

67. Mark Aulisio, "Why Did Hospital Ethics Committees Emerge in the US?," *AMA Journal of Ethics* 18 (2016): 546–553.

68. Stuart J. Youngner, David L. Jackson, Claudia Coulton, Barbara W. Juknialis, and Era M. Smith, "A National Survey of Hospital Ethics Committees," *Critical Care Medicine* 11 (1983): 902–905.

69. Glenn McGee, Joshua Spanogle, Arthur L. Caplan, and David A. Asch, "A National Study of Ethics Committees," *American Journal of Bioethics* 1, 4 (2001): 60–64.

70. Ellen Fox, Sarah Myers, and Robert A. Pearlman, "Ethics Consultation in United States Hospitals: A National Survey," *American Journal of Bioethics* 7 (2007): 13–25.

71. Joint Commission on Accreditation of Healthcare Organizations, "Patient Rights," in *Accreditation Manual for Hospitals, 1992* (Oakbrook Terrace, IL: Joint Commission on Accreditation of Healthcare Organizations, 1993), 1–16.

72. John C. Fletcher and Diane E. Hoffman, "Ethics Committees: Time to Experiment with Standards," *Annals of Internal Medicine* 120 (1994): 335–338.

73. George Annas and Michael Grodin, "Hospital Ethics Committees, Consultants, and Courts," *AMA Journal of Ethics* 18 (2016): 554–559.

74. Fatemeh Hajibabaee, Soodabeh Joolaee, Mohammad Ali Cheraghi, Pooneh Salari, and Patricia Rodney, "Hospital/Clinical Ethics Committees' Notion: An Overview," *Journal of Medical Ethics and History of Medicine* 9, 17 (2016), https://www.ncbi.nlm.nih.gov/pmc/articles/PMC5432947/pdf/JMEHM-9-17.pdf.

75. Margaret R. Moon, "The History and Role of Institutional Review Boards: A Useful Tension," *Virtual Mentor* 11 (2009): 311–316.

76. National Research Act, P.L. 93–348 (July 12, 1974), https://www.govinfo.gov/content/pkg/STATUTE-88/pdf/STATUTE-88-Pg342.pdf.

77. Todd W. Rice, "The Historical, Ethical, and Legal Background of Human-Subjects Research," *Respiratory Care* 53 (2008): 1325–1329.

78. Stephen G. Post, "The IRB, Ethics, and the Objective Study of Religion in Health," *IRB: Ethics and Human Research* 17, 5–6 (1995): 8–11; and Laurence J. O'Connell, "Religious Perspectives and the Work of the Ethics Committee," *HEC Forum* 7 (1995): 205–210.

79. "ASBH History," American Society for Bioethics and Humanities, http://asbh.org/about/history.

80. "Bioethics and Humanities Academic Programs," American Society for Bioethics and Humanities, http://asbh.org/professional-development/academic-programs.

81. "Graduate Bioethics Education Programs Results," Association of Bioethics Program Directors (2019), https://www.bioethicsdirectors.net/graduate-bioethics-education-programs-results/.

82. Warren T. Reich, ed., *Encyclopedia of Bioethics* (New York: Free Press, 1978).

83. Bruce Jennings, ed., *Encyclopedia of Bioethics*, 4th ed. (Farmington Hills, MI: Macmillan Reference USA, 2014).

84. Martin Marty, quoted in Bruce Buursma, "Medical Ethics and Religion: New Center Hopes to Reconcile Questions, Conflicts," *Chicago Tribune* (May 4, 1986).

85. See the special issue, "Theology and Bioethics," of the *Journal of Medicine and Philosophy* (June 1992), especially the lead article, Lisa Sowle Cahill, "Theology and Bioethics: Should Religious Traditions Have a Public Voice?," *Journal of Medicine and Philosophy* 17 (1992): 263–272.

86. Guinn, *Handbook of Bioethics and Religion*.

87. Numerous monographs were published, including material on Anabaptist, Buddhist, Christian Science, Episcopal, Islamic, Jehovah's Witness, Jewish, Latter-Day Saint, Lutheran, Orthodox Christian, Presbyterian, Roman Catholic, Seventh-day Adventist, United Church of Christ, and United Methodist traditions.

88. Elliot N. Dorff, *The Jewish Tradition: Religious Beliefs and Health Care Decisions* (Chicago: Park Ridge Center, 1996).

89. A set of fifteen teaching monographs and case studies—each akin to a "grand rounds" session on topics such as euthanasia, genetic screening, organ donation, cloning, stem-cell research, and abortion—was produced from 1988 to 2009 by the Union

of American Hebrew Congregations (later the Union of Reform Judaism), initially through its Committee on Bio-Ethics, then through its Department of Jewish Family Concerns.

90. Tom L. Beauchamp and James F. Childress, *Principles of Biomedical Ethics*, 7th ed. (New York: Oxford University Press, 2013); and T. L. Beauchamp, "Methods and Principles in Biomedical Ethics," *Journal of Medical Ethics* 29 (2003): 269–274.

91. Beauchamp and Childress, *Principles of Biomedical Ethics*, quotations 13.

92. Ibid.

93. Ibid.

94. Beauchamp, "Methods and Principles in Biomedical Ethics," quotations 269.

95. Raymond J. Deveterre, "The Principled Approach: Principles, Rules, and Actions," in *Meta Medical Ethics: The Philosophical Foundations of Bioethics*, ed. Michael A. Grodin (Dordrecht, Netherlands: Kluwer Academic Publishers, 1995), 27–47.

96. Critiques of the four-principles model, and principlism in general, have been published (e.g., Clouser and Gert, "A Critique of Principlism"), as well as a countercritique (B. Andrew Lustig, "The Methods of 'Principlism': A Critique of the Critique," *Journal of Medicine and Philosophy* 17 (1992): 487–510). Similarly, casuistry has been critiqued and counter-critiqued (Carson Strong, "Critiques of Casuistry and Why They Are Mistaken," *Theoretical Medicine and Bioethics* 20 (1999): 395–411).

97. Mark J. Cherry and Ana Smith Iltis, eds., *Pluralistic Casuistry: Balancing Moral Arguments, Economic Realities, and Political Theory* (Dordrecht, Netherlands: Springer, 2007).

98. Raanan Gillon, "Defending the Four Principles Approach as a Good Basis for Good Medical Practice and Therefore for Good Medical Ethics," *Journal of Medical Ethics* 41 (2015): 111–116.

99. Ibid., 111.

100. Ibid., 115.

101. Aasim J. Padela, "Medical Ethics in Religious Traditions: A Study of Judaism, Catholicism, and Islam," *Journal of the Islamic Medical Association* 38 (2006): 106–117.

102. John F. Peppin, Mark J. Cherry, and Ana Iltis, eds., *Religious Perspectives in Bioethics* (New York: Taylor and Francis, 2004).

103. Anna E. Westra, Dick L. Willems, and Bert J. Smit, "Communicating with Muslim Parents: 'The Four Principles' Are Not as Culturally Neutral as Suggested," *European Journal of Pediatrics* 168 (2009): 1383–1387.

104. Steinberg, *Encyclopedia of Jewish Medical Ethics*, especially the entries on "Ethics, Jewish," 380–389, and "Ethics, Secular," 389–402. The principles are important within Judaism, says Steinberg, yet interpreted differently (386), and anyway, "Judaism in general prefers the *casuistic approach* to resolve halakhic questions [in medical ethics]" (385).

105. See chapters on Roman Catholicism, Anglicanism, Judaism, Islam, Buddhism, and secular humanism in Raanan Gillon, ed., *Principles of Health Care Ethics* (Chichester, UK: Wiley, 1994).

106. Sahin Aksoy and Ali Tenik, "The 'Four Principles of Bioethics' as Found in 13th-Century Muslim Scholar Mawlana's Teachings," *BMC Medical Ethics* 3 (2002), doi.org/10.1186/1472-6939-3-4.

107. Avraham Steinberg, "A Jewish Perspective on the Four Principles," in Gillon, *Principles of Health Care Ethics*, 65–74.

108. Padela, "Medical Ethics in Religious Traditions," 115.

109. Edmund D. Pellegrino and David C. Thomasma, *Helping and Healing: Religious Commitment in Health Care* (Washington, DC: Georgetown University Press, 1997).

110. Mackler, *Introduction to Jewish and Catholic Bioethics*.

111. Hauerwas, *God, Medicine, and Suffering*; and Post, *Encyclopedia of Bioethics*, 3rd ed.

112. Edmund D. Pellegrino and David C. Thomasma, *The Christian Virtues in Medical Practice* (Washington, DC: Georgetown University Press, 1996).

113. Elliot N. Dorff, *Matters of Life and Death: A Jewish Approach to Modern Medical Ethics* (Philadelphia: Jewish Publication Society, 1998); and Jakobovits, *Jewish Medical Ethics*.

114. Steinberg, *Encyclopedia of Jewish Medical Ethics*.

115. S. Cromwell Crawford, *Hindu Bioethics for the Twenty-First Century* (Albany: State University of New York Press, 2003).

116. James Hughes, "Buddhist Bioethics," in *Principles of Health Care Ethics*, 2nd ed., ed. Richard E. Ashcroft, Angus Dawson, Heather Draper, and John R. McMillan (West Sussex, UK: John Wiley and Sons, 2007), 127–134.

117. Abdulazziz Sachedina, *Islamic Biomedical Ethics: Principles and Application* (New York: Oxford University Press, 2009).

118. Devinder Singh Chahal, "Sikh Perspectives on Bioethics," in Peppin et al., *Religious Perspectives in Bioethics*, 211–220.

119. Jonathan Chan, "Daoism and Bioethics: Daoda Jin's Doctrine of Naturalness and the Principle of Non-Action," in Peppin et al., *Religious Perspectives in Bioethics*, 221–231.

120. H. Tristram Engelhardt Jr., *Bioethics and Secular Humanism: The Search for a Common Morality* (London: SCM Press; Philadelphia: Trinity Press International, 1991).

121. Earl E. Shelp, ed., *Secular Bioethics in Theological Perspective* (Dordrecht, Netherlands: Kluwer Academic Publishers, 1996); and Mark J. Cherry, "The Scandal of Secular Bioethics: What Happens When the Culture Acts as If There Is No God?," *Christian Bioethics* 23 (2017): 85–99.

122. See "Section Five: Religious Contexts of Psychiatric Ethics," in John Z. Sadler, C. W. Van Staden, and K. W. M. Fulford, eds., *The Oxford Handbook of Psychiatric Ethics*, vol. 1 (New York: Oxford University Press, 2015).

123. Guinn, *Handbook of Bioethics and Religion*.

124. Camenisch, *Religious Methods and Resources in Bioethics*.

125. Peppin et al., *Religious Perspectives in Bioethics*.

126. Dena S. Davis and Laurie Zoloth, eds., *Notes from a Narrow Ridge: Religion and Bioethics* (Hagerstown, MD: University Publishing Group, 1999).

127. An early discussion: Robert M. Sade, "Medical Care as a Right: A Refutation," *New England Journal of Medicine* 285 (1971): 1288–1292.

128. Dan E. Beauchamp, "Public Health as Social Justice," *Inquiry* 13 (1976): 3–14; and Aaron L. Mackler, "Judaism, Justice, and Access to Health Care," *Kennedy Institute for Ethics Journal* 1 (1991): 143–161.

129. Paul Farmer, *Pathologies of Power: Health, Human Rights, and the New War on the Poor* (Berkeley: University of California Press, 2003).

130. Laurie Zoloth, *Health Care and the Ethics of Encounter: A Jewish Discussion of Social Justice* (Chapel Hill: University of North Carolina Press, 1999).

131. Potter, "Bioethics, the Science of Survival."

132. Michael D. Rozier, "Structures of Virtue as a Framework for Public Health Ethics," *Public Health Ethics* 9 (2016): 37–45.

133. Jeff Levin, "Jewish Ethical Themes That Should Inform the National Healthcare Discussion: A Prolegomenon," *Journal of Religion and Health* 51 (2012): 589–600.

134. A revised version appeared in *Judaism and Health: A Handbook of Practical, Professional, and Scholarly Resources*, ed. Levin and Prince, 336–351, 394–397.

135. Daniel B. Rubin, "A Role for Moral Vision in Public Health," *Hastings Center Review* 40, 6 (2010): 20–22. Rubin considers bioethics and public health as "largely estranged" (20).

136. Michael D. Rozier, "When Populations Become the Patient," *Health Progress* 98, 1 (2017): 5–8.

137. Solomon R. Benatar, "Just Healthcare beyond Individualism: Challenges for North American Bioethics," *Cambridge Quarterly of Healthcare Ethics* 6 (1997): 397–415.

138. Rita Charon, "Narrative Medicine: A Model for Empathy, Reflection, Profession, and Trust," *JAMA* 286 (2001): 1897–1902; John L. Coulehan, Frederic W. Platt, Barry Egener, Richard Frankel, Chen-Tan Lin, Beth Lown, and William H. Salazar, "'Let Me See If I Have This Right . . . ': Words That Build Empathy," *Annals of Internal Medicine* 135 (2001): 221–227; and Jodi Halpern, "What Is Clinical Empathy?," *Journal of General Internal Medicine* 18 (2003): 670–674.

139. Eric J. Cassel, "The Relief of Suffering," *Archives of Internal Medicine* 143 (1973): 522–523.

140. John Bowker, *Problems of Suffering in Religions of the World* (Cambridge: Cambridge University Press, 1970).

141. Timothy E. Quill, Ira R. Byock, and the ACP-ASIM End-of-Life Care Consensus Panel, "Responding to Intractable Terminal Suffering: The Role of Terminal Sedation and Voluntary Refusal of Food and Fluids," *Annals of Internal Medicine* 132 (2000): 408–414; and Gilbert Meilaender, "On Removing Food and Water: Against the Stream," *Hastings Center Report* 14, 6 (1984): 11–13.

142. Bowker, *Problems of Suffering in Religions of the World*

143. Ibid., 1.

144. Center for Medical Humanities, Compassionate Care, and Bioethics, Stony Brook University (2018), https://www.stonybrook.edu/commcms/bioethics/.

145. Ibid.

146. Beth A. Lown, Julie Rosen, and John Marttila, "An Agenda for Improving Compassionate Care: A Survey Shows about Half of Patients Say Such Care Is Missing," *Health Affairs* 30 (2011): 1772–1778.

147. Andrew Tomkins, Jean Duff, Atallah Fitzgibbon, Azza Karam, Edward J. Mills, Keith Munnings, Sally Smith, Shreelata Rao Seshadri, Avraham Steinberg, Robert Vitillo, and Philemon Yugi, "Controversies in Faith and Health Care," *Lancet* 386 (2015): 1776–1785.

148. Richard A. McCormick, "To Save or Let Die: The Dilemma of Modern Medicine," *JAMA* 229 (1974): 172–176.

149. *Roe et al. v. Wade*, District Attorney of Dallas County: Appeal from the United States District Court for the Northern District of Texas, 410 U.S. 113 (1973), No. 70-18, Supreme Court of the United States (Decided December 22, 1973), http://cdn.loc.gov/service/ll/usrep/usrep410/usrep410113/usrep410113.pdf.

150. Thomas H. Murray, "Ripples: What to Expect When You Serve on a Bioethics Commission," *Hastings Center Report* 47, 3 (2017): S54–S56, quotation S56.

151. Paul Ramsey, "Shall We 'Reproduce'?: I. The Medical Ethics of In Vitro Fertilization," *JAMA* 220 (1972): 1346–1350; and Paul Ramsey, "Shall We 'Reproduce'?: II. Rejoinders and Future Forecast," *JAMA* 220 (1972): 1480–1485.

152. Lord Riddell, "Ethics of Abortion, Sterilization, and Birth Control," *British Medical Journal* 1, 3706 (1932): 106.

153. Raymond S. Duff and A. G. Campbell, "Moral and Ethical Dilemmas in the Newborn Nursery," *New England Journal of Medicine* 289 (1973): 890–894.

154. Reproductive Health Act, S. 240/A. 21 (January 9, 2019), https://legislation.nysenate.gov/pdf/bills/2019/S240.

155. Catholic News Service, "Cardinal Dolan Rejects Call for Gov. Cuomo's Excommunication over New Abortion Law," *America: The Jesuit Review* (January 29, 2019), https://www.americamagazine.org/politics-society/2019/01/29/cardinal-dolan-rejects-call-gov-cuomos-excommunication-over-new.

156. Disagreement on abortion among Christian denominations is described in Alan Brown, "Christianity," in Morgan and Lawton, *Ethical Issues in Six Religious Traditions*, 216–282, esp. 248–251.

157. Steinberg, *Encyclopedia of Jewish Medical Ethics*, 7–8.

158. Moshe Zemer, *Evolving Halakhah: A Progressive Approach to Traditional Jewish Law* (Woodstock, VT: Jewish Lights, 1999).

159. Dena S. Davis, "Methods in Jewish Bioethics," in Camenisch, *Religious Methods and Resources in Bioethics*, 109–126, 116.

160. Fred Rosner, "Abortion," in *Modern Medicine and Jewish Ethics* (Hoboken, NJ: KTAV, 1986), 139–160. Rulings by a minority of rabbis relax these stringencies, but according to Rosner, they have been "vigorously denounced by most rabbinic authorities" (151).

161. Daniel B. Sinclair, *Jewish Biomedical Law: Legal and Extra-Legal Dimensions* (Oxford: Oxford University Press, 2003), 17.

162. J. David Bleich, "Abortion in Halakhic Literature," in *Jewish Bioethics*, augmented ed., ed. Fred Rosner and J. David Bleich (Hoboken, NJ: KTAV Publishing House, 2000), 155–196 (originally published in *Tradition* 10, 2 (1968): 72–120).

163. Fred Rosner and Moses D. Tendler, *Practical Medical Halachah*, 2nd ed. (Jerusalem: Feldheim Publishers, 1980), 35–36, includes a compilation of *t'shuvot* sponsored by the Association of Orthodox Jewish Scientists.

164. Bleich, "Abortion in Halakhic Literature," esp. "Basis of the Prohibition," 156–163.

165. David M. Feldman, "Abortion: The Jewish View," in *Life and Death Responsibilities in Jewish Biomedical Ethics*, ed. Aaron L. Mackler (New York: Jewish Theological Seminary of America, 2000), 196–203.

166. Fred Rosner, "The Jewish Attitude toward Abortion," *Tradition* 10, 2 (1968): 48–71.

167. Walter Jacob, *Contemporary American Reform Responsa* (New York: Central Conference of American Rabbis, 1987), 26–27; and Also Jacob, "Responsibilities for Fetal Life: Abortion," in Mackler, *Life and Death Responsibilities in Jewish Biomedical Ethics*, 193–231.

168. Rosner, "The Jewish Attitude toward Abortion," 65.

169. Steinberg, *Encyclopedia of Jewish Medical Ethics*, 19.

170. See "Abortion," in Sinclair, *Jewish Biomedical Law*, 12–67. The author, an Orthodox rabbi and attorney, is on the faculty of Fordham University School of Law.

171. David M. Feldman, *Health and Medicine in the Jewish Tradition*: L'Hayyim—*To Life* (New York: Crossroad, 1986), 82.

172. Fred Rosner, *Biomedical Ethics and Jewish Law* (Hoboken, NJ: KTAV, 2001), 186.

173. See "Fetal Indications for Abortion," in Steinberg, *Encyclopedia of Jewish Medical Ethics*, 10–12.

174. Seen in the statement on abortion from the politically and religiously progressive Reconstructionist movement (see David A. Teutsch, *Bioethics: Reinvigorating the Practice of Contemporary Jewish Ethics* (Wyncote, PA: Reconstructionist Rabbinical College, 2005)).

175. Feldman, *Health and Medicine in the Jewish Tradition*, 90.

176. Immanuel Jakobovits, "Jewish Views on Abortion," in Rosner and Bleich, *Jewish Bioethics*, 139–154, 139 (chapter originally appeared in D. T. Smith, ed., *Abortion and the Law* (Cleveland: Western Reserve University Press, 1965, 1967)).

177. Ibid., 139–140.

178. Feldman, *Health and Medicine in the Jewish Tradition*, 89.

179. Peggy Morgan, "Buddhism," in Morgan and Lawton, *Ethical Issues in Six Religious Traditions*, 61–177, esp. 88–89.

180. Werner Menski, "Hinduism," in Morgan and Lawton, *Ethical Issues in Six Religious Traditions*, 1–60, esp. 36–37.

181. Azim Nanji, "Islam," in Morgan and Lawton, *Ethical Issues in Six Religious Traditions*, 283–344, esp. 314–315.

182. Eleanor Nesbitt, "Sikhism," in Morgan and Lawton, *Ethical Issues in Six Religious Traditions*, 118–167, esp. 142–143.

183. Brown, "Christianity," 248–249.

184. James Rachels, "Active and Passive Euthanasia," *New England Journal of Medicine* 292 (1975): 78–80.

185. Johann Legemaate and Ineke Bolt, "The Dutch Euthanasia Act: Recent Legal Developments," *European Journal of Health Law* 20 (2013): 451–469.

186. Todd May, "Would Human Extinction Be a Tragedy?," *New York Times* (December 17, 2018), https://www.nytimes.com/2018/12/17/opinion/human-extinction-climate-change.html.

187. Joshua E. Perry, "Biblical Biopolitics: Judicial Process, Religious Rhetoric, Terri Schiavo, and Beyond," *Health Matrix* 16 (2006): 553–630.

188. Timothy E. Quill, "Terri Schiavo—A Tragedy Compounded," *New England Journal of Medicine* 352 (2005): 1630–1633.

189. Joshua E. Perry, Larry R. Churchill, and Howard S. Kirshner, "The Terri Schiavo Case: Legal, Ethical, and Medical Perspectives," *Annals of Internal Medicine* 143 (2005): 744–748.

190. Ronald Cranford, "Facts, Lies, and Videotapes: The Permanent Vegetative State and the Sad Case of Terri Schiavo," *Journal of Law, Medicine and Ethics* 33 (2005): 363–371, 366.

191. Leaders of the religious right—including the Southern Baptist Convention's Richard Land, Focus on the Family's James Dobson, the Family Research Council's Tony Perkins, and Operation Rescue's Randall Terry—denounced the courts' disposition of the case, accusing them of fostering a culture of death and eroding the sanctity of life, and obscenely compared the judges to murderers, Nazis, and Ku Klux Klansmen (see Perry, "Biblical Biopolitics").

192. For a legal chronology of the case, see Perry, "Biblical Biopolitics" and Lois Shepherd, "Terri Schiavo: Unsettling the Settled," *Loyola University Chicago Law Journal* 37 (2006): 297–341.

193. Robert L. Fine, "From Quinlan to Schiavo: Medical, Ethical, and Legal Issues in Severe Brain Injury," *Baylor University Medical Center Proceedings* 18 (2005): 303–310, 310.

194. Quill, "Terri Schiavo—A Tragedy Compounded," 1633.

195. Kalman J. Kaplan, "Zeno, Job and Terry [*sic*] Schiavo: The Right to Die versus the Right to Live," *Ethics and Medicine* 23 (2007): 95–102.

196. T. Koch, "The Challenge of Terri Schiavo: Lessons for Bioethics," *Journal of Medical Ethics* 31 (2005): 376–378.

197. Robert J. Blendon, John M. Benson, and Melissa J. Hermann, "The American Public and the Terri Schiavo Case," *Archives of Internal Medicine* 165 (2005): 2580–2584.

198. See the sections on euthanasia in the chapters in Morgan and Lawton, *Ethical Issues in Six Religious Traditions*. See also Hans-Henrik Bülow, Charles L. Sprung, Konrad Reinhart, Shirish Prayag, Bin Du, Apostolos Armaganidis, Fekri Abroug, and Mitchell M. Levy, "The World's Major Religions' Points of View on End-of-Life Decisions in the Intensive Care Unit," *Intensive Care Medicine* 34 (2008): 423–430.

199. H. Tristram Engelhardt Jr. and Ana Smith Iltis, "End-of-Life: The Traditional Christian View," *Lancet* 366 (2005): 1045–1049.

200. Elliot N. Dorff, "End-of-Life: Jewish Perspectives," *The Lancet* 366 (2005): 862–865.

201. Mackler, *Introduction to Jewish and Catholic Bioethics*, 85–119.

202. Baruch Brody, "Jewish Reflections on Life-and-Death Decision Making," in Pellegrino and Faden, *Jewish and Catholic Bioethics*, 17–24, 20.

203. Feinstein, *Responsa of Rav Moshe Feinstein,* 1:53.

204. Steinberg, *Encyclopedia of Jewish Ethics*, 1058.

205. Baruch A. Brody and Amir Halevy, "Is Futility a Futile Concept?," *Journal of Medicine and Philosophy* 20 (1995): 123–144.

206. James Wind, "What Can Religion Offer Bioethics? ," *Hastings Center Report* 20 (1990): 18–20.

207. Ibid., 18.

208. Ibid.

Chapter 8

1. Hinduism, Buddhism, Sikhism, and Islam have focused on discrete clinical procedures (e.g., abortion, euthanasia), and less on healthcare policy or public health (Peggy Morgan and Clive A. Lawson, eds., *Ethical Issues in Six Religious Traditions,* 2nd ed. (Edinburgh: Edinburgh University Press, 2007)).

2. Mackler, *Introduction to Jewish and Catholic Bioethics*, 191–192.

3. Elliot N. Dorff, *Matters of Life and Death: A Jewish Approach to Modern Medical Ethics* (Philadelphia: Jewish Publication Society, 2003), 281.

4. Edmund D. Pellegrino, "Toward an Expanded Medical Ethics: The Hippocratic Ethic Revisited," in *Cross-Cultural Perspectives in Medical Ethics,* 2nd ed., ed. Robert M. Veatch (1973; Sudbury, MA: Jones and Bartlett, 2000), 41–53, 47.

5. Pellegrino and Faden, *Jewish and Catholic Bioethic*); and Zoloth, *Health Care and the Ethics of Encounter.*

6. Health Security Act, H.R. 3600, 113th Congress (November 20, 1993), https://www.gpo.gov/fdsys/pkg/BILLS-103hr3600ih/pdf/BILLS-103hr3600ih.pdf.

7. Peter Swenson and Scott Greer, "Foul-Weather Friends: Big Business and Health Care Reform in the 1990s in Historical Perspective," *Journal of Health Politics, Policy & Law* 27 (2002): 605–638.

8. Vicente Navarro, "Looking Back at the Future: Why Hillarycare Failed," *International Journal of Health Services* 38 (2008): 205–212.

9. Rod Howrigon, "How Did We Get Here?," *Journal of Medical Practice Management* 33 (2017): 5.

10. Collin Robertson, "The American Health Care Debate: An Unfinished Lesson in Politicking," *Policy Options* (November 2009), 31–36, esp. 34, http://irpp.org/wp-content/uploads/sites/2/assets/po/health-care/robertson.pdf.

11. Membership was kept mostly secret, as were its deliberations.

12. Lisa Klug, "Rabbi Adds Voice to Ethics Panel Advising Health Care Task Force: Insurance: Elliot Dorff Hopes Group Headed by First Lady Hillary Rodham Clinton Will Provide a Medical Plan Using a Communitarian Approach," *Los Angeles Times* (May 16, 1993), http://articles.latimes.com/1993-05-16/news/we-36245_1_task-force.

13. United Synagogue of Conservative Judaism, "Judaism and Health Care Reform," A United Synagogue Position Paper (April 1993), http://uscj2004.aptinet.com/Judaism_and_Health_C5336.html.

14. "A Framework for Comprehensive Health Care Reform: Protecting Human Life, Promoting Human Dignity, Pursuing the Common Good: A Resolution of the Catholic Bishops of the United States, June 1993," in *Pastoral Letters and Statements*

of the United States Catholic Bishops: vol. 6: *1989–1997,* ed. Patrick W. Carey (Washington, DC: National Conference of Catholic Bishops, United States Catholic Conference, 1998), 519–526.

15. Ibid.

16. "Health and Health Care: A Pastoral Letter of the American Catholic Bishops, November 19, 1981" (Washington, DC: United States Catholic Conference, 1982), http://www.usccb.org/issues-and-action/human-life-and-dignity/health-care/upload/health-and-health-care-pastoral-letter-pdf-09-01-43.pdf.

17. John XXIII, *Pacem in Terris: Encyclical of Pope John XXIII on Establishing Universal Peace in Truth, Justice, Charity, and Liberty, April 11, 1963,* quotation I.11, http://w2.vatican.va/content/john-xxiii/en/encyclicals/documents/hf_j-xxiii_enc_11041963_pacem.html.

18. "The USCCB and Health Care Reform," United States Conference of Catholic Bishops, June 2010, http://www.usccb.org/issues-and-action/human-life-and-dignity/health-care/upload/health-care-reform-summary-2010.pdf.

19. Hugh Heclo, "Religion and Public Policy: An Introduction," *Journal of Policy History* 13 (2001): 1–18.

20. Ram A. Cnaan, with Stephanie C. Boddie, Femida Handy, Gaynor Yancey, and Richard Schneider, *The Invisible Caring Hand: American Congregations and the Provision of Welfare* (New York: New York University Press, 2002).

21. David J. O'Brien, *American Catholics and Social Reform: The New Deal Years* (New York: Oxford University Press, 1968).

22. Stanley W. Carlson-Thies, "Charitable Choice: Bringing Religion Back into American Welfare," special issue on "Religion, Politics, Policy," ed. Hugh Heclo, *Journal of Policy History* 13 (2001): 109–132, 110.

23. Louise W. Knight, *Jane Addams: Spirit in Action* (New York: W. W. Norton and Co., 2010).

24. Ibid., 51.

25. Julian E. Zelizer, *The Fierce Urgency of Now: Lyndon Johnson, Congress, and the Battle for the Great Society* (New York: Penguin, 2015).

26. Barend A. de Vries, *Champions of the Poor: The Economic Consequences of Judeo-Christian Values* (Washington, DC: Georgetown University Press, 1998).

27. Jonathan Gruber and Daniel M. Hungerman, "Faith-Based Charity and Crowd-Out during the Great Depression," *Journal of Public Economics* 91 (2007): 1043–1069.

28. Edmund F. Haislmaier, Robert E. Moffit, Nina Owcharenko, and Alyene Senger, "A Fresh Start for Health Care Reform," *Heritage Foundation Backgrounder* 2970 (2014): 1–16, 1.

29. Earlier Republican legislation includes Sen. John Chafee's Health Equity and Access Reform Act of 1993 (S. 1770, 103rd Congress), with bipartisan support, and Sen. Michael Enzi's Ten Steps to Transform Health Care in America Act (S. 1783, 110th Congress).

30. E.g., Jason Linkins, "A Brief History of the Republican Alternative to Obamacare: Your Sunday Morning Conversation," *Huffington Post* (March 2, 2014), https://www.huffingtonpost.com/2014/03/02/republican-alternative-to-obamacare_n_4877100.html.

31. Patient Protection and Affordable Care Act, P.L. 111-148, 124 STAT. 119 (March 23, 2011), http://www.gpo.gov/fdsys/pkg/PLAW-111publ148/pdf/PLAW-111publ148.pdf; and Health Care and Education Reconciliation Act of 2010, P.L. 111–152, 124 STAT. 1029 (March 20, 2010), http://www.gpo.gov/fdsys/pkg/PLAW-111publ152/pdf/PLAW-111publ152.pdf.

32. Barack Obama, "United States Health Care Reform: Progress to Date and Next Steps," *JAMA* 316 (2016): 525–532.

33. White House Office of Faith-Based and Community Initiatives, *Compassion in Action Roundtable: Community-Based Solutions for Health Needs* (Washington, DC: The White House, 2008).

34. Ibid., 3.

35. Ibid.

36. Ibid.

37. Jay Hein, "Better Health . . . for More People . . . at Less Cost," *Communities in Action: Reforming the Health Care System from the Inside Out*, A Report for the U.S. Bureau of Primary Healthcare (October 2001), https://folio.iupui.edu/bitstream/handle/10244/309/hein.bhpc.pdf?sequence=1, 21.

38. CDC/ATSDR, *Engaging Faith Communities as Partners in Improving Community Health* (Atlanta: Centers for Disease Control and Prevention, Public Health Practice Office, 1999).

39. Ibid., 1.

40. "Book of Resolutions: Health Care for All in the United States," United Methodist Church (2016), http://www.umc.org/what-we-believe/health-care-for-all-in-the-united-states.

41. "ELCA Assembly Hearing Discusses Health Care Proposal," Evangelical Lutheran Church in America (August 25, 1999), http://www.elca.org/News-and-Events/3636?_ga=2.45561383.2012974723.1530669929-293971445.1530669929.

42. Evangelical Lutheran Church in America, "Health Care Reform," Social Policy Resolution CA09.04.18 (2009), http://download.elca.org/ELCA%20Resource%20Repository/Health_Care_ReformSPR09.pdf?_ga=2.32087550.1331255625.1530670647-159177688.1530670647.

43. The Office of the General Assembly, *Life Abundant: Values, Choices, and Health Care—The Responsibility and Role of the Presbyterian Church (U.S.A.)* (Louisville, KY: Presbyterian Church [U.S.A.], 1988), https://www.presbyterianmission.org/wp-content/uploads/8-life-abundant-1988.pdf.

44. The Office of the General Assembly, *Resolution on Christian Responsibility and a National Health Plan* (Louisville, KY: Presbyterian Church [U.S.A.], 1991).

45. The Office of the General Assembly, *Life Abundant*, 35.

46. The Office of the General Assembly, *Resolution on Christian Responsibility and a National Health Plan*.

47. Ginna Bairby, "The Backstory: Healthcare, Christianity, and the Presbyterian Church (U.S.A.)," *Unbound: An Interactive Journal of Christian Social Justice* (February 20, 2014), http://justiceunbound.org/carousel/the-backstory-healthcare-christianity-and-the-presbyterian-church-u-s-a/.

48. Southern Baptist Convention, "Resolution on Health Care Reform" (1994), http://www.sbc.net/resolutions/594/resolution-on-health-care-reform.

49. Ibid.

50. Ibid.

51. Southern Baptist Convention, "On Protecting Religious Liberty" (2012), http://www.sbc.net/resolutions/1223/on-protecting-religious-liberty.

52. The Episcopal Church ratified two Acts of Convention advocating for comprehensive, universal, national healthcare: "Urge Passage of a Universal Health Care Program," Resolution Number 2009-D048, in General Convention, *Journal of the General Convention of . . . The Episcopal Church, Anaheim, 2009* (New York: General Convention, 2009), 360–361; and "Urge Advocacy for Comprehensive Health Care Coverage," Resolution Number 2009-C071, in General Convention, *Journal of the General Convention of . . . The Episcopal Church, Anaheim, 2009* (New York: General Convention, 2009), 177.

53. The United Church of Christ passed a resolution aimed at combating "health care injustice" through universal healthcare: "Resolution Reaffirming Universal Health Care," United Church of Christ (2000), http://www.ucc.org/justice_health_resolution-reaffirming. This action reaffirmed a document from 1991.

54. At its 2009 Convention, the Mennonite Church USA adopted a "Resolution on Healthcare Access: Next Step"; see http://anabaptistwiki.org/mediawiki/index.php?title=Resolution_on_Healthcare_Access:_Next_Step_(Mennonite_Church_USA,_2009). This was in follow-up to earlier statements on healthcare access (in 2005) and healthcare policy (in 2007).

55. In 2009 the presiding bishop of the Church of God in Christ issued a pastoral statement endorsing the Obamacare legislation, but voiced disapproval of public coverage of abortion (Adrienne S. Gaines, "COGIC Endorses Health Reform Bill," *Charisma Magazine* (September 28, 2009), https://www.charismamag.com/site-archives/570-news/featured-news/6893-cogic-endorses-health-reform-bill).

56. The Church of the Brethren passed a resolution in 1992 calling for a national health plan: Church of the Brethren General Board, "Resolution on Health Care in the United States" (March 1992), http://www.brethren.org/about/statements/1992-health-care.pdf.

57. At its 2007 General Assembly, the Christian Church (Disciples of Christ) approved an Item for Reflection and Research affirming universal access to healthcare as a matter of social justice: "Concerning the Ethical Provision of Health Care in a Religiously Pluralistic Society," Item for Reflection and Research No. 0730 (2007), https://disciples.org/wp-content/uploads/ga/pastassemblies/2007/resolutions/0730.pdf.

58. Louay Safi, "Towards Fair, Inclusive, and Efficient Health Care System," Islamic Society of North America (August 28, 2009), https://web.archive.org/web/20150529235739/http://www.isna.net/uploads/1/5/7/4/15744382/isnahealthcarereformpaper2009.pdf.

59. Levin, "Jewish Ethical Themes That Should Inform the National Healthcare Discussion."

60. Zoloth, *Health Care and the Ethics of Encounter*.

61. Ibid., 221.

62. Union for Reform Judaism, "Health Insurance," Resolutions (2007), https://urj.org/what-we-believe/resolutions/health-insurance.

63. Union of American Hebrew Congregations, "Reform of the Health Care System," Resolutions (1993), https://urj.org/what-we-believe/resolutions/reform-health-care-system.

64. United Synagogue of Conservative Judaism, "Judaism and Health Care Reform."

65. Rabbinical Council of America, "Health Care Reform 1999" (June 1, 1999), http://www.rabbis.org/news/article.cfm?id=100998.

66. Ibid.

67. Agudath Israel of America, "Health Care Reform [Letter to President Obama] " (August 19, 2009), http://daledamos.blogspot.com/2009/08/agudath-israel-weighs-in-onhealth-care.html.

68. Ibid.

69. Agudath Israel of America, *Federal Agenda 2015* (New York: Agudath Israel of America, 2015), http://agudathisrael.org/federal-agenda-2015-mission-to-washington/.

70. The Jewish Federation of North America hosted a Health and Long-Term Care Workgroup (Alexia Kelley, "Dialogue with the Jewish Federations of North America on Health Care Reform," The White House (July 12, 2010), https://obamawhitehouse.archives.gov/blog/2010/07/12/dialogue-with-jewish-federations-north-america-health-care-reform). Other documents are found at: "Health & Long Term Care Reform Documents and Implementation," The Jewish Federations of North America (2011), https://web.archive.org/web/20150313084848/https://www.jewishfederations.org/page.aspx?id=235364.

71. The Jewish Council on Public Affairs has passed several resolutions regarding health-care and social services, including the Hillarycare era's "Principles on National Health Care Coverage" (June 28, 1993), http://www.jewishpublicaffairs.org/principles-on-national-health-care-coverage; and the Bush-era "Health Care Coverage" (February 24, 2003), http://www.jewishpublicaffairs.org/health-care-coverage/.

72. B'nai B'rith International, "Healthcare Repair: A B'nai B'rith Agenda for Reform" (2009), https://web.archive.org/web/20090604045749/http://www.bnaibrith.org/healthcare_principles.cfm.

73. National Council of Jewish Women, "Health Care Reform Talking Points" (August 2009), https://web.archive.org/web/20110105091313/http://www.ncjw.org/media/PDFs/rsrcehealthcarereformtps0809.pdf.

74. See the documents archived at Jewish Federations of North America, "Health & Long-Term Care Resource Center" (2018), https://jewishfederations.org/about-jfna/washington-office/health-long-term-care-resource-center.

75. Margaret Gibelman and Sheldon R. Gelman, "The Promise of Faith-Based Social Services: Perception versus Reality," *Social Thought* 22 (2003): 5–23. Whether the eventual legislation clearly reflected religious values or instead was a product of a dealmaking process sidetracked in the weeds of political calculation is a separate issue.

76. E.g., "Faith-Based Initiative," Theocracy Watch (April 2006), http://www. theocracywatch.org/faith_base.htm. This article begins, "Under the Bush administration, our country is experiencing a major transformation from a secular to a religious government. The President's faith-based initiative is central to this transformation."

77. Personal Responsibility and Work Opportunity Reconciliation Act of 1996, P.L. 104–193, 110 STAT. 2105 (August 22, 1996). https://www.congress.gov/104/plaws/publ193/PLAW-104publ193.pdf.

78. Ibid., quotation 110 STAT. 2162.

79. Ram A. Cnaan and Stephanie C. Boddie, "Charitable Choice and Faith-Based Welfare: A Call for Social Work," *Social Work* 47 (2002): 224–235, 224.

80. See the Actions Overview for "H.R.3734—Personal Responsibility and Work Opportunity Reconciliation Act of 1996," https://www.congress.gov/bill/104th-congress/house-bill/3734/actions. Senator Ashcroft offered a follow-up bill, the Charitable Choice Expansion Act of 1999, that died in committee (see https://www. govtrack.us/congress/bills/106/s1113).

81. George W. Bush, "Executive Order 13198 of January 29, 2001: Agency Responsibilities with Respect to Faith-Based and Community Initiatives," *Federal Register* 66 (2001): 8497–8498; and George W. Bush, "Executive Order 13199 of January 29, 2001: Establishment of White House Office of Faith-Based and Community Initiatives," *Federal Register* 66 (2001): 8499–8500.

82. Barack H. Obama, "Executive Order 13498 of February 5, 2009: Amendments to Executive Order 13199 and Establishment of the President's Advisory Council for Faith-Based and Neighborhood Partnerships," *Federal Register* 74 (2009): 6533–6535.

83. For additional background, see Jay Hein, *The Quiet Revolution: An Active Faith That Transforms Lives and Communities* ([U.S.]: Waterfall Press, 2014); and Jeff Levin and Jay Hein, "A Faith-Based Prescription for the Surgeon General: Challenges and Recommendations," *Journal of Religion and Health* 51 (2012): 57–71.

84. Hein, *The Quiet Revolution*, 25.

85. Robert G. Brooks and Harold G. Koenig, "Crossing the Secular Divide: Government and Faith-Based Organizations as Partners in Health," *International Journal of Psychiatry in Medicine* 32 (2002): 223–234.

86. Hein, *The Quiet Revolution*.

87. George W. Bush, "Executive Order 13279 of December 12, 2002: Equal Protection of the Laws for Faith-Based and Community Organizations," *Federal Register* 67 (2002): 77141–77144, 77141.

88. Levin and Hein, "A Faith-Based Prescription for the Surgeon General," 62–63.

89. Cnaan and Boddie, "Charitable Choice and Faith-Based Welfare."

90. Bush, "Executive Order 13279 of December 12, 2002," 77142, emphasis added.

91. Tommy G. Thompson, "Participation in Department of Health and Human Services Programs by Religious Organizations: Providing for Equal Treatment of All Department of Health and Human Services Program Participants," 45 CFR Parts 74, 87, 92, and 96 (RIN 0991-AB34), *Federal Register* 69 (2004): 42586–42595.

92. Ibid., 42586.

93. Ibid., 42587–42592.

94. Barack H. Obama, "Executive Order 13559 of November 17, 2010: Fundamental Principles and Policymaking Criteria for Partnerships with Faith-Based and Other Neighborhood Organizations," *Federal Register* 75 (2010): 71319–71323, 71320, emphasis added.

95. Carl H. Esbeck, "A Constitutional Case for Government Co-Operation with Faith-Based Social Service Providers," *Emory Law Journal* 46 (1997): 1–41; and Ira C. Lupu and Robert W. Tuttle, "The Faith-Based Initiative and the Constitution," *DePaul Law Review* 55 (2005): 201–317. An opposing view was presented by David Saperstein, "Public Accountability and Faith-Based Organizations: A Problem Best Avoided," *Harvard Law Review* 116 (2003): 1353–1396, yet once the Obama administration was in power he accepted an appointment to the office's advisory council.

96. Vee Burke, "Comparison of Proposed Charitable Choice Act of 2001 with Current Charitable Choice Law," *CRS Report for Congress*, Order Code RL31030 (June 22, 2001) (Washington, DC: Congressional Research Service, Library of Congress, 2001).

97. Melissa Rogers and E. J. Dionne Jr., *Serving People in Need, Safeguarding Religious Freedom: Recommendations for the New Administration on Partnerships with Faith-Based Organizations* (Washington, DC: Brookings Institution, 2008). Bipartisan support for religion in the public square has been largely underreported (see A. James Reichley, *Religion in American Public Life* (Washington, DC: Brookings Institution, 1985)).

98. Lew Daly, "Why 'Faith-Based' Is Here to Stay," *Policy Review* 57 (2009): 31–46.

99. Donald J. Trump, "Executive Order 13831 of May 3, 2018: Establishment of a White House Faith and Opportunity Initiative," *Federal Register* 83 (2018): 20715–20717.

100. Ibid., 20716.

101. Jane E. Norton, "Removing Barriers for Religious and Faith-Based Organizations to Participate in HHS Programs and Receive Public Funding," 21 CFR Chapter I, 42 CFR Chapters 1 and IV, and 45 CFR Subtitle A and Subtitle B, Chapters II, III, IV, X, and XIII (HHS-9928-RFI), *Federal Register* 82 (2017): 49300–49302.

102. "The Center for Faith and Opportunity Initiatives (Partnership Center)," U.S. Department of Health and Human Services, https://www.hhs.gov/about/agencies/iea/partnerships/index.html.

103. Trump, "Executive Order 13831 of May 3, 2018," 20715.

104. "About the President's Advisory Council on Faith-Based and Neighborhood Partnerships," Office of Faith-Based and Neighborhood Partnerships, The White House, https://obamawhitehouse.archives.gov/administration/eop/ofbnp/about/council.

105. White House Office of Faith-Based and Community Initiatives, *The Quiet Revolution: The President's Faith-Based and Community Initiative: A Seven-Year Progress Report* (Washington, DC: The White House, 2008); White House Office of Faith-Based and Community Initiatives, *Innovations in Compassion: The Faith-Based and Community Initiative: A Final Report to the Armies of Compassion* (Washington, DC: The White House, 2008); and White House Office of Faith-Based

and Neighborhood Partnerships, *Partnerships for the Common Good: A Partnership Guide for Faith-Based and Neighborhood Organizations* (Washington, DC: The White House, 2011).

106. White House Office of Faith-Based and Community Initiatives, *Compassion in Action Roundtable: Faith-Based and Community Strategies to Promote Healthy Families* (Washington, DC: The White House, 2008).

107. Johnson, *Objective Hope*; and Baylor Institute for Studies of Religion, *Not by Faith or Government Alone: Rethinking the Role of Faith-Based Organizations* (Waco, TX: Baylor University, 2008).

108. Byron R. Johnson, "Introduction," in *Not by Faith or Government Alone*, 1.

109. President's Advisory Council on Faith-Based and Neighborhood Partnerships, *A New Era of Partnerships: Report of Recommendations to the President* (Washington, DC: The White House, 2010).

110. Ibid., 119.

111. White House Office of Faith-Based and Community Initiatives, *The Quiet Revolution*, and *Innovations in Compassion*; and White House Office of Faith-Based and Neighborhood Partnerships, *Partnerships for the Common Good*, and *A New Era of Partnerships*.

112. Eric Goosby, Mark Dybul, Anthony A. Fauci, Joe Fu, Thomas Walsh, Richard Needle, and Paul Bouey, "The United States President's Emergency Plan for AIDS Relief: A Story of Partnerships and Smart Investments to Turn the Tide of the Global AIDS Pandemic," *Journal of Acquired Immune Deficiency Syndromes* 60, Suppl. 3 (2012): S51–S56; and Charles B. Holmes, John M. Blandford, Nalinee Sangrujee, Scott R. Stewart, Amy DuBois, Tyler R. Smith, Julia C. Martin, Ann Gavaghan, Caroline A. Ryan, and Eric Goosby, "PEPFAR'S Past and Future Efforts to Cut Costs, Improve Efficiency, and Increase the Impact of Global HIV Programs," *Health Affairs* 31 (2012): 1553–1560.

113. Pam Das, "Mark Dybul: US Global AIDS Coordinator in Charge of PEPFAR," *The Lancet* 369 (2007): 1161.

114. Mark Dybul, "Lessons Learned from PEPFAR," *Journal of Acquired Immune Deficiency Syndromes* 52, Suppl. 1 (2009): S12–S13, quotation S12.

115. Mark Dybul, "How to Save Lives by Breaking All the Rules," *Foreign Policy* (September 22, 2009), https://foreignpolicy.com/2009/09/22/how-to-save-lives-by-breaking-all-the-rules/.

116. Ibid.

117. Ibid.

118. Ibid.

119. A 2013 evaluation report commissioned from the Institute of Medicine noted that PEPFAR had been "globally transformative," over time shifting its emphasis from "providing services directly to providing technical assistance, building capacity, and strengthening systems" among partner countries (Institute of Medicine, "Evaluation of PEPFAR," *Report Brief* (February 2013), quotations 4, 3, http://nationalacademies.org/hmd/~/media/Files/Report%20Files/2013/PEPFAR/PEPFAR_RB.pdf).

120. *PEPFAR: 2018 Annual Report to Congress: 15 Years of Saving Lives through American Generosity and Partnership* (Washington, DC: U.S. Department of State, Office of the U.S. Global AIDS Coordinator and Health Diplomacy, 2008).

121. Levin and Hein, "A Faith-Based Prescription for the Surgeon General," and its follow-up, Levin, "Engaging the Faith Community for Public Health Advocacy."

122. Jeff Levin, "An Antipoverty Agenda for Public Health: Background and Recommendations," *Public Health Reports* 132 (2017): 431–435.

123. John Blevins, *Christianity's Role in United States Global Health and Development Policy: To Transfer the Empire to the World* (New York: Routledge, 2019).

124. Saroj Jayasinghe, "Faith-Based NGOs and Healthcare in Poor Countries: A Preliminary Exploration of Ethical Issues," *Journal of Medical Ethics* 33 (2007): 623–626.

125. Ibid., 623.

126. Ibid.

127. Ibid., 625.

128. M. C. Marazzi, G. Guidotti, G. Liotta, and L. Palombi, *DREAM: An Integrated Faith-Based Initiative to Treat HIV/AIDS in Mozambique: Case Study*, Perspectives and Practice in Antiretroviral Treatment (Geneva: World Health Organization, 2005).

129. Ibid.

130. "Executive Summary: Appreciating Assets: Mapping, Understanding, Translating and Engaging Religious Health Assets (RHAs) in Zambia and Lesotho," HIV/AIDS Programme, World Health Organization (February 8, 2007), http://www.who.int/hiv/mediacentre/executivesummaryARHAP.pdf?ua=1.

131. Ibid.

132. Searching for "faith-based" on the WHO website (http://www.who.int/en/) yields over fifteen hundred hits, including official documents and program descriptions. In most cases, these do not reference formal faith-based programs—religious NGOs are simply partners in larger efforts. But in some instances, substantive partnerships are described.

133. Manoj Kurian, "The Role of WCC's Health and Health Programme in a Changing World," *Contact* 193 (September 2011): 2–3.

134. "Interchurch Medical Assistance (IMA)," The Partnership for Maternal, Newborn & Child Health, World Health Organization (2018), http://www.who.int/pmnch/about/members/database/ima/en/.

135. "IMA World Health Joins Africa's Christian Health Associations to Focus on Sustainable Development Goals," IMA World Health (2017), https://imaworldhealth.org/achap2017/.

136. Tedros Adhanom Ghebreyesus, "The 70th Anniversary of the World Council of Churches," Director-General's Office, World Health Organization (June 16, 2018), http://www.who.int/dg/speeches/2018/world-council-churches/en/.

137. Ibid.

138. Ibid.

139. Ibid.

140. Gary Bandy, Alan Crouch, Claudine Haenni, Paul Holley, Carole Jane Larsen, Sian Penlington, Nicholas Price, and Carolyn Wilkins, *Building from Common Foundations: The World Health Organization and Faith-Based Organizations in Primary Healthcare*, ed. Ted Karpf and Alex Ross (Geneva, Switzerland: World Health Organization, 2008).

141. *WHO Traditional Medicine Strategy: 2014–2023* (Geneva: World Health Organization, 2013).

142. "About Us," CCIH: Christian Connections for International Health, http://www.ccih.org/about-us/.

143. Douglas Huber, Evelyn Rong Yang, Judith Brown, and Richard Brown, *International Family Planning: Christian Actions and Attitudes: A Survey of Christian Connections for International Health Member Organizations* (McLean, VA: CCIH, 2008).

144. "Religion and Public Health," Yale Divinity School (2018), https://divinity.yale.edu/admissions-aid/application-instructions-and-requirements/joint-applications/religion-public-health.

145. "Dual Degree: Public Health and Theology," Candler School of Theology, Emory University (2018), http://candler.emory.edu/academics/degrees/public-health/index.html.

146. World Faiths Development Dialogue, *Global Health and Africa: Assessing Faith Work and Research Priorities: Full Report* (London: World Faiths Development Dialogue and Tony Blair Faith Foundation, 2012), 3. A concise summary is contained in Lynn Aylward and Katherine Marshall, "Health in Africa and Faith Communities: What Do We Need to Know?," *Policy Brief* 9 (2013): 1–4, https://s3.amazonaws.com/berkley-center/130618WFDDPolicyBriefHealthAfricaFaithCommunitiesWhatDoWeNeedKnow.pdf.

147. World Faiths Development Dialogue, *Global Health and Africa*, 3.

148. Katherine Marshall, "Development and Religion: A Different Lens on Development Debates," *Peabody Journal of Education* 76 (2001): 339–375; Katherine Marshall, "Religion and Global Development: Intersecting Paths," in *Religious Pluralism, Globalization, and World Politics*, ed. Thomas Banchoff (New York: Oxford University Press, 2008), 195–228; and Katherine Marshall and Marisa Van Saanen, *Development and Faith: Where Mind, Heart, and Soul Work Together* (Washington, DC: World Bank, 2007).

149. Katherine Marshall and Sally Smith, "Religion and Ebola: Learning from Experience," *The Lancet* 386 (2005): e24–e25; and Azza Karam, Julie Clague, Katherine Marshall, and Jill Oliver, "The View from Above: Faith and Health," *The Lancet* 386 (2015): e22–e24.

150. Katherine Marshall, "Message from the Executive Director," in *World Faiths Development Dialogue: 2017 Annual Report* (Washington, DC: World Faiths Development Dialogue, 2018), 2–3, 2.

151. World Faiths Development Dialogue, *Global Health and Africa*.

152. Ibid., 11.

153. Ibid., 8.

154. Ibid.

155. Ibid., 72.

156. Ibid., quotation 8, emphasis added.

157. Aylward and Marshall, "Health in Africa and Faith Communities," 2.

158. World Faiths Development Dialogue, *Global Health and Africa*, 35–37.

159. Ibid., quotations 69.

160. "Ahimsa Forum," Ahimsa Fund, http://www.ahimsa-fund.com/ahimsa-forum/.

161. *Ahimsa Round Table 2013: Global Health and Faith based Communities: Final Report* (Lyon, France: Ahimsa Fund, 2013), http://www.ahimsa-fund.com/wp-content/uploads/2013/07/ART2013_Final-report1.pdf.

162. *Ahimsa Round Table 2015: Global Health and Faith-Inspired Communities: Final Report* (Lyon, France: Ahimsa Fund, 2015), http://www.ahimsa-fund.com/wp-content/uploads/2015/09/ART2015_Final-Report.pdf.

163. Jean-François de Lavison, "Editorial," *Ahimsa Fund Newsletter* (May 25, 2018), https://us6.campaign-archive.com/?u=b89bf3e2367f95d26794de257&id=79090038ec.

164. Holman, *Beholden*.

165. Ibid., 23.

166. Ibid., 11.

167. Brian J. Grim and Melissa E. Grim, "The Socio-Economic Contribution of Religion to American Society: An Empirical Analysis," *Interdisciplinary Journal of Research on Religion* 12 (2016): 1–31, http://www.religjournal.com/pdf/ijrr12003.pdf.

168. Ibid., 27.

169. Robert L. Mole and Dale M. Mole, *For God and Country: Operation Whitecoat: 1954–1973* (Brushton, NY: Reach Services, 1998).

170. Phillip R. Pittman, Sarah L. Norris, Kevin M. Coonan, and Kelly T. McKee Jr., "An Assessment of Health Status among Medical Research Volunteers Who Served in the Project Whitecoat Program at Fort Detrick, Maryland," *Military Medicine* 170 (2005): 183–187.

171. "The Politics of Liberty," in Malcolm Bull and Keith Lockhart, *Seeking a Sanctuary: Seventh-day Adventism and the American Dream*, 2nd ed. (Bloomington: Indiana University Press, 1989), 182–198.

172. Pittman et al., "An Assessment of Health Status among Medical Research Volunteers Who Served in the Project Whitecoat Program at Fort Detrick, Maryland."

173. Krista Thompson Smith, "Adventists and Biological Warfare," *Spectrum* 25, 3 (1996): 35–50.

174. James H. Jones, *Bad Blood: The Tuskegee Syphilis Experiment*, new and exp. ed. (New York: Free Press, 1993).

175. John Marks, *The Search for the Manchurian Candidate: The CIA and Mind Control: The Secret History of the Behavioral Sciences* (New York: W. W. Norton and Co., 1979).

176. Ninian Smart, *Dimensions of the Sacred: An Anatomy of the World's Beliefs* (Berkeley: University of California Press, 1996), esp. chapter 5, "The Ethical and Legal Dimension," 196–214.

177. National Religious Partnership for the Environment, http://www.nrpe.org/.

178. Mark A. Shibley and Jonathon L. Wiggins, "The Greening of Mainline American Religion: A Sociological Analysis of the National Religious Partnership for the Environment," *Social Compass* 44 (1997): 333–348.

179. Jeff Levin, "Ebola: Epidemiology's Challenge to Theology," *Syndicate* 2, 1 (2015): 3–8.

180. Christoph Benn, "Guest Introduction: Faith and Health in Development Contexts," *Development in Practice* 27 (2017): 575–579. See also the remainder of the special issue containing this article.

181. Jeff Levin and Ellen L. Idler, "Islamophobia and the Public Health Implications of Religious Hatred," *American Journal of Public Health* 108 (2018): 718–719.

182. Hugh Heclo and Wilfred M. McClay, eds., *Religion Returns to the Public Square: Faith and Policy in America* (Baltimore: Johns Hopkins University Press, 2003).

183. Wilson Carey McWilliams, "American Democracy and the Politics of Faith," in Heclo and McClay, *Religion Returns to the Public Square*, 143–162.

184. Hugh Heclo, "An Introduction to Religion and Public Policy," in Heclo and McClay, *Religion Returns to the Public Square*, 3–30, 3.

185. Ibid., 11–13, 12.

186. Ibid., quotations 18.

187. Ibid.

188. Ibid., 20.

189. Andrew Tomkins, Jean Duff, Atallah Fitzgibbon, Azza Karam, Edward J. Mills, Keith Munnings, Sally Smith, Shreelata Rao Seshadri, Avraham Steinberg, Robert Vitillo, and Philemon Yugi, "Controversies in Faith and Health Care," *The Lancet* 386 (2015): 1776–1785.

Chapter 9

1. Levin, "The Discourse on Faith and Medicine," 277.

2. On the medical profession's "dominance, autonomy and authority" over health and healthcare: Dianna T. Kenney and Barbara Adamson, "Medicine and the Health Professions: Issues of Dominance, Autonomy and Authority," *Australian Health Review* 15 (1992): 319–334.

3. John T. S. Madeley and Zsolt Enyedi, eds., *Church and State in Contemporary Europe: The Chimera of Neutrality* (London: Frank Cass, 2003).

4. Peter Conrad, "Medicalization and Social Control," *Annual Review of Sociology* 18 (1992): 209–232.

5. Ibid., 213–214.

6. M. J. D. Roberts, "The Society for the Suppression of Vice and Its Early Critics, 1802–1812," *Historical Journal* 26 (1983): 159–176.

7. Heidi Rimke and Alan Hunt, "From Sinners to Degenerates: The Medicalization of Morality in the 19th Century," *History of the Human Sciences* 15 (2002): 59–88.

8. Ibid., 79, 80.

9. Ibid., 65.

10. Ibid., 64.

11. Conrad, "Medicalization and Social Control," 214.

12. Rodney Stark, "Secularization R.I.P.," *Sociology of Religion* 60 (1999): 249–273; and Peter L. Berger, "Secularism in Retreat," *National Interest* 46 (1996/1997): 3–12.

13. Levin, "The Discourse on Faith and Medicine."

14. Ibid.

15. Levin, "Restoring the Spiritual"; and James Giordano, "Quo Vadis?: *Philosophy, Ethics, and Humanities in Medicine* Preserving the Humanistic Character of Medicine in a Biotechnological Future," *Philosophy, Ethics, and Humanities in Medicine* 4 (2009): 12.

16. Articles began appearing in the 1970s: e.g., M. S. M. Watts, "Orthodox Medicine— Humanistic Medicine—Holistic Health Care," *Western Journal of Medicine* 131 (1979): 463.

17. Alan Barnard and Margarete Sandalowski, "Technology and Humane Nursing Care: (Ir)reconcilable or Invented Difference?," *Journal of Advanced Nursing* 34 (2001): 367–375.

18. For respective Republican and Democratic viewpoints, see Hein, *The Quiet Revolution*; and Rogers and Dionne, *Serving People in Need, Safeguarding Religious Freedom*.

19. Levin, "Engaging the Faith Community for Public Health Advocacy."

20. Sheila Suess Kennedy and Wolfgang Bielefeld, "Government Shekels without Government Shackles?: The Administrative Challenges of Charitable Choice," *Public Administration Review* 62 (2002): 4–11.

21. Eleanor Clift, "Federal Faith-Based Office Less Controversial, but Still Stirs Discussion," TheNonProfitTimes (November 7, 2016), http://www.thenonprofittimes.com/news-articles/federal-faith-based-offices-less-controversial-still-stir-discussion/.

22. Support for and opposition to the office alternates depending upon the party in power. E.g., ThinkProgress, the news arm of the Center for American Progress, a progressive beltway think tank, decried "dismantling" of the Obama administration's faith-based initiative by the Trump administration ("Trump Is Dismantling Obama's Religion Initiatives: He's Replacing Them with Unofficial Evangelical Advisers," ThinkProgress (October 10, 2017), https://thinkprogress.org/trump-dismantling-obamas-religion-initiatives-49d89df9b0e4/). Yet they expressed opposition to a faith-based office under President Bush, labeling the concept as legally and Constitutionally "problematic" ("State of the Union: Faith-Based Initiative," Center for American Progress (January 21, 2004), https://www.americanprogress.org/issues/religion/news/2004/01/21/493/state-of-the-union-faith-based-initiative/).

23. The Trump administration continues its predecessors' work in facilitating participation of FBOs in partnership with DHHS (see Department of Health and Human Services, "Removing Barriers for Religious and Faith-Based Organizations to Participate in HHS Programs and Receive Public Funding," HHS-9928-RFI, *Federal Register* 82 (2017): 49300–49302).

24. As listed on the White House website, https://www.whitehouse.gov/.

25. "About Faith-Based and Neighborhood Partnerships," U.S. Department of Health and Human Services (October 26, 2017), https://www.hhs.gov/about/agencies/iea/

partnerships/about-the-partnership-center/index.html. Its official description states that it works in collaboration with twenty-seven DHHS agencies.

26. Bush, "Executive Order 13198 of January 29, 2001"; Bush, "Executive Order 13199 of January 29, 2001"; Bush, "Executive Order 13279 of December 12, 2002"; and Obama, "Executive Order 13498 of February 5, 2009."

27. Michelle Dibadj, "The Legal and Social Consequences of Faith-Based Initiatives and Charitable Choice," *Southern Illinois University Law Journal* 26 (2002): 529–557; Vernadette Ramirez Broyles, "The Faith-Based Initiative, Charitable Choice, and Protecting the Free Speech Rights of Faith-Based Organizations," *Harvard Journal of Law and Public Policy* 26 (2003): 315–353; Linda C. McClain, "Unleashing or Harnessing 'Armies of Compassion'?: Reflections on the Faith-Based Initiative," *Loyola University Chicago Law Journal* 39 (2008): 361–426; Steven K. Green, "'A Legacy of Discrimination'?: The Rhetoric and Reality of the Faith-Based Initiative: Oregon as a Case Study," *Oregon Law Review* 84 (2005): 725–777; and Stanley W. Carlson-Thies, "Faith-Based Initiative 2.0: The Bush Faith-Based and Community Initiative," *Harvard Journal of Law and Public Policy* 32 (2009): 931–947.

28. Rogers and Dionne, *Serving People in Need, Safeguarding Religious Freedom*.

29. *Americans United v. PRISON FELLOWSHIP*, 555 F. Supp. 2d 988 (S.D. Iowa 2008)," U.S. District Court for the Southern District of Iowa (May 19, 2008), https://law. justia.com/cases/federal/district-courts/FSupp2/555/988/2460159/.

30. *Burwell v. Hobby Lobby Stores, Inc.*, 573 U.S. ___ (2014), Supreme Court of the United States (Decided June 30, 2014), https://supreme.justia.com/cases/federal/us/573/13-354/.

31. Kristin M. Roshelli, "Religiously Based Discrimination: Striking a Balance between a Health Care Provider's Right to Religious Freedom and a Woman's Ability to Access Fertility Treatment without Facing Discrimination," *St. John's Law Review* 83 (2009): 977–1016.

32. Religious Freedom Restoration Act of 1993, Public Law 103-141, 107 STAT. 1488 (November 16, 1993), https://www.gpo.gov/fdsys/pkg/STATUTE-107/pdf/STATUTE-107-Pg1488.pdf.

33. International Religious Freedom Act of 1998, Public Law 105-292, 112 STAT. 2787 (October 27, 1998), https://www.congress.gov/105/plaws/publ292/PLAW-105publ292.pdf.

34. Charitable choice is a provision (Sec. 104) of the Personal Responsibility and Work Opportunity Reconciliation Act of 1996, Public Law 104-193, 110 STAT. 2105 (August 22, 1996), https://www.congress.gov/104/plaws/publ193/PLAW-104publ193.pdf.

35. The pertinent clause of P.L. 104-193 is a single paragraph, "Nondiscrimination Against Religious Organizations" (Sec. 104 (c)), stating that "religious organizations are eligible, on the same basis as any other private organization, as contractors to provide assistance, or to accept certificates, vouchers, or other forms of disbursement, under any program described in subsection (a)(2) so long as the programs are implemented consistent with the Establishment Clause of the United States Constitution."

36. Brett H. McDonald, "The Liberal Case for *Hobby Lobby*," *Arizona Law Review* 57 (2015): 777–822.

37. Ibid., quotations 779.

38. "Dershowitz: Hobby Lobby Decision Is 'Monumentally Insignificant,' " Real Clear Politics Video (July 1, 2014), https://www.realclearpolitics.com/video/2014/07/01/dershowitz_hobby_lobby_decision_is_monumentally_insignificant.html.

39. At a panel titled "Beyond *Hobby Lobby*: What Is at Stake with the HHS Contraceptive Mandate?," held in Washington, DC, March 24, 2014. See Kathleen Parker, "Hobby Lobby Case Creates Unexpected Allies in Alan Dershowitz and Kenneth Starr," *Washington Post* (March 25, 2014), https://www.washingtonpost.com/opinions/kathleen-parker-hobby-lobby-case-creates-unexpected-allies-in-alan-dershowitz-and-kenneth-starr/2014/03/25/3e9d0936-b45a-11e3-8cb6-284052554d74_story.html.

40. Bennett and Hale, *Building Healthy Communities through Medical-Religious Partnerships*.

41. Gunderson and Cochrane, *Religion and the Health of the Public*.

42. World Faiths Development Dialogue, *Global Health and Africa*.

43. Levin, "An Antipoverty Agenda for Public Health."

44. Michael Marmot and Richard G. Wilkinson, eds., *Social Determinants of Health* (Oxford: Oxford University Press, 1999).

45. Levin, "An Antipoverty Agenda for Public Health," 431.

46. Ibid., 432.

47. Gapminder, "World Health Chart" (2018), https://www.gapminder.org/fw/world-health-chart/.

48. Adam Wagstaff, "Poverty and Health Sector Inequalities," *Bulletin of the World Health Organization* 80 (2002): 97–105.

49. Ibid., 102.

50. John W. Selsky and Barbara Parker, "Cross-Sector Partnerships to Address Social Issues: Challenges to Theory and Practice," *Journal of Management* 31 (2005): 849–873.

51. Lester M. Salomon and Helmut K. Anheier, "The Civil Society Sector," *Society* 34 (1997): 60–65.

52. Levin, "An Antipoverty Agenda for Public Health," 431.

53. Ibid., 432.

54. David Satcher, "The Prevention Challenge and Opportunity," *Health Affairs* 25 (2006): 1009–1011.

55. Bennett and Hale, *Building Healthy Communities through Medical-Religious Partnerships*.

56. Levin, "Faith-Based Initiatives in Health Promotion," and "Faith-Based Partnerships for Population Health."

57. Jeff Levin, "Healthcare Reform ≠ Public Health Reform: On Pathogens, Poverty, and Prevention," *Global Advances in Health and Medicine* 7 (2018): 1–5.

58. George W. Bush, *Rallying the Armies of Compassion* (Washington, DC: Executive Office of the President, 2001), https://archives.hud.gov/reports/rally.pdf.

59. HHS Strategic Plan: FY 2014–2018, U.S. Department of Health and Human Services (March 10, 2014), https://aspe.hhs.gov/system/files/pdf/258821/StrategicPlanFY2014-2018.pdf.

60. Strategic Plan FY 2018–2022, U.S. Department of Health and Human Services (February 28, 2018), https://www.hhs.gov/about/strategic-plan/index.html.

61. Office of Global Affairs (OGA), U.S. Department of Health and Human Services (June 14, 2016), https://www.hhs.gov/about/agencies/oga/index.html.

62. *The Global Strategy of the U S. Department of Health and Human Services* (Washington, DC: U.S. Department of Health and Human Services, Office of Global Affairs, 2012), https://www.hhs.gov/sites/default/files/hhs-global-strategy.pdf.

63. Ibid., 14.

64. Global Health Security Agenda, *Implementing the Global Health Security Agenda: Progress and Impact from U.S. Government Investments* (February 2018), https://www.ghsagenda.org/docs/default-source/default-document-library/global-health-security-agenda-2017-progress-and-impact-from-u-s-investments.pdf.

65. Healthy People 2020, Office of Disease Prevention and Health Promotion (April 4, 2018), https://www.healthypeople.gov/.

66. Levin, "Engaging the Faith Community for Public Health Advocacy," 377.

67. Ibid., 379.

68. E.g., Levin, "Engaging the Faith Community for Public Health Advocacy," and "Faith-Based Initiatives in Health Promotion."

69. Levin, "Faith-Based Partnerships for Population Health."

70. Secretary's Advisory Committee on National Health Promotion and Disease Prevention Objectives for 2030, *Report #2: Recommendations for Developing Objectives, Setting Priorities, Identifying Data Needs, and Involving Stakeholders for Healthy People 2030* (2018), https://www.healthypeople.gov/sites/default/files/Advisory_Committee_Objectives_for_HP2030_Report.pdf.

71. Ibid., 9.

72. Levin and Hein, "A Faith-Based Prescription for the Surgeon General."

73. Ibid., 58–60.

74. Ibid.

75. Ibid., 65.

76. Ibid., 65–67.

77. Levin, "Engaging the Faith Community for Public Health Advocacy," 380.

78. Satcher, "Opening Address."

79. "U.S. Surgeon General to Headline White House/HHS Faith-Based Conference in New Orleans," HHS Press Office (June 2, 2011), http://standardnewswire.com/news/771546296.html.

80. Stephen G. Post, Christine M. Puchalski, and David B. Larson, "Physicians and Patient Spirituality: Professional Boundaries, Competency, and Ethics," *Annals of Internal Medicine* 132 (2000): 578–583.

81. Timmins et al., "The Role of the Healthcare Chaplain."

82. Ibid., 87.

83. Ibid., 93.

84. Michael Owen, "The Church, Not the NHS, Should Be Funding Hospital Chaplains" [Letter], *Nursing Standard* 28, 9 (2013): 32.

85. Ibid.

86. Mark Burleigh, "NHS Chaplains Are Professional Members of the Healthcare Team" [Letter], *Nursing Standard* 28, 13 (2014): 35.

87. Association of Professional Chaplains (APC), *Standards of Practice for Professional Chaplains* (October 22, 2015), http://www.professionalchaplains.org/Files/ professional_standards/standards_of_practice/Standards_of_Practice_for_ Professional_Chaplains_102215.pdf.

88. Annelieke Damen, Allison Delaney, and George Fitchett, "Research Priorities for Healthcare Chaplaincy: Views of U.S. Chaplains," *Journal of Healthcare Chaplaincy* 24 (2018): 57–66.

89. Association of Professional Chaplains (APC), *Standards of Practice for Professional Chaplains*, 2.

90. Fitchett et al., "Evidence-Based Chaplaincy Care: Attitudes and Practices in Diverse Healthcare Chaplain Samples."

91. John J. Gleason, "An Emerging Paradigm in Professional Chaplaincy," *Chaplaincy Today* 14 (1998): 9–14.

92. See Research, HealthCare Chaplaincy Network (2018), https://healthcarechaplaincy. org/research.html).

93. Mary Martha Thiel and Mary Redner Robinson, "Physicians' Collaboration with Chaplains: Difficulties and Benefits," *Journal of Clinical Ethics* 8 (1997): 94–103.

94. Ford and Tartaglia, "The Development, Status, and Future of Healthcare Chaplaincy," 677.

95. Wendy Cadge and Julia Bandini, "The Evolution of Spiritual Assessment Tools in Healthcare," *Society* 52 (2015): 430–437.

96. Ford and Tartaglia, "The Development, Status, and Future of Healthcare Chaplaincy," 676.

97. Ibid., 676–677.

98. Ibid., 676.

99. De Vries et al., "Lost in Translation," 23.

100. Ibid.

101. Ibid., 25.

102. Ibid., 24–26.

103. Jeffrey Cohen, "How Is Chaplaincy Marginalised—By Our Faith Communities and by Our Institutions and Can We Change It?," *Religions* 9 (2018): 24, doi:10.3390/ rel9010024.

104. Harold G. Koenig, Margot Hover, Lucille B. Bearon, and James L. Travis III, "Religious Perspectives of Doctors, Nurses, Patients, and Families," *Journal of Pastoral Care* 45 (1991): 254–267.

105. Rosemary Kennedy Chapin, Devyani Chandran, Julie F. Sergeant, and Terry L. Koenig, "Hospital to Community Transitions for Adults: Discharge Planners and Community Service Providers' Perspectives," *Social Work in Health Care* 53 (2014): 311–329.

106. Laura Rydholm, Rajean Moone, Lisa Thornquist, Wanda Alexander, and Vicki Gustafson, "Care of Community-Dwelling Older Adults by Faith Community Nurses," *Journal of Gerontological Nursing* 34, 4 (2008): 18–29.

107. Rosalee C. Yeaworth and Ronnette Sailors, "Faith Community Nursing: Real Care, Real Cost Savings," *Journal of Christian Nursing* 31 (2014): 178–183.

108. Robert G. Anderson and John L. Young, "The Religious Component of Acute Hospital Treatment," *Hospital and Community Psychiatry* 39 (1988): 528–533.

109. "Hospital's Transition Program Coordinates Care throughout the Continuum," *Hospital Case Management* 23 (2015): 19–21.

110. Giancarlo Luccetti, Alessandra Lamas Granero Lucchetti, and Christina M. Puchalski, "Spirituality in Medical Education: Global Reality?," *Journal of Religion and Health* 51 (2012): 3–19.

111. Kenneth A. Rasinski, Youssef G. Kalad, John D. Yoon, and Farr A. Curlin, "An Assessment of US Physicians' Training in Religion, Spirituality, and Medicine," *Medical Teacher* 33 (2011): 944–945.

112. Anita J. Tarzian, Lucia D. Wocial, and the ASBH Clinical Ethics Consultation Affairs Committee, "A Code of Ethics for Health Care Ethics Consultants: Journey to the Present and Implications for the Field," *American Journal of Bioethics* 15, 5 (May 2015): 38–51.

113. Fox et al., "Ethics Consultation in United States Hospitals."

114. Numbers and Sawyer, "Medicine and Christianity in the Modern World," especially the discussion of the "secularization of medical theory," 139.

115. Puchalski and Ferrell, *Making Health Care Whole*.

116. Farr A. Curlin, Ryan E. Lawrence, Marshall H. Chin, and John D. Lantos, "Religion, Conscience, and Controversial Practices," *New England Journal of Medicine* 356 (2007): 593–600.

117. Quill, "Terri Schiavo—A Tragedy Compounded."

118. Christine M. Puchalski, "Spirituality and Health: The Art of Compassionate Medicine," *Hospital Physician* 37, 3 (2001): 30–36.

119. Ibid., 35.

120. Quoted from " 'I Swear by Apollo Physician . . . ': Greek Medicine from the Gods to Galen," trans. Michael North, *Greek Medicine* (Washington, DC: History of Medicine Division, National Library of Medicine, National Institutes of Health, 2002). https://www.nlm.nih.gov/hmd/greek/greek_oath.html.

121. Keith G. Meador, "Redeeming Medicine," in *Christian Reflection: A Series in Faith and Ethics,* 22: *Health* (Waco, TX: Baylor University Center for Christian Ethics, 2007), 81–86.

122. Ibid., quotations 85.

123. On the "pro" side: Dossey, *Prayer Is Good Medicine*; on the "con" side: Paul A. Offit, *Bad Faith: When Religious Belief Undermines Modern Medicine* (Philadelphia: Perseus Books, 2015).

124. E.g., Sloan, *Blind Faith*.

125. E.g., Farr A. Curlin, John D. Lantos, Chad J. Roach, Sarah A. Sellergren, and Marshall H. Chin, "Religious Characteristics of U.S. Physicians: A National Review," *Journal of General Internal Medicine* 20 (2005): 629–634.

126. Matthews with Clark, *The Faith Factor*.

127. Ibid., 17–18.

128. King, *Faith, Spirituality, and Medicine*.

129. Megan Best, Phyllis Butow, and Ian Oliver, "Do Patients Want Doctors to Talk about Spirituality?: A Systematic Literature Review," *Patient Education and Counseling* 98 (2015): 1320–1328.

130. King, *Faith, Spirituality, and Medicine*.

131. David R. Hodge, "A Template for Spiritual Assessment: A Review of the JCAHO Requirements and Guidelines for Implementation," *Social Work* 51 (2006): 317–326.

132. Teo Forcht Dagi, "Prayer, Piety, and Professional Propriety: Limits on Religious Expression in Hospitals," *Journal of Clinical Ethics* 6 (1995): 274–279, 278.

133. Quoted in "GPs Can Pray with Patients—As Long as It's 'Tactful'" [Press release], Christian Medical Fellowship (July 28, 2011), https://www.cmf.org.uk/advocacy/pressrelease/?id=108.

134. Michael J. Balboni, Amenah Babar, Jennifer Dillinger, Andrea C. Phelps, Emily George, Susan D. Block, Lisa Kachnic, Jessica Hunt, John Peteet, Holly G. Prigerson, Tyler J. VanderWeele, and Tracy A. Balboni, "'It Depends': Viewpoints of Patients, Physicians, and Nurses on Patient-Practitioner Prayer in the Setting of Advanced Cancer," *Journal of Pain and Symptom Management* 41 (2011): 836–847.

135. Religious Freedom Project, *Report of the Georgetown Symposium on Religious Freedom and Healthcare Reform, March 22, 2012*, Berkley Center for Religion, Peace and World Affairs (Washington, DC: Georgetown University, 2012).

136. Claire E. Brolan, Peter S. Hill, and Gorik Ooms, "'Everywhere but Not Specifically Somewhere': A Qualitative Study on Why the Right to Health Is Not Explicit in the Post-2015 Negotiations," *BMC International Health and Human Rights* 15 (2015): 22f, doi:10.1186/s12914-015-0061-z.

137. David S. Oderberg, "Declaration in Support of Conscientious Objection in Health Care," University of Reading, (2018), https://research.reading.ac.uk/conscientious-objection-in-health-care-declaration/.

138. Quoted from "FAQS," ibid., https://research.reading.ac.uk/conscientious-objection-in-health-care-declaration/faqs/.

139. Quoted from "Declaration," ibid., https://research.reading.ac.uk/conscientious-objection-in-health-care-declaration/declaration/.

140. Wesley J. Smith, "The 'Medical Conscience' Civil Rights Movement," *First Things* (March 30, 2018), https://www.firstthings.com/web-exclusives/2018/03/the-medical-conscience-civil-rights-movement.

141. Jide Nzelibe, "Strategic Globalization: International Law as an Extension of Domestic Political Conflict," *Northwestern University Law Review* 105 (2011): 635–687.

142. Lawrence O. Gostin, Eric A. Friedman, Kent Buse, Attiya Waris, Moses Mulumba, Mayowa Joel, Lola Dare, Ames Dhai, and Devi Sridhar, "Towards a Framework Convention on Global Health," *Bulletin of the World Health Organization* 91 (2013): 790–793.

143. Ibid., 791.

144. Kate Garland Holmes and James C. Garland, "The Clash of Rights: Explaining Attitudes toward a Religious Exemption to the HHS Contraception Mandate," *PS: Political Science and Politics* 51 (2018): 358–369.

145. Kegler et al., "Facilitators, Challenges, and Collaborative Activities in Faith and Health Partnerships to Address Health Disparities," 666.

146. Peterson et al., "Key Elements for Church-Based Health Promotion Programs," 408.

147. Johnson, *Objective Hope.*

148. Levin, "Engaging the Faith Community for Public Health Advocacy," 379. See also Bopp and Fallon, "Health and Wellness Programming in Faith-Based Organizations"; and Markens et al., "Role of Black Churches in Health Promotion Programs."

149. Levin, "Engaging the Faith Community for Public Health Advocacy," 379. See also DeHaven et al., "Health Programs in Faith-Based Organizations."

150. E.g., Campbell et al., "Church-Based Health Promotion Interventions."

151. E.g., Newlin et al., "A Methodological Review of Faith-Based Health Promotion Literature."

152. Kegler et al., "Facilitators, Challenges, and Collaborative Activities in Faith and Health Partnerships to Address Health Disparities."

153. Ibid., 671–675.

154. Ibid., 669–671.

155. Gunderson and Cochrane, *Religion and the Health of the Public*; and Bennett and Hale, *Building Healthy Communities through Medical-Religious Partnerships.*

156. Goldmon and Roberson, "Churches, Academic Institutions, and Public Health: Partnerships to Eliminate Health Disparities."

157. Levin, "An Antipoverty Agenda for Public Health."

158. See Preuss, *Biblical and Talmudic Medicine.*

159. Satcher, "Opening Address," 3.

Index